the complete
Migraine health, diet guide & cookbook

Practical solutions for managing migraine and headache pain + **150** recipes

Susan Hannah,
BA, BScH

with
Dr. Lawrence Leung,
Medical Advisor, MBBChir,
BChinMed, FRCGP, CCFP

and
Elizabeth Dares-Dobbie,
BSc, BEd, RD, MA

Robert
ROSE

For complete cataloguing information, see page 336.

Disclaimer
This book is a general guide only and should never be a substitute for the skill, knowledge, and experience of a qualified medical professional dealing with the facts, circumstances, and symptoms of a particular case.

The nutritional, medical, and health information presented in this book is based on the research, training, and professional experience of the authors, and is true and complete to the best of their knowledge. However, this book is intended only as an informative guide for those wishing to know more about health, nutrition, and medicine; it is not intended to replace or countermand the advice given by the reader's personal physician. Because each person and situation is unique, the authors and the publisher urge the reader to check with a qualified health-care professional before using any procedure where there is a question as to its appropriateness. A physician should be consulted before beginning any exercise program. The authors and the publisher are not responsible for any adverse effects or consequences resulting from the use of the information in this book. It is the responsibility of the reader to consult a physician or other qualified health-care professional regarding his or her personal care.

This book contains references to products that may not be available everywhere. The intent of the information provided is to be helpful; however, there is no guarantee of results associated with the information provided. Use of brand names is for educational purposes only and does not imply endorsement.

The recipes in this book have been carefully tested by our kitchen and our tasters. To the best of our knowledge, they are safe and nutritious for ordinary use and users. For those people with food or other allergies, or who have special food requirements or health issues, please read the suggested contents of each recipe carefully and determine whether or not they may create a problem for you. All recipes are used at the risk of the consumer. We cannot be responsible for any hazards, loss, or damage that may occur as a result of any recipe use. For those with special needs, allergies, requirements, or health problems, in the event of any doubt, please contact your medical adviser prior to the use of any recipe.

Design and Production: Daniella Zanchetta/PageWave Graphics Inc.
Editors: Bob Hilderley, Senior Editor, Health; and Sue Sumeraj, Recipes
Copy editor: Sheila Wawanash
Proofreader: Kelly Jones
Indexer: Gillian Watts
Illustrations: Kveta (Three in a Box)

We acknowledge the financial support of the Government of Canada through the Book Publishing Industry Development Program (BPIDP) for our publishing activities.

Published by Robert Rose Inc.
120 Eglinton Avenue East, Suite 800, Toronto, Ontario, Canada M4P 1E2
Tel: (416) 322-6552 Fax: (416) 322-6936
www.robertrose.ca

Printed and bound in Canada

1 2 3 4 5 6 7 8 9 MI 21 20 19 18 17 16 15 14 13

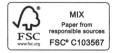

This book is dedicated to all people
whose lives are disrupted by headaches.

Contents

continued...

Introduction

"I'm very brave generally," he went on in a low voice: "only today I happen to have a headache." (Tweedledum)
– Lewis Carroll, *Through the Looking Glass and What Alice Found There*

For people who suffer from migraine, tension and cluster headaches, it is hard to imagine a time when they were pain free and able to enjoy a high-quality lifestyle without fear of being bothered by a headache. Headaches can dominate your life, threatening your performance in the workplace and disturbing your family life. How many times have you called in to report you cannot come to work because of a migraine? How many times have you postponed events with your children because of a tension headache? How often has a cluster headache prevented you from enjoying a dinner party or other activities with your friends, or the fear of having a headache discouraged you from pursuing social and physical activities?

Despite the prevalence of migraine, tension and cluster headaches in the Western world, and a growing mountain of research into their causes and cure, headaches still challenge the medical community. But while there is no one cause or a specific cure for headache, identifying headache triggers, appropriate medications, Western- and alternative-based therapies, lifestyle strategies and diet management strategies have been seen to reduce headache frequency, intensity and duration. Research has shown that for some people, these headaches can be associated with high levels of histamines in the body, which for some can be managed effectively by understanding what triggers headaches and following a specific nutrition and diet program.

The Complete Migraine Health, Diet Guide & Cookbook provides basic information to help you understand the characteristics of the three most common primary headaches and leads you through steps intended to help prevent your headaches, reduce headache symptoms or rescue you from your headaches when they occur. This program culminates in the presentation of a set of diet plans and recipes based on the histamine hypothesis.

> Headaches can dominate your life, threatening your performance in the workplace and disturbing your family life.

> Research has shown that for some people, these headaches can be associated with high levels of histamines in the body.

Part 1 of *The Complete Migraine Health, Diet Guide & Cookbook* will help you

- Identify the signs and symptoms for migraine, cluster and tension headaches
- Discover the triggers that cause headaches
- Understand the medical tests for diagnosing headaches

Part 2 of *The Complete Migraine Health, Diet Guide & Cookbook* will help you

- Understand the various treatments traditionally used by physicians and other health-care providers, including the use of prescription medications, physiotherapy and surgery
- Weigh the benefits and risks of alternative treatments, such as acupuncture, body-mind medicine and medicinal herbs
- Understand the role of nutrition and diet in the management of headaches

Part 3 of *The Complete Migraine Health, Diet Guide & Cookbook* helps you

- Make lifestyle changes to eliminate or reduce headaches, especially changes in your eating habits
- Adopt a healthy meal plan that focuses on enjoying low-histamine foods and eliminating foods that increase the risk of headache
- Select from among 150 recipes as you develop 28-day meal plans

> Make lifestyle changes to eliminate or reduce headaches, especially changes in your eating habits

The authors of *The Complete Migraine Health, Diet Guide & Cookbook* bring together a unique collection of education, experience and skills to guide and support people who suffer from migraine, cluster and tension headaches.

Susan Hannah, former research associate at the Centre of Studies in Primary Care in the Department of Family Medicine at Queen's University, has developed her expertise in health-related research and writing while preparing reports about disease states, such as colon cancer, arthritis, and motion disorders, as well as writing journal articles and conference abstracts. She suffers from cluster headaches.

Dr. Lawrence Leung is the medical advisor for this book and an associate professor in the Department of Family Medicine at Queen's University, a widely published medical research scientist and a practicing physician of Western and traditional Chinese medicine. Dr. Leung's focus is on chronic pain syndromes and their treatment with acupuncture and related modalities. He has helped many patients who suffer from primary headaches improve their quality of life dramatically. He suffers from migraines himself.

Elizabeth Dares-Dobbie, a consulting Registered Dietitian at the Department of Family Medicine at Queen's University for over five years, is passionate about improving patients' quality of life through evidence-based nutritional care. As a registered dietitian and nutrition consultant, Elizabeth has expertise in providing care for diabetes, hypertension, cholesterol management, geriatric nutrition, gastroenterology and food allergies. Elizabeth holds a Bachelor of Education and a master's degree in Educational Psychology, has taught nutrition for life science students, completed research in cognitive learning and design, and delivered evidence-based presentations on health and nutrition topics for health-care practitioners and for special interest groups. Elizabeth is a member of Dietitians of Canada, the Consultant Dietitians Network and the Ontario College of Dietitians. She is counted among migraine sufferers.

Recent advances in medicine have significantly improved the success of care for primary headaches, so we encourage you to consult your health-care team about your headaches. There is no replacement for a proper consultation with your family physician. Of particular importance, any child with headache should be under the care of a family physician. Overall improvement in quality of life requires a more comprehensive approach that includes lifestyle changes and diet therapy, and may include surgery or medication, depending on each individual's situation. Although no diet or nutritional supplement has been proven to cure primary headaches, this book reviews foods that have a positive impact on the frequency, intensity and duration of headaches, leading to better self-management. The authors hope that this book will equip you with the information you need to better manage your condition and to inspire you to make good nutrition a priority in your life.

Susan Hannah
Lawrence Leung
Elizabeth Dares-Dobbie

> The authors hope that this book will equip you with the information you need to better manage your condition and to inspire you to make good nutrition a priority in your life.

Part 1

Understanding Migraine, Cluster and Tension Headaches

Chapter 1
Who Gets Migraine, Cluster and Tension Headaches?

CASE HISTORY
Workday Headaches

Jane is a 30-something-year-old office administrator who suffers from migraine headaches. Recently, her headache attacks have increased to about 10 episodes a month and become more severe. The over-the-counter ibuprofen she has been using for years no longer provides effective relief, and the pain and discomfort have forced her to take several days off work.

Jane was diagnosed with migraine headache when she was a teenager, soon after her menstrual cycle began. Her mother also suffers from headaches, though not as frequently or severely as Jane, whose migraines still occur a few days before and during her menstrual period and more often at the end of the workday. The office where Jane works as a manager is busy and she spends a lot of time at her computer. She eats breakfast on a regular basis but finds that she often doesn't have time to stop for lunch and keeps going on coffee and sugary snacks. She works full time and takes college-level classes two nights a week. She cannot afford the time for exercise, even though she has a free health club membership through her workplace. Friday evenings are usually her time to unwind with a few glasses of red wine, either at home or with friends, but the rest of the weekend is generally spoiled with headache and nausea.

Jane is concerned about these changes in her headaches and has become somewhat depressed. She has booked a visit with her family physician, hoping to find better ways of managing her headaches.

M any people suffering from headaches are not properly diagnosed. Headaches are often described in the medical literature as "underestimated, under-recognized and undertreated." Part of the problem in understanding headaches is that their presenting symptoms are not always well differentiated from other conditions with similar symptoms. Before seeking treatment strategies, identifying the kind of headache you have is a good place to start.

Kinds of Headaches
Primary Headaches

Primary headaches are among the most common complaints that send people to visit their doctors. These headaches occur without any clearly defined reason (in medical language, they are called idiopathic) and are not due to any underlying problems of the body systems, which is why imaging or blood tests will usually come back as normal. Doctors generally reckon that primary headaches may be related to how the brain maintains its *physiological* equilibrium rather than to abnormalities of the brain structure itself. Primary headaches include migraine, cluster and tension-type headaches. Migraine and cluster headaches are the two most common disabling headache disorders for people with chronic pain.

Immune System Glossary

Allergen: Any substance that causes an allergic reaction.

Antigen: Any molecule that causes an immune response, such as antibody production.

Aura: Blind spots, random flashes of light and tingling sensations in the hands and face.

Histamine: A molecule (made in the body or consumed as part of the diet) that is released in the body as part of the immune response. Regulates physiological function in the gut and acts as a neurotransmitter to dilate blood vessels and increase movement in and out of blood vessels.

Pathogen: Any disease-producing agent, but especially a bacterium, virus or other microorganism.

Kinds of Primary Headaches

Migraine headaches or attacks are defined as two main types — with aura or without aura — but there are several sub-types of migraine as well:

- Familial hemiplegic migraine (FHM), which has several subsets (aura type)
- Sporadic hemiplegic migraine (aura type)
- Retinal migraine (aura type)
- Chronic migraine
- Hormone-related migraine

This book discusses the symptoms of the most common forms of migraine.

Cluster headache is also called

- Histamine headache: Headache that results from histamine toxicity.
- Migrainous neuralgia: A formal name for cluster headache.
- Horton's headache: A type of cluster headache named for American neurologist Bayard T. Horton (1895–1980).
- Alarm clock headache: The kind of headache that wakes you up on a regular basis in the middle of the night.

Tension-type headache (TTH) is also called

- Tension and muscle contraction headache: Headache that results in pain from muscular contraction.
- Psychomyogenic headache: An earlier name for tension headache.
- Ordinary headache: The most common form of headache.
- Idiopathic headache: Headache with no known cause.
- Psychogenic headache: Another archaic name for tension-type headache.
- Stress headache: Headache caused by stress that can be relieved by reducing stress.
- Essential headache: Yet another seldom-used name for tension-type headache.

Secondary Headaches

Secondary headaches arise from other, coexisting conditions, such as brain tumors, aneurysms or autoimmune, infective or inflammatory diseases, and may require more urgent diagnosis and early surgical or medical treatment. This type of headache usually will not resolve until the actual cause is properly diagnosed and treated.

Location of the Three Primary Headache Types: Where Does It Hurt?

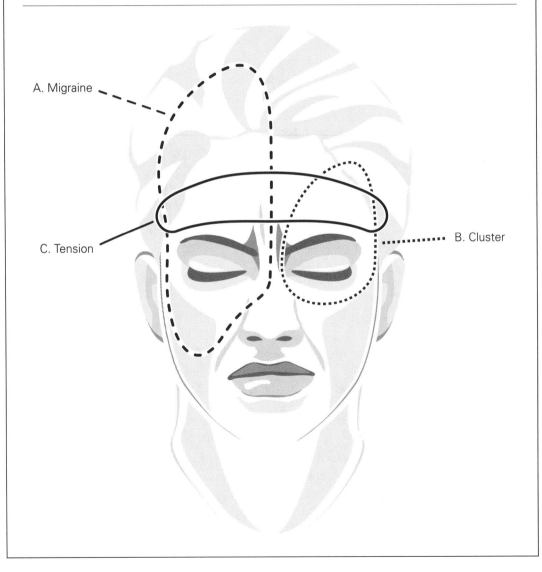

A. Migraine

C. Tension

B. Cluster

Location, prevalence, and brief description of the three primary headache disorder types

A. Migraine

- Almost always located on one side of the head, recurrent, lifelong for many people.
- Pain level is moderate to severe.
- For some people, the activation of a deep-brain mechanism is thought to cause the release of substances in the tissues surrounding the nerves and blood vessels in your head.
- The cause of migraine is under debate — whether nerve-related, vascular-related or both — but environmental triggers along with family history, or genetics, are likely involved.
- Attack symptoms may include a warning phase with symptoms of flashing lights in the eyes, nausea or even numbness of the face (for people who have migraine with aura). May be made worse by normal daily physical tasks. Typically lasts anywhere from a few hours up to 2 to 3 days. Frequency of attacks can be as few as one per year or as many as one per week; the average is one to two times per month or more for the chronic type. For children, attacks tend to be shorter, but abdominal symptoms more likely.

B. Cluster Headache (CH)

- For most people, cluster headaches happen in groups, or clusters, and follow a cyclical pattern.
- Cluster headache pain is usually felt on one side of the head only, around the eye and the temple area.
- Pain level is severe to excruciating (described as worse than childbirth).
- Affects <1 in 1000 adults, but 6 men for every woman is affected.
- Typically affects adults >20 years old.
- Because of its cyclical nature, cluster headache is thought to be caused by a dysfunction in the back of the hypothalmus (in the brain), responsible for our internal clock.
- Attack symptoms: frequent recurring, brief but extremely severe headache, typically including pain around the eye, tearing, redness, runny nose or blocked nose on the affected side only; for some, the eyelid may droop. Includes episodic and chronic forms.

C. Tension Headache (TTH)

- Usually, located on both sides of the head, close to the temple area and around the eye. Can be episodic (70% of some populations) or chronic (1% to 3% of adults).
- Pain level is mild to moderate (rarely severe). Feels like a tight band of pressure around the forehead and may also affect the neck.
- Can be stress-related or associated with neck problems (musculoskeletal).
- Episodic type usually lasts a few hours to several days.
- Chronic type is known to not let up, and is more disabling than the episodic form of TTH.

Prevalence and Incidence

Because of the high levels of disability and financial costs to our society, primary headache disorders are considered a major health concern. These headaches deprive individuals of work satisfaction, reduce their take-home pay due to days of work lost and destroy quality time with their family, to say nothing of the physical and psychological effects of chronic pain experienced by these persons. It also translates to financial losses and setbacks in our economy from lost productivity and increased sick benefits.

WHO Facts

In October 2012, the World Health Organization (WHO) published a report called *Headache Facts* that tallies our knowledge of this disorder.

Demographic
- About half of adults across the globe had a serious headache in the one-year period studied. One out of 10 of those headaches were migraines.
- Headache disorders are a worldwide health problem for all ages, races, income levels and geographic regions. In particular, women are three times more likely than men to have a migraine attack.

Diagnosis
- Around the world, health professionals diagnose migraine and tension headache in only about 4 out of 10 of the people who truly suffer from these disorders. Diagnostic accuracy for migraine increases with income category, but tension headaches show no such income-related trend.

Migraine Attacks
- The most common age of onset for migraine attacks is from 30 to 39 years old, but in 5% to 10% of cases, onset occurs at 18 years or younger.
- Migraine attacks usually decrease as people age, especially for women after their menopause. Unfortunately, one out of three women with migraine continue to have migraine, or even increased attacks, during or post-menopause.
- Migraines are known to be hereditary.
- Depression, anxiety, stressful events, snoring, head trauma, medication overuse (pain relievers or analgesics), specific food sensitivity, and caffeine use are also some of the factors that may bring on migraine attacks.

Tension Headaches

- Tension headache is the most common headache experienced.
- More women than men (90% compared to 70%) have tension headaches at some point in their lives.
- Although the causes of tension headaches are not fully understood, they may include interactions between muscle contractions, along with mental and emotional factors.

Cluster Headaches

- Cluster headaches are more rare (1% of the population), with more men affected than women. Sufferers usually get their first cluster headache when they are between 20 and 40 years old.
- One woman for every six men gets a cluster headache.
- Cluster headaches are often experienced by several different members within a family. For a small percentage of sufferers (5%), the condition might be hereditary.

Associated Conditions

- For some people, dealing with primary headaches on a long-term basis may increase their risk of other health problems. For example, people who suffer from migraines or any other severe headaches are much more likely to suffer from depression.

Q. What's my risk of developing a migraine headache?

A. If you are female, you are three times more likely to get migraine than a man. Some types of migraine may start in the first or second decade of life, but frequency often decreases with age. Although many women who suffer from migraine find that the attacks stop after menopause, one-third of women who get migraines still have them after menopause, and for some in this smaller group, the frequency of headaches even increases. The most common age for migraine attacks is between 30 and 39 years old, but it also affects 5% to 10% of children 18 years and younger.

Signs and Symptoms

For family physicians to correctly diagnosis and manage your headaches, they need to differentiate the signs and symptoms of your condition. One way of doing so is to keep a log of your actual headache symptoms, frequency and intensity. This will help to rule out any other possible reason for your headaches.

Signs and Symptoms for Migraine, Cluster and Tension-Type Headaches

Type of Headache	Signs and Symptoms
Migraine	Headache that happens on a regular basis and is 4 to 72 hours in duration
	For many people, described as pain on one side that pulsates
	Pain is described as ranging from moderate to severe
	With or without nausea
	Possible pain from exposure to light (photophobia)
	Pain can be made worse by normal daily physical activities
	About one in five people with migraines experiences an aura prior to migraine onset (auras are non-pain symptoms that may have visual or other sensory content; they may also differ from one attack to another)
Cluster	Severe one-sided pain, usually in the eye area or on one side of the head
	Pain is usually on the same side during each cluster attack
	Headache often lasts from 15 to 180 minutes
	Frequency of attack ranges from once every 48 hours to eight times a day
	Pain location is on the same side as all other symptoms
	Possible tearing of the eye on the affected side
	Possible congestion or runny nose, forehead and facial sweating, drooping eyelids or eyelid swelling on the same side
	Possible restlessness or agitation because of excruciating pain
	Attacks happen in clusters on a periodic basis, with some extended headache-free periods (from weeks to years) in between
	Some people with cluster headaches (10% to 15%) do not have long periods of remission

Type of Headache	Signs and Symptoms
Tension	Infrequent headaches that last from just minutes to days
	Pain is usually on both sides of the head, with a classic band-like or tightening nature
	Usually not worsened by physical activity
	May be able to continue with normal daily activities
	Nausea is not a typical symptom
	Possible light sensitivity (called photophobia)
	Possible sound sensitivity (called phonophobia)
	When occurring daily, causes serious chronic pain with disability and significantly affects quality of life
	Chronic tension-type headache is the most challenging to treat due to increased sensitivity to pain in the central nervous system (more widely felt around the head), as well as in local areas, such as the temples or jaw line.

Source: Adapted from World Health Organization, *Headache Facts*.

Defining Your Headache

Worksheet

Complete this worksheet to see if you have migraine or tension-type headache. Learning to recognize differences between migraines and tension-type headaches may help you and your health-care team to diagnose and manage your headaches better. Just giving your condition a name can be reassuring. You may find that your symptoms will improve.

Instructions

1. Columns A and B show symptoms that are commonly seen for migraines and tension-type headaches.
2. Identify your symptoms and mark them with a checkmark or an X in column C, then compare them with the list of migraine and tension-type headaches.
3. Decide whether symptoms in column A or B most closely resemble your symptoms.
4. If you find you have symptoms in both columns, you may have both types of primary headaches.
5. Discuss your headache symptoms with your family physician, especially if they are getting more severe in duration or intensity, or you are experiencing new symptoms.

Symptom	A Migraine	B Tension-Type	C Your Symptoms
Intensity and Quality of Pain			
Mild to moderate pain intensity	✓	✓	
Severe pain intensity	✓		
Intense throbbing and pounding and/or disabling	✓		
Disturbing but not disabling		✓	
Constant ache		✓	
Duration			
From 30 minutes to 7 days		✓	
From 4 to 72 hours	✓		
Location of Pain on Head			
One side	✓		
Both sides	✓	✓	
Associated Symptoms			
Nausea or vomiting	✓		
Light and/or sound intolerance	✓		
Aura before headache begins (visual symptoms)	✓		

Source: Adapted from The American Headache Society, "Information for Patients," www.achenet.org.

Chapter 2
Possible Causes and Triggers

> ## CASE HISTORY
> ### Migraine Control
>
> Kara has been getting migraines since she was 4 years old. She has gone to many emergency rooms for help with severe migraines. CAT scans and MRIs have been used to find the source of her headaches. She has volunteered for several research studies, trying out new medications for migraine. Despite these efforts, at 27 years old, she still doesn't know why she gets migraines.
>
> Kara's emotional pain has become as severe and debilitating as her physical pain. Kara reports that she has considered suicide to get away from the migraine pain. She has also lost her social life. She feels that her family and friends don't understand that migraines need to be taken seriously. As she says, "I wouldn't wish this pain on my very worst enemy." When she was a child, she never got to stay at her friends' overnight or go to concerts because her parents were afraid she would get a migraine. Now, she has a baby boy and worries that he will get migraines too. Her mother, grandmother and aunt get migraines. She feels as if migraines control her life.

Many people who do not suffer from migraines, tension-type headaches or cluster headaches may joke that the symptoms are not physically real, but rather are all in the head. Not so. Primary headaches are recognized by the World Health Organization as a distinct neurobiological disease that is potentially lifelong and affects women and men of all ages throughout the world, and are caused by biological or neuronal dysfunction that leads to pain. There is good reason for research that explores the anatomy and biology of migraine if we are to understand the pathophysiology — the causes and course — of these headaches and plan an effective program for headache prevention and management.

Contributing Factors in Primary Headaches

- Genetic predisposition
- Common triggers
- Immune response
- Inflammation
- Neurovascular reaction
- Neurolimbic reaction
- Nitrous oxide circulation
- Hormone imbalance
- Histamine overload

Q. What does pathophysiology mean?

A. Physiology is the term used to describe the study of the structure and function of anatomical systems that lead to normal bodily processes, such as digestion, respiration (breathing), and movement. Pathophysiology is the study of these systems when they go wrong, resulting in illness with symptoms such as nausea and vomiting, high blood sugar, and headaches.

Genetic Predisposition

Medical scientists and geneticists have been looking at families with members who have migraine to determine which genes are involved. Knowing that a single gene or a suite of genes that appear together in someone's genetic makeup when they have a disease or condition helps to identify when someone is at higher risk or has a genetic predisposition for getting that disease. Research about genes involved with migraine and other primary headaches could lead to improved therapies, and if a damaged gene is found, a cure for migraine may be within reach.

Genetic predisposition is a known factor for cluster headaches and frequent episodic or chronic tension headaches. Looking at your family history for primary headaches will help you understand whether there is a higher chance that you will also get these headaches.

Did You Know?

New Genes

In 2010, a gene regulating potassium channels was found to relate to migraine with aura. Potassium channels are vital to maintain a nerve cell at the resting state, and mutations in these potassium channel genes can lead to easily excited nerve cells that set off the pain process of migraine. More research needs to be done to understand how to safely treat genetic conditions related to migraine.

Genetic Risk in Migraine

Understanding the genetic risks helps health-care providers test appropriately for conditions related to migraine with aura. Genes involved in regulating the vascular system are also possibly related to migraines. For people who suffer from migraine with aura, the associated gene also predisposes to stroke.

Cluster Headaches and Histamine

Recent reports have shown that people who suffer from cluster headaches often have a higher risk for sensitivities to biogenic amines, such as histamine or tyramine, which are found in certain foods. This is why cluster headaches are also called histamine headaches. A low-histamine diet could give you some relief from your headaches by reducing their frequency, intensity, and duration. Moreover, people who suffer from cluster headaches also have a frequency-dependent risk of depression. That is, the more cluster headaches they experience, the higher their risk for depression.

Common Triggers

Triggers are external or internal factors that may initiate primary headaches, either by exposure or withdrawal, by themselves or in combination with other factors. Triggers are also called precipitating or provoking factors and usually occur within 48 hours before any attack. Stress, missing meals, dehydration, alcohol, food sensitivities and sleep patterns are possible triggers for all three primary headaches — migraine, cluster, and tension-type.

External Triggers

Allergens: Food allergy may be a trigger for persistent migraines for some people, but not all. Evaluation by an allergist will help to identify whether your headaches are caused by an allergy.

Antigens: A substance that causes our body's immune system to produce antibodies against it, such as sensitivities to specific foods or to chemical products, may be the cause of primary headaches.

Behavioral: Habits such as drinking red wine or beer, staying up late on Friday nights, oversleeping on weekends, exercising strenuously and skipping meals are all known triggers for primary headaches.

Chemical: Exposure to perfumes, soaps or gasoline may trigger primary headaches for some people.

Dietary: Sensitivities to specific foods, consuming foods containing tyramine, histamine, histamine liberators or diamine oxidase (DAO) blockers, or taking drugs that block enzymes, could trigger primary headaches for some people with insufficient enzyme activity or dysfunctions.

Environmental: On a daily basis, we are bombarded by environmental factors such as changes in temperature or altitude, perfume from flowers, gas from swamps, pollen from plants and trees, the clothing we wear, the shampoo and soap we use, the noise or smoke from city streets or the bright sun coming in our windows. Any of these could be a potential trigger for primary headaches.

Some drugs: Medications given to relieve pain from primary headaches may cause rebound headaches for some people if directions for dosage are not followed.

Internal Triggers

Stress (most common): Stress can trigger headaches in several ways. First, it can cause muscles to tighten in the neck, shoulders and head, leading to tension headaches. As well, adrenaline from stressful situations can release histamine from mast cells and result in inflammation and pain around nerves in the head.

Emotional stress: Crying can trigger primary headaches by releasing stress hormones, reducing the amount of oxygen taken in, or placing stress or pressure on veins and arteries in your head and brain.

Sleep disturbance: For people who are prone to headaches, too little or too much sleep or changes in sleep patterns may affect hormones such as serotonin or cortisol and trigger primary headaches.

Sleep and stress for migraine with aura: Many of the same factors that trigger migraine without aura also have an impact on migraine with aura, such as stress, bright lights, fatigue and changes in sleep patterns.

Environmental factors for migraine without aura: Intense physical activity, changes in the barometric pressure, sun glare and bright lights can trigger headaches.

Sex hormones (neurosteroids and ovarian steroids): For women, the chance of having a migraine, having migraine more often or having more severe migraine is higher when their hormones fluctuate, such as during first menstruation, pregnancy and menopause.

Medications: Oral contraceptives and vasodilator medications (nitroglycerin) are examples of medications that can trigger migraine headaches.

> Adrenaline from stressful situations can release histamine from mast cells and result in inflammation and pain around nerves in the head.

Cluster Headaches

Although cluster headaches are thought to be associated with the circadian rhythm that governs distinct periods, there are still contributing factors that could trigger a headache within that period:

Stress: Activation of the inflammation cascade through the release of stress hormones may trigger a cluster headache during a headache period.

Smoking: Also known as a trigger for cluster headache during a headache cycle.

Alcohol: Drinking alcohol during a cluster headache cycle will cause or worsen a headache.

Napping: The circadian rhythm connection of cluster headaches means that napping can act as a trigger.

Extreme variations in temperature: Fluctuations in temperature can act as a trigger.

Elevated temperatures, from hot baths to hot days: Although a hot bath is seen as a headache relief, for some people, it may trigger a cluster headache.

Exercise: Many people suffer from cluster headache following strenuous exercise. Finding your limit in terms of exertion and time will help reduce frequency.

Exposure to histamines, through food or perfumes or chemicals: Cluster headaches are also called histamine headaches.

Bright light: Bright light can be a trigger for cluster headaches during a cycle.

Tension Headaches

For tension headaches, triggers may work differently than for the other primary headaches. Physical stress causing tightness in muscles may act as a trigger for tension headaches. This is also true for emotional stress, depression or anxiety. Physical behaviors that can trigger headaches include awkward working positions, being forced to hold the same position for long periods, poor posture overall and clenching your jaws. These behaviors can be changed.

Immune Response

The anatomical and biochemical structures and processes that cause migraine attacks are not yet fully understood, and scientists have held different positions. Among the most popular is the theory that migraines arise when pain-producing pro-inflammatory chemicals are released, as the result of a signal indicating a disturbance in the immune system, and then act on certain nerves and blood vessels within the head. When the blood vessels dilate in response to these chemicals, they exert pressure on the pain-sensitive nerves, which results in pain. The pro-inflammatory chemicals can also travel to other areas in the body, either close by (via nerves) or far from the point of origin (via the bloodstream), and give rise to other symptoms, such as visual disturbances, vomiting and intolerance to sound and light.

Immune Functions

Our immune system functions through an intricate network of chemicals, proteins and cells, both in the blood and locally in the various tissues. This system detects and destroys harmful organisms of various sizes, including bacteria, viruses, fungi and parasites, as well as others that invade our bodies every minute. The immune system also picks up and clears our body's own cells that have become abnormal (that is, cancerous). Normally, a state of dynamic balance called homeostasis exists within our immune system so we remain free of disease. When our immune system moves away from this balance, we give in to a state of hypoactive immunity (resulting in infections or cancer) or hyperactive immunity (resulting in autoimmune diseases or chronic pain).

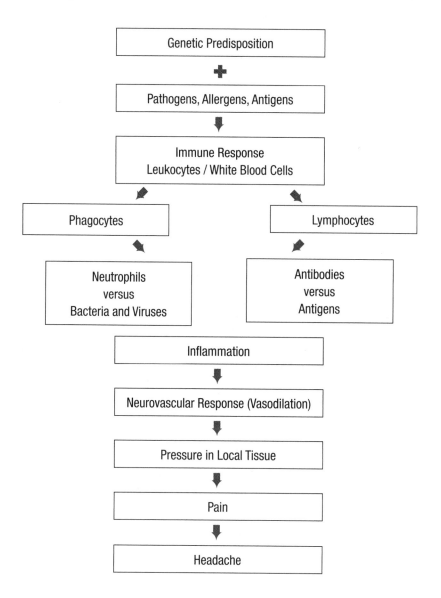

Immunity Cascade

If you are genetically predisposed to migraine and come under attack from pathogens, allergens or antigens, your immune system responds by deploying leukocytes, which produce antibodies to counterattack. Inflammation of tissues can result during this conflict, which in turn can affect nerve endings and blood vessels and result in pain.

Leukocytes

Our immune system includes leukocytes, also known as white blood cells. After being manufactured in the bone marrow, leukocytes travel through the blood and lymphatic circulation system to reside in various locations, such as the thymus gland, spleen, lymph nodes and bone marrow, where they are ready for action against invaders. Phagocytes and lymphocytes are two forms of leukocyte cells.

Phagocytes and Lymphocytes

Phagocytes surround and digest foreign bodies or harmful bacteria and viruses into smaller molecules called antigens. The neutrophil is the most common of the many forms of phagocytes. It seeks out bacteria to destroy.

Lymphocytes identify and respond to antigens presented by the phagocytes. Two types of lymphocytes, B cells and T cells, are both produced in the bone marrow. B cells stay and mature in the bone marrow, where they track down antigens and alert other network lymphocytes (mainly T cells) about the invaders. T cells are lymphocytes that travel from the bone marrow to the thymus gland and mature there. T cells travel through the body to destroy antigens and other mutated cells that have been identified by the B cells. Together, the B and T cells provide an effective grid to protect the body from the potential harm of foreign bodies and pathogens.

Antibodies

Special proteins called antibodies are produced by the B cells in response to stimulation by an antigen. The antibody tags onto the specific antigens, which usually originate from the invading pathogens. The antibodies themselves do not destroy the antigens or pathogens but instead stimulate the B and the T cells to destroy the tagged enemy. As part of the immune system network, antibodies help neutralize toxins or poisons that have been identified. Antibodies also activate a protein group called the complement system to become part of the network that destroys molecules that are harmful to the body.

Inflammation

Inflammatory chemicals are released upon activation of the immune system network (see the section on histamine overload, page 39) when a potentially harmful event is identified — an infection, an irritant, a physical injury or an alien molecule. This pro-inflammatory action by the immune system has two goals: first, to enhance the odds of destroying the injurious agent; and, second, to set the stage for the healing process.

Mast Cells

Mast cells circulate in the body close to the blood vessels and nerves as immature cells and are triggered by T cells to mature. Mast cells become part of the inflammatory cascade when they are activated by antigens and release histamine. Histamine release causes local swelling (called edema), increased warmth and redness. Histamine irritates nerve endings, leading to itching or pain.

Did You Know?

Vasoactive Amines

For people who suffer from vascular headaches, they may be caused by vasoactive amines, such as tyrosine or histamine, that are either made in the body or part of the food we eat.

The Three Stages of the Inflammatory Response

The inflammatory response has three stages. Especially important for understanding migraine is the role histamine plays during the inflammation process.

1. *Vasodilation:* Harm done to the body's tissues results in the local release of three chemicals — histamine, bradykinin and prostaglandin — by the damaged tissue, either into the bloodstream or the tissue environment. These chemicals cause the local blood capillaries to dilate, which increases the total blood flow to the target area. At the same time, these chemicals cause the dilated blood vessels to leak clear fluid (plasma) into surrounding tissue, which causes local swelling and pain.

2. *Phagocytosis:* A local cell-to-cell domino effect (called a cascade of events) occurs where a variety of protein and hormone molecules (kinins and prostaglandins), each with a different role, attract and activate certain phagocytes and leukocytes to deal with the damaged tissue. Increased blood flow, plasma and accumulation of local pro-inflammatory chemicals result in redness, heat and swelling of the affected tissues — referred to as the classic triad of symptoms for inflammation.

3. *Tissue repair:* The activated leukocytes clean up any dead cells. Leukocytes themselves may also die during this inflammatory event, and may in turn be digested, which contributes to the production of pus (white blood cells and blood plasma). Pus is usually present at the site of bacterial infection.

Neurovascular System

The nervous system is a collection of nerve cells (neurons) that conduct nerve impulses to coordinate (send, receive and process) information instantly throughout the body. It is also responsible for making muscle movements in the limbs and gut, and further acts as the master control unit (computer) for the body. The nervous system is also central to understanding migraine pathophysiology. Inflammatory chemicals released around the nerves and blood vessels in the brainstem may lead to dilation, constriction and pain.

The nervous system is broadly divided into the central nervous system (brain and spinal cord) and the peripheral nervous system (all nerves and their network outside the brain and spinal cord). The brain is the crux of our nervous system and is protected by the skull. The spinal cord is an extension of the brain. It protects the nerve roots and sends off nerve fibers to reach all parts of the body. The cell bodies of neurons group together to form ganglia, which are often located outside the brain and spinal cord. As a convention, the term "peripheral nervous system" refers to all distal nervous tissues, inclusive of the nerve ganglia.

Anatomy of a Headache

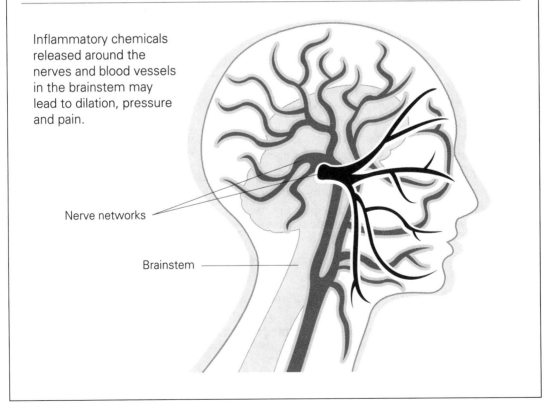

Inflammatory chemicals released around the nerves and blood vessels in the brainstem may lead to dilation, pressure and pain.

Nerve networks

Brainstem

Nerve Cells

The ability to receive and send impulses makes it possible to convey information from one part of the body to another. Sensory cells receive stimuli through different neurons, and these stimuli range from slow and generalized (not very particular) to fast and highly specific.

Each nerve cell contains a nucleus and at least one axon and dendrite. Dendrites are short extensions of the cell body that receive stimuli, while the single elongated extension (the axon) transmits signals from the region of the cell body to connect with other neurons via synapses in a kind of one-way logical junction for signal conduction. Some of the neurons end on muscle, which results in muscle contractions, while others synapse with intermediary neurons inside the spinal cord to form a reflex arc to fine-tune muscle movements. The skin also contains neurons that end as sensors for specific signals, such as pain, cold, heat or pressure.

Nerve Network

Cranial nerves exit from the brain through openings in the skull. In a similar fashion, the peripheral nerves travel from the spinal cord through the spaces between the vertebrae of the spine. Both cranial and spinal nerves convey impulses to and from the central nervous system. Most peripheral nerves are mixed, with both sensory and motor components. They carry sensory messages from the body to the brain and in turn send messages from the brain to the body for muscle activity. The 12 cranial and 31 spinal nerves run in pairs, one supplying each side of the body. Cranial nerves travel to the head and neck only, except for the vagus nerve, which extends to the chest and abdomen. Cranial nerves manage muscle functions of the head, eyes, face, tongue and larynx, as well as chewing and swallowing. The spinal nerves extend to the other parts of the body to reach the extremities.

Did You Know?

Oversensitive Nerves

Some people feel pain more acutely than others, and the nerves that signal pain can sometimes be oversensitive. Biofeedback or other relaxation techniques may help to reduce pain for these people.

Autonomic Nervous System

Alongside the peripheral nervous system is the autonomic nervous system, which keeps the body in balance (called homeostasis) and manages the respiratory, circulatory, digestive and urogenital systems through the sympathetic and parasympathetic nervous systems. The autonomic nervous system connects with the central nervous system at the brainstem. The sympathetic system is responsible for stress responses, while the parasympathetic system puts the body into rest and relaxation mode — together managing the fight or flight response to internal and external stress.

Although we cannot exert conscious control over the autonomic nervous system, fluctuating hormone levels in our bodies act as messengers to effect changes. Any damage to this system could have an overall negative impact on health. Since stress is a trigger for all primary headaches, understanding the relationship between our nervous systems may help you understand why learning to reduce stress in your life could help you manage and reduce your headaches.

The Autonomic Nervous System

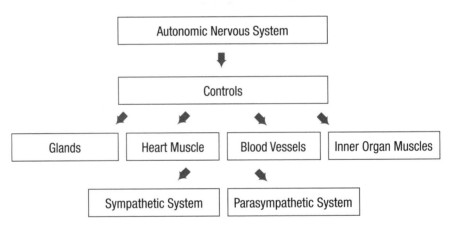

Metabolism

All chemical reactions that keep your cells and the body in a living state are collectively referred to as metabolism and can be classified as catabolic (breaking down of molecules for energy) or anabolic (building up of molecules from simpler compounds). Metabolism is a dynamic balance between anabolic and catabolic reactions and, without it, life ends. Our thyroid gland secretes the hormone thyroxine, which sets the pace of metabolism. Nutrients from our diet provide the building blocks for our body to metabolize into chemical and heat energy to meet our daily requirements.

Types of Nutrients

Food consists of macronutrients (carbohydrates, fatty acids and proteins) and micronutrients (minerals, vitamins, amino acids and essential fats and lipids). Essential nutrients are the vitamins and minerals necessary for the constant building, maintenance and repair of tissues. Although normal metabolism provides some of the essential nutrients needed for optimum health, not every essential nutrient can be synthesized by our bodies, so some essential fatty acids, amino acids, vitamins and most of the minerals are required as part of a healthy diet. Each person's requirements for essential nutrients to maintain good health are unique.

Enzymes

The countless catabolic and anabolic biochemical reactions that happen inside our bodies are mediated by special protein molecules called enzymes. Enzymes are the catalysts that make it possible for metabolism to happen efficiently. Biochemical reactions grouped with relevant enzymes achieve physiological goals to form metabolic pathways, and different metabolic pathways link up and react with each other to form bodily systems. When an enzyme becomes dysfunctional — for example, if the diamine oxide enzyme that breaks down histamine is unable to maintain an appropriate balance — many of our body systems may be profoundly affected.

Nervous System Disorders

Nervous system problems and behavioral problems are difficult to separate because they function through the same structure. Problems such as poisoning, metabolic defects, vascular disorders or inflammation involve either the nerve cells themselves or the elements that support them. In disorders such as migraine, tests have not revealed any sign of damage to the nervous system. This finding suggests some hope for improved quality of life through lifestyle changes.

Vascular Reactions

Since there is no physical sign of biological damage in people who have migraine attacks, it is difficult to say whether it is a problem with either the vascular or the neural system that causes migraine symptoms. Recent functional imaging techniques have shown, however, that both mechanisms — thus called neurovascular mechanisms — are in fact involved. Different areas of the brain are now known to be specific to headache types. The brainstem, for example, is where episodic migraines are triggered. Recent research suggests that primary headaches may soon be diagnosed based on the pattern of brain activation seen in imaging, leading to more effective therapies.

Cluster Headache and the Hypothalamus

The overall cause, or etiology, of cluster headaches is still not fully understood. Cluster headaches are periodic in nature, they occur on a regular basis over a 24-hour period, and the cyclic pattern also follows the seasons, suggesting involvement of our brain's biological clock — located in the hypothalamus, deep in the brain. Current theories suggest that abnormalities of the hypothalamus may explain the cyclic nature of cluster headaches. The back of the hypothalamus responds to signals from many different organs and systems in your body: light; smells; sex steroids; corticosteroids; neural signals from the heart, stomach and reproductive organs; autonomic messages; blood-borne stimuli (hormones); and stress. The variety of signals received by this area of the brain may help to explain the range of triggers during a cluster period.

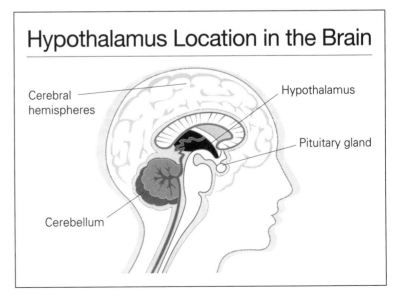

Hypothalamus Location in the Brain

Cerebral hemispheres

Hypothalamus

Pituitary gland

Cerebellum

Tension Headache and Inflammation

Tension headache pain may result from stress and tight muscles in your neck, jaw, lower skull and forehead. How often these headaches occur will depend on the frequency and level of stressful events during the day.

Repeated and sustained muscle tension in your scalp and nearby areas (the pericranial myofascial tissues) could increase the level of the central nervous system's response to the pain signals. A person with tension headache would experience increased pain from the same sensory signal that is not painful for a patient without tension headache. Not getting relief from physical or emotional stress or tight muscles can change episodic tension headaches into chronic tension headache.

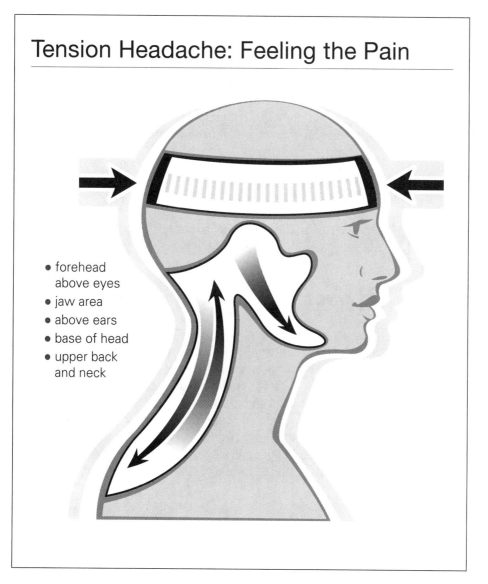

Tension Headache: Feeling the Pain

- forehead above eyes
- jaw area
- above ears
- base of head
- upper back and neck

Nitric Oxide

Nitric oxide is a quick-acting, cell-to-cell chemical messenger in the nervous system that affects how and when a migraine might begin and how it proceeds. Made by many different kinds of cells, nitric oxide acts in several ways, depending on its location. Since it travels very short distances and doesn't last long, a signal is sent to the specific body location to make nitric oxide where the reaction is to take place:

1. The inside cell layer of an artery, called the endothelium, carries blood from the heart to the tissues. When nitric oxide is made in the endothelium, it is carried from cell to cell quickly, moving past the membrane of the artery to the muscle cells below. The nitric oxide relaxes the muscle cells, making them dilate. This reaction regulates blood pressure and where blood is distributed in the body.

2. Nitric oxide is produced in white blood cells (macrophages) and fights infection from bacteria and parasites with the large amounts of toxins produced.

3. Nitric oxide is also produced by many nerve cells that function as signaling molecules. This forms the basis of regulation of quite a number of bodily functions (for example, behavior and gastrointestinal function).

Studies have also suggested a possible role for nitric oxide in the development of tension-type headaches. Generalized heightened sensitivity to pain is present in chronic tension-type headache, but the ability to inhibit nitric oxide is lost. The use of chemicals that block nitric oxide, called nitric oxide synthase inhibitors, could possibly become part of future treatment plans.

Stress Reactions

Stress is an ancient bodily response to predators or life-threatening situations that would have triggered a fight or flight response meant to protect your life and your family. Today, stress is still a physical, emotional and mental response to real or perceived threats and challenges in everyday life. Examples of daily stress include getting your family out the door in the morning, driving in heavy traffic, carrying a big workload, balancing your budget and taking care of your aging parents, to name a few.

Hormonal Mechanisms

Like the immune response, the stress response leads to vascular changes that might result in migraine. Stress activates the hypothalamus (a small area at the bottom of the brain) to raise an alarm that releases a variety of hormones into the bloodstream. The alarm also stimulates the adrenal glands (sitting on top of each kidney) to release a flood of hormone messengers, such as adrenaline and cortisol. Adrenaline prepares your body for fight or flight by increasing your blood pressure, heart rate and energy supplies, while cortisol, called the primary stress hormone, pulls sugars from storage into the bloodstream, increases the use of glucose in your brain and prepares the body for quick tissue repair. During the fight or flight response, cortisol also turns off unneeded body functions to save energy, shutting down the digestive and reproductive systems and altering immune system responses. Once the threat is over, your body's regulation system returns all processes to normal activity levels. If stress is a constant factor in your life, the fight or flight mechanism continues to dominate your bodily functions.

Stress-Associated Pain

The stress response is a known trigger for people with primary headaches. Stress initiates pain perception in the central brain, increasing the neurotransmitter messages that start headaches for many people. Over time, it also amplifies the sensitivity of nerve endings, a phenomenon called the wind-up effect. Stress can also increase the intensity and duration of each headache and hasten the progression of headaches from episodic to chronic.

Histamine Overload and Intolerance

Histamine is a vasoactive (affecting the blood vessels) amine formed in the body from the amino acid histidine. Histamine is stored in mast cells, which are scattered throughout the connective tissues of your body. During an immune response, histamine starts a chain of events that ultimately causes blood vessels to expand, leading to symptoms that may include headache, rash, skin irritation, congestion in the ear and nose, and contraction of the airways. In some instances, the response may rapidly escalate to an anaphylactic reaction, which can be fatal and must be treated as an emergency.

For some people, vasodilation is also the cause of migraine and tension-type headaches.

The histamine load in the body is increased by the high-histamine foods we tend to favor in the Western diet. Once the body overloads with histamine, migraine symptoms or other symptoms appear, typically slowly. A small amount of histamine will not cause a response — it is the total amount of histamine in excess of the body's requirements that can result in a migraine. Determining your overload, or intolerance level, for histamine is important for managing migraine headaches, as is determining the histamine content of common foods. For some people, avoiding high-histamine foods will help prevent migraine headaches.

High-Histamine Foods to Avoid

This list of 10 common foods that are high in histamine is excerpted from a more extensive list in Part 3 (page 146).

1. Matured cheeses, such as extra-old Cheddar
2. Sausages, cold cuts, ham
3. Fish (tuna, mackerel, anchovy, canned fish)
4. Oranges, grapefruit, strawberries
5. Fermented foods (sauerkraut, pickles, tamari)
6. Red wine vinegar, balsamic vinegar, white wine vinegar
7. Alcoholic beverages
8. Some vegetables (spinach, tomatoes)
9. Shellfish
10. Processed foods

Food Allergies and Sensitivities

Food poisoning, allergies, intolerances and sensitivities can also trigger migraine headaches. Only you can figure out which foods are healthy and healing for you and which foods are headache triggers, alone or in combination.

Food Poisoning

Food poisoning is an adverse reaction that happens only as a specific result of improper storage, processing or contamination of food. You could eat the same food on other occasions and not have this reaction again.

10 Most Common Food Allergens

- Peanuts
- Tree nuts
- Seafood
- Milk
- Eggs
- Soy foods
- Wheat
- Sesame seeds
- Sulfites
- Mustard

Food Allergy

Food allergy is different from food poisoning. A food allergy happens every time you eat that food or type of food, which sets off a body-wide immune reaction and can be life-threatening. Food allergy reactions can range from mild skin itch to acute swelling of the face and neck with difficulty in breathing. Such severe allergic reaction is called anaphylaxis and is fatal if not treated urgently. People with serious food allergies carry injectable epinephrine as a life-saver and must avoid contact with their allergens for their entire lives. It is very important to be checked for food allergies if you suspect you have one.

Food Sensitivity and Intolerance

Some people think they may have a food allergy when in fact they are suffering from a food sensitivity or intolerance. Food sensitivity, or intolerance, is an adverse reaction (like an upset stomach) that happens every time you eat a particular food or type of food. The difference between food allergy and food

Q. What causes food intolerance?

A. A shortage of digestive enzymes or improperly working digestive enzymes can be the cause of many illnesses, including food intolerances. Enzymes are the nuts and bolts for every biochemical reaction and function in our body, and digestive enzymes break down all the foods we eat. The molecules that remain are used as nutrients to build, repair and replace tissues and are the source of the energy that drives our bodies.

intolerance is that allergies are caused by a direct reaction from the immune system in response to a particular ingredient in the food, while food intolerances may or may not directly involve immune response.

Lactose intolerance is an example where a person experiences bloating, pain and gas every time they drink milk or eat milk-based products. Along with lactose intolerance, people are commonly sensitive to wheat (and other grains that contain gluten), sugar in honey and fruit (a particular glucose) and corn products.

While people can be tested for food allergies with recordable positive or negative results, it is more difficult to test for sensitivities. Often, no allergic response is seen from testing the immune system. Some people overcome their sensitivity to a particular food after removing the food from their diet for some time, followed by a gradual re-exposure over time.

> Some people overcome their sensitivity to a particular food after gradual re-exposure over a period of time.

Common Foods Suspected of Triggering Migraine

Vegetables: onions, snow peas, pickles, sauerkraut, canned vegetable soup

Fruit: avocados, red plums

Nuts: tree nuts, nut spreads

Beans: lima, navy and pinto beans

Legumes: peanuts, peanut butter

Meat: aged, cured, processed or canned meats

Dairy products: aged cheese, buttermilk, sour cream

Flavorings and additives: meat tenderizer, soy sauce, monosodium glutamate (MSG), tyramine, nitrates, caffeine (intake or withdrawal), brewer's yeast

Chapter 3
How Are Migraine, Cluster and Tension Headaches Diagnosed?

CASE HISTORY
Hormone Trigger

Beth's life has been affected by migraine attacks since she was very young. Going to bed in a dark room was the only way she could get through an attack. As an adult, her identified triggers are hormonal changes around her period, bright light (natural or artificial), flickering lights, dehydration, missed meals, any alcohol, loud or irritating noise, chemical odors, stress or tense muscles. With her migraines, Beth also experiences dizziness and nausea.

The number of migraine attacks Beth experiences ranges from eight to as many as 20 per month. She has a few close friends who have stuck by her, but her social life has certainly suffered.

Several of Beth's family members (sisters and a grandmother) also get migraines.

Beth has been prescribed several medications to give her some relief from her symptoms, but is now looking for new headache management strategies.

If you are suffering from headaches that significantly interfere with your daily routine, whether they are occasional or daily, you should consult your family doctor. The usual starting point is a careful symptom-by-symptom clinical evaluation to consider all possible disorders (forming a list of differential diagnoses) before the most likely diagnosis is arrived at. The current headache guidelines used by physicians agree that the diagnosis of headache is entirely clinical. Investigations, whether blood tests or imaging, may not be necessary if you do not show signs of abnormality of the brain or the central nervous system.

Patient History

Your physician or health-care provider will take a careful history of your headache profile. Here are some sample questions you might be asked:

When did the headache first start (in terms of days/months/years)?

_____

How did your headache start (did you have a head injury)?

_____

Has your headache stayed the same as time has gone by?

_____

How has it changed over time?

_____

How often do the headaches appear?

_____

How long do they last?

_____

How severe is the pain (on a scale of 1 to 10)?

_____

Are there any associated symptoms?

_____

What have you been doing to relieve the headache pain?

_____

How effective have any treatments been?

_____

Family History

In addition to your personal medical history, your health-care provider will ask about the health of your family, especially your parents. Your history and your family history by themselves can provide enough information for a diagnosis of primary headache. Even so, symptoms of possible secondary headache should be tested in all patients to rule out more urgent conditions.

Clinical Reasoning

Health-care providers follow a standard course of clinical reasoning as they diagnose health conditions. The flow chart below illustrates the clinical reasoning involved in diagnosing primary and secondary headaches, starting with your first visit to your doctor and, depending on what is discovered during your medical history and assessment, what further tests may be required and what therapies may be recommended.

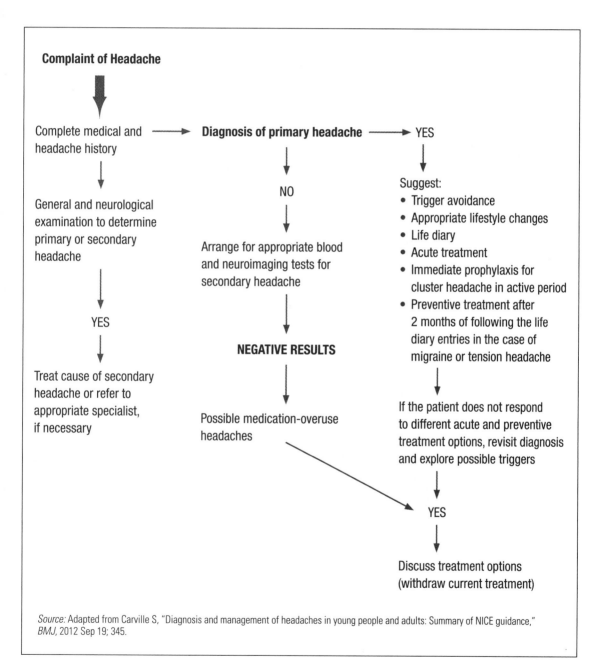

Complaint of Headache

Complete medical and headache history → **Diagnosis of primary headache** → YES

General and neurological examination to determine primary or secondary headache

YES

Treat cause of secondary headache or refer to appropriate specialist, if necessary

NO

Arrange for appropriate blood and neuroimaging tests for secondary headache

NEGATIVE RESULTS

Possible medication-overuse headaches

Suggest:
- Trigger avoidance
- Appropriate lifestyle changes
- Life diary
- Acute treatment
- Immediate prophylaxis for cluster headache in active period
- Preventive treatment after 2 months of following the life diary entries in the case of migraine or tension headache

If the patient does not respond to different acute and preventive treatment options, revisit diagnosis and explore possible triggers

YES

Discuss treatment options (withdraw current treatment)

Source: Adapted from Carville S, "Diagnosis and management of headaches in young people and adults: Summary of NICE guidance," *BMJ*, 2012 Sep 19; 345.

Diagnostic Criteria for Migraine, Tension, and Cluster Headaches

To assist your health-care provider in arriving at a clear diagnosis, you may be asked to complete a symptom questionnaire. This will help to distinguish migraine from tension and cluster headaches.

Classification Criteria for Migraine

A. Five or more attacks that include symptoms as described in points B to D below

B. Headache attacks lasting 4 to 72 hours (not treated or no improvement with treatment)

C. Headache with two or more of these symptoms:
1. Pain is felt on one side of the head (unilateral location)
2. Pain is felt as a pulse (pulsating quality)
3. Pain is of moderate to severe pain intensity
4. Pain is worsened by walking, climbing stairs, etc; may lead to inactivity

D. During headache, one or more of these symptoms:
1. Nausea, vomiting
2. Unable to tolerate light or unable to tolerate sound (but not both)

E. Not caused by another disorder

Classification Criteria for Migraine with Aura

A. Two or more attacks with symptoms as described in points B and C below

B. At least one fully reversible aura symptom:
1. Sensory
2. Visual
3. Motor
4. Speech and/or language
5. Retinal
6. Brainstem

C. Two or more of these symptoms:
1. One or more aura-related symptom (noted in B), with a gradual increase in 5 or more minutes and with at least 2 of the symptoms happening one after another
2. Any aura-related symptom that occurs for 5 to 60 minutes
3. One or more aura-related symptom that is one-sided
4. Headache occurs with or follows aura-related symptoms within an hour

D. Transient ischaemic attack has been ruled out, and no other ICHD-3 diagnosis better fits the group of aura-related symptoms

Classification Criteria for Cluster Headache

A. Five or more attacks with symptoms as described in points B to D below

B. Severe or extremely severe one-sided pain in one eye, behind one eye or on one side of the head (orbital, supraorbital, temporal) that lasts from 15 to 180 minutes if not treated

C. One or both of the following points:
   1. Headache has one or more of these symptoms:
      a) Red eye and/or tear flow (ipsilateral conjunctival injection and/or lacrimation) on one side only
      b) Nasal congestion and/or runny nose (rhinorrhea) on one side only
      c) Eyelid swelling (edema) on one side only
      d) Sweating of forehead and face
      e) Flushing of forehead and face
      f) Feeling of fullness in the ear
      g) Increase and/or decrease in pupil size (miosis and/or ptosis) on one side only
   2. Restlessness/agitation (pacing to escape the pain)

D. Frequency of headache attacks: one every other day to as many as eight per day

E. Not caused by another disorder

Classification Criteria for Tension Headache

A. At least 10 episodes that happen an average of less than 1 day a month with symptoms as described in points B to D below

B. Duration of 30 minutes to as long as 7 days

C. Headaches with two or more of the following symptoms:
   1. Pain is felt on both sides of the head (bilateral location)
   2. Band-like pain of a pressing or tightening (non-pulsing) feeling
   3. Pain is of mild to moderate pain intensity
   4. Pain is not made worse by everyday physical activity (walking or climbing stairs)

D. Including these symptoms:
   1. No nausea or vomiting
   2. Unable to tolerate light or unable to tolerate sound (but not both)

E. Not caused by another disorder

Source: Adapted from International Headache Classification (ICHD-III beta, 2013), http://ihs-classification.org/en/.

Diagnostic Criteria

Guidelines to assist health-care professionals with the diagnosis of primary and secondary headaches have been developed by research centers that specialize in headaches, such as the International Headache Society. Recommendations for decision-making and treatment strategies are based on the best available evidence-based research and include the experience and opinions of headache and pain experts who have clinical experience.

Diagnostic Processes

- Signs and Symptoms
- Family History
- Physical Examination
- Triggers and Factors
- Comorbidities
- Differential Diagnosis
- Prognosis
- Treatment Options

Q. What questions should I ask during my first meeting with my doctor?

A. It's a good idea to prepare some questions to ask your doctor about your headaches. Here are some ideas. Take a copy of this page with you and write down any other questions on another sheet before your appointment. Don't trust yourself to remember them. Write them down.

Questions about symptoms:

- Are my headaches symptoms of other health problems?
- Can you tell me what makes my headache different from other types of headaches?

Possible questions about treatment:

- What kinds of treatments are usually given for these headaches?
- How can I control these headaches? Will changing my lifestyle or going on a diet make a difference?
- Do you know of any cures for this type of headache?
- Are there any risks to this treatment?
- Should I go right to emergency if I have any side effects from this treatment?
- Is this treatment better for me because of another health issue that I have?
- How long does this treatment work? Does it work right away?
- How long do you think I will need to take this treatment?
- Are there any side effects from taking this treatment for a long time?
- Will I always keep taking this treatment dose?

Sometimes, your doctor or nurse might have information that will help you and your family cope with your headaches:

- Where do people go for support for this kind of headache? Are there any organizations in this community?
- Do you have any information about my headaches that I could share with my family?
- Will this headache continue to affect my work, studies and social life? What can I do to improve this?
- What can I expect to happen with these headaches as I get older? Will it ever go away?
- My wife would like to know if there is something she could be doing to help me with these headaches. Do you have any suggestions?
- Could I speak to a social worker about my headaches?

Women might have other concerns as well:

- Should I still take the same dose when I have my period?
- Will this treatment make my cramps better? Or worse?
- Will I need to switch to another birth control method because of this treatment?
- What can I expect?
- Is there a danger of blood clots from this treatment?
- Will this treatment be dangerous if I get pregnant?

Chapter 4
Other Associated Conditions

CASE HISTORY
Comorbid Asthma

Shirley will be 40 years old in October. She was diagnosed with migraines in her early 20s and has been struggling with them ever since. Shirley has sensitivities to chemical products such as soaps, cleaners, and perfumes. Several years ago, she had pneumonia that lasted for several months, even though she was on antibiotics twice. At the end of the second prescription, her family physician prescribed puffers for Shirley, since she was showing signs and symptoms of asthma as well.

These days, Shirley is exhausted and struggling to breathe, using her maintenance puffer to keep her airways open but still needing care for emergency medication for the asthma once and sometimes twice yearly. Her doctor has explained that her risk of asthma was higher because she had migraines. It's a lot to cope with, having several migraines a month that keep her at home in bed in a quiet room with the curtains drawn for at least a day, and then having to deal with the inconvenience of puffers and the terror that accompanies the asthma attacks, which leave her breathless. She misses work several days a month and is grateful that her supervisor appreciates her skills rather than counting her sick days.

People who have migraine attacks are diagnosed with other illnesses more often than are people who don't. These other illnesses are then considered to be associated, or comorbid, with the migraines. Identifying comorbidities is important because it may lead to a better understanding of migraine pathophysiology and improve treatment strategies. Epilepsy, fibromyalgia and irritable bowel syndrome are among the most common and concerning comorbidities of migraine.

Epilepsy

If you suffer from migraine attacks, your risk of having an epileptic seizure is higher than for people who do not have migraines.

Shared Symptoms

Migraine and epilepsy share many symptoms:

- Disturbed sensation (including vision, hearing and taste)
- Abnormal mood or mental function
- Attacks are episodic
- Glutamate, an excitatory neurotransmitter molecule, plays a role in both conditions

Genetic Affinities

Research has shown a higher risk of epilepsy for people with migraine and has identified common genes for migraine and epilepsy for some people. Genetic mutations are associated with familial hemiplegic migraine (FHM) and epileptic seizures in family members, and for some people, seizures can happen during or soon after a migraine attack (a condition called migralepsy). Insights into the common nervous system pathways that cause epilepsy and migraine may suggest new treatment approaches for both conditions.

Treatment

Identifying comorbidities can help health-care providers make better therapeutic choices, first by treating the two conditions with a single appropriate drug (for example, divalproex sodium or topiramate may treat both epilepsy and migraine) or by being aware of some issues that relate to one or the other condition and so choosing to not use specific treatments (for example,

Common Medical Conditions Comorbid with Migraine

Stroke	Different kinds of heart- and brain-related illnesses are associated with migraine. Some are related to migraine with aura, while others are associated only with migraine without aura. If you suffer from migraine with aura, you have a higher risk of having a stroke, whether you are a man or a woman. This is not the case if you have migraine without aura. Your doctor may make treatment decisions based on this information, and especially if there is a family history of stroke.
Subclinical vascular brain lesions	Inflammatory or vasoactive molecules, which affect blood vessel diameter when released into the brain's blood vessels during migraine attacks, can damage vascular cell walls and cause stroke or other medical issues. People with migraine (and particularly those who experience aura) also have a reduced ability to heal the inner layer of the vascular system, increasing their risk of vascular diseases.
Coronary heart disease	People who have migraine with aura have a higher risk of coronary heart disease if they also have high levels of total cholesterol. Women and men who suffer from migraine with and without aura have higher risk for myocardial infarction. Genetic risk factors may be a mechanism linking migraine and cardiovascular diseases.
Hypertension	People with chronic migraines have double the risk of having hypertension.
Psychiatric diseases	Anxiety, panic disorder, depression, bipolar disorder, and suicide have all been associated with migraine.
Restless legs syndrome	Restless legs syndrome (RLS) affects both sensory and motor functions, and their pathways. Some research has shown that RLS is more common in people with migraine than in people with tension or cluster headache, perhaps because of shared central nervous system pathways.
Obesity	Obesity is linked with migraines; the higher their body mass index (BMI), the more likely a person will suffer from migraines.
Fibromyalgia	Fibromyalgia is diagnosed more often in people who get migraines.
Epilepsy	Research has identified common genes for migraine and epilepsy.
Asthma	A high percentage of people with chronic migraines also have asthma.
Irritable bowel syndrome	Reports of data from a national U.S. health-care plan also show that people with migraine are more likely to have IBS.

tricyclic antidepressants may lower the seizure threshold for epilepsy). Some anti-epileptic drugs are effective for preventing migraine headaches, likely because genetic or environmental factors (such as a head injury) cause brain hyperexcitability that can lead to either condition. In addition, since anti-epileptic medication (such as valproic acid) has been found to be effective against cluster headaches, you could reason that epilepsy and cluster headaches share the same pathophysiology.

Fibromyalgia

Several chronic pain disorders, notably fibromyalgia, are associated with migraine. Headache frequency appears to be a strong predictor for musculoskeletal pain. People with headache have reported that they suffer more from musculoskeletal pain than people without headache.

Irritable Bowel Syndrome

Migraine also shares many epidemiological, psychosocial and pathophysiological symptoms with irritable bowel syndrome (IBS) and gluten sensitivity. Research suggests that ongoing stressful events can make the central nervous system hypervigilant and over-responsive to future events. The enteric, or gastrointestinal, nervous system of a genetically predisposed person may also become overly sensitive to stress. Reports of data from a national U.S. health-care plan also show that people with migraine are more likely to have IBS.

Other Comorbidities

- Tension Headache
- Insomnia
- Cluster Headache
- Sinusitis
- Malignancy
- Diabetes Mellitus
- Glaucoma
- Depression

Part 2

Managing Primary Headaches

Chapter 5
Lifestyle Changes

CASE HISTORY
Big Changes

Birjit is 52 years old and was first diagnosed with migraine headache when she was 14. Her headache attacks usually last from 1 to 3 days. At long last, she decided to explore management strategies beyond the over-the-counter medications she had been taking for years. On the advice of her doctor, Birjit made some lifestyle changes. She began doing stretches first thing in the morning, five days a week. She found that walking outside or using a treadmill was something that worked with her schedule, and she was able to keep the intensity level below the level that could trigger a headache. She had one session with an exercise trainer who had experience with headache issues and tried following a diet that excluded foods that might trigger her headaches. Finally, Birjit started visiting a massage therapist once a month and met with a psychologist for cognitive behavioral counseling. After work, Birjit would find a quiet place and listen for 10 to 15 minutes to a relaxation tape that the counselor had given her. Her bedroom was kept at a lower temperature and ventilation was improved.

Birjit was able to follow most of this protocol for 6 months, with some deviation in the diet. She did gain some relief from her headaches — they were rarely happening, and when they did, were much shorter and not nearly as intense. Birjit lost 10 pounds (4.5 kg) and said she felt happier in general. She was sleeping fewer hours (closer to 8 than 10) and felt refreshed in the morning, able to get out of bed to do her stretching. Carrying an attractive water bottle filled with coconut water was her sure way to stay hydrated. In retrospect, Birjit said it was difficult to make these lifestyle changes; she did well initially but easily lapsed into old habits. Working with your doctor or other health professional to stay motivated with your lifestyle changes can make all the difference. For Birjit, the most important change has been her mental aspect. She feels "much improved" and more in control of her life.

Unfortunately, there is no silver bullet, no one absolutely reliable remedy for curing primary headache. The aim of managing the symptoms of primary headache is to relieve the pain by eliminating the triggers and counteracting the factors that cause migraine. These strategies include lifestyle changes, medications, physiotherapies, botanical medicines and dietary therapy, specifically a diet of foods that are low in histamine content.

Making Changes

These aims can only be achieved if headache patients are willing to adjust their attitude toward their illness and to change key elements of their lifestyle.

Stages of Change

1. **Acceptance.** Perhaps you have not yet come to terms with your headaches, thinking that they will one day go away and never come back. Wishful thinking and denial won't do much to help you manage chronic pain.

2. **Education.** Learn about the condition. Solicit information from all available sources so you can recognize the symptoms and understand the medical diagnosis. An informed patient has the best chance for recovery.

3. **Action.** Do what you can to manage the condition yourself, using appropriate individual-directed lifestyle changes, such as stress reduction strategies and improved sleep habits.

4. **Assistance.** Turn to health-care professionals for other healing modalities, such as medical doctors for the use of medications and registered dieticians for dietary therapy.

Lifestyle Counseling

> A healthy and scheduled lifestyle may be the key to managing your headaches.

A healthy and scheduled lifestyle may be the key to managing your headaches. Keeping a journal over a period of time may help you see areas of your life that could be contributing to your headaches, such as diet, meal schedule, fluid intake, exercise, sleep patterns or excessive stress at the workplace or at home. Discussions with your health-care team about making changes in these lifestyle habits can help you put together a plan that keeps you motivated. Having options for therapy strategies along with the medication therapy prescribed by your doctor makes it easier to manage your headaches.

Primary Headache Management Modalities

Because there is no one cure for primary headache, treatment tends to be holistic, bringing together, or integrating, a wide range of treatment strategies, or modalities. These modalities all contribute to the PARR treatment goals (see Chapter 6):

- Lifestyle counseling
- Pharmaceutical medications
- Physiotherapies
- Surgery
- Complementary and alternative therapies
- Nutritional and herbal supplements
- Dietary therapy

Stress Management

Of the various lifestyle factors that lead to the onset of primary headache, stress can be reduced, if not eliminated, by adopting specific strategies. Failure to manage stress leads to fatigue and exhaustion, which creates a hormone imbalance and leaves you prone to infection. If you address stress now, these imbalances and responses can be prevented, avoided or at least reduced. Educating patients about stress avoidance and teaching coping mechanisms helps them gain control of their pain and prevent further headaches.

Strategies for Reducing Stress

1. Eat a healthy, nutritious diet.
2. Exercise regularly — but be sure it is an enjoyable activity for you.
3. Have a safe and trusted ear for venting your stress-related concerns.
4. Stay organized to make the most efficient use of your time.
5. Be prepared to ask for help (perhaps professional). Someone else may know an easier way to move that mountain!
6. Learn to relax by using breathing exercises, guided imagery and other anti-stress strategies.

Sleep Hygiene

At one time, troubled sleep was thought to be the cause of headaches and good sleep was seen as the cure. If only it were that easy. Poor sleep is certainly another lifestyle factor that can trigger primary headache, however, and improving your sleep hygiene can help prevent and reduce headache pain.

If you are having trouble getting enough sleep and you have headaches, you are not alone. Sleep pattern disturbances are a major trigger for primary headache, with too little, too much or disrupted sleep all increasing the risks of chronic headache. The reverse is also true, that migraine, cluster and tension headaches can cause sleep fragmentation, loss of sleep and oversleeping. Of these factors, waking frequently during the night is directly related to headache severity. Sleeping issues can also indicate other health problems, so they should always be assessed by your doctor.

Sleep Mechanisms

Headache pain comes from collected signals of the sensory receptors that travel to the amygdala and the mesolimbic centers (higher/emotional centers) of the brain. These brain regions learn to "turn up or turn down the noise volume from pain signals" based on other factors (emotions, anxiety, the degree of attention or distraction, past experience, memories). The mesolimbic center also sends out messages to the rest of the body through the hypothalamus. Body temperature, blood pressure, appetite, sexual responses and circadian rhythm (including sleep) are all controlled by the hypothalamus. Along with coordinating behavior, the amygdala also maintains autonomic responses, such as the fight or flight stress response. In a similar way, stress can trigger sleep disturbances and headaches or make them worse.

Strategies for Improving Your Sleep Hygiene

1. Just as a parent does for young children, knowing they need sleep to grow, it is important for you to establish a regular sleep pattern. Go to bed and get up at the same time every day to support your circadian rhythm (sleep-wake cycles).

2. If you find that you are tossing and turning for more than 15 minutes, get out of bed and do something relaxing under dim lighting (not looking at a television or computer screen). Go back to bed when you feel sleepy.

3. Limit afternoon naps to prevent waking in the middle of the night, but a nap of around 10 to 30 minutes before 3 p.m. will not interfere with your nightly slumber.

4. Stop eating a few hours before you go to bed (easy if you are following a regular sleep schedule), but don't go to bed hungry either. Planned snacks early in the evening are part of a well-thought-out meal plan.

5. Limit fluid intake, nicotine, alcohol and caffeine close to bedtime or suffer the consequences of disrupted sleep and possible headache attacks.

6. Exercise. Tiring your body physically will lead to better-quality sleep. We are physical creatures, and as such, require physical exercise on a daily basis. Exercising earlier in the day works better than pre-bedtime workouts, which may increase your mental activity at a time when you need to wind down — true even for something as calm as tai chi.

7. Create your own special space for good-quality sleep. Think cool, dark and quiet for sleep success. We learn so much from our pets. Watch a dog prepare to go to bed — it will circle and circle, wrapping its body this way and that to find the perfectly comfortable place and position to sleep.

8. Reduce noise and light. Some items that may be useful to achieve your sleep goals are blinds, shades or curtains to darken your room, a fan or window that opens slightly to keep it cool, and comfortable earplugs. Sleep on whatever style of mattress and pillow suits your needs.

9. If you share your bed with a partner, child or pets, be sure you have enough space. Establish limits that allow you to get the sleep you need.

10. In the same way that you have your children wash their face and hands or have a bath, brush their teeth and read a nighttime story, establish a ritual for yourself that helps you relax and prepare your body for sleep. Examples include a warm bath or shower, soothing music or reading under dimmed lights. Using electronic media with bright screens close to bedtime may interfere with your circadian rhythms and make it difficult to fall asleep.

11. Manage your stress as part of your bedtime ritual. If you are not already discussing ways to manage your stress with your doctor, now may be the time for that visit.

12. As part of your bedtime ritual, list the concerns that are keeping you awake at night and leave that list in another room besides your bedroom. This may help you enjoy a peaceful night's sleep.

Eating Habits

Missing a meal or irregular meal schedules can increase the risk of headaches. After a meal, most of the food we eat is metabolized into glucose, the form of sugar that is used as fuel for our bodies. The sensation of hunger from missing a meal is due to a drop in the level of glucose in the bloodstream (called hypoglycemia), which raises stress levels in the body. Low blood sugar causes a flood of events in the body. More insulin is released to pull glucose from storage to be used by the body. Insulin is a hormone needed to change glucose into glycogen for storage and is produced by the pancreas, an endocrine gland located behind the stomach, but irregularities in the supply of this hormone create a host of problems, including insulin resistance, metabolic syndrome and diabetes. Some of the physical responses to high insulin levels include tremors of the hand or body (often most intensely at night), sweating anywhere on the body (also most intensely at night), a pounding heart, mental and physical fatigue, decreased focus and headaches.

Other meal-related issues that may cause headaches include following an extreme diet that may exclude an entire food group, such as carbohydrates or protein; overindulging in a particular food, such as salt; or not including a food that you may be physically dependent upon, such as caffeine from tea or coffee. Regular meals and snacks based on a diet plan built from nutritious, healthy foods will help to maintain a regular supply of fuel for your body and brain.

> Regular meals and snacks based on a diet plan built from nutritious, healthy foods will help to maintain a regular supply of fuel for your body and brain.

Strategies for Preventing Hypoglycemia and Hyperglycemia

Hypoglycemia

1. Eat every 2 to 3 hours, either a meal or a snack. Never skip meals and always carry a snack with you if you are away from home.

2. Food choices should include carbohydrates that are digested slowly (for example, apples, pears, large-flake and steel-cut oatmeal, milk, yogurt, nuts and seeds, legumes); protein to maintain steady blood sugar (lean meat, poultry, fish, low-fat cheese, eggs, nuts and yogurt); and soluble fiber to slow the digestion rate (oatmeal, psyllium, flax seeds, barley, legumes, sweet potatoes, citrus).

Hyperglycemia

1. Moderate exercise (brisk walking, for example) for 30 minutes five out of every seven days will help to control hyperglycemia.

2. If you are considered overweight or obese, reaching your optimal weight will reduce your risk of hyperglycemia.

Dehydration

Two-thirds of our body weight is water, with about 70% inside the cells, roughly 20% in the spaces that surround our cells and only about 10% in the bloodstream. The brain, with 85% water content, requires more water. Maintaining the water level of your body is key to staying healthy. If you are healthy, matching how much water you take in to how much you lose (this includes how much you sweat) on a daily basis will ensure sufficient water levels. If you do not watch your hydration, however, dehydration may result and can trigger headaches, as well as incontinence, constipation or urinary tract infections (UTIs), or worse, renal stones and even renal disease.

If you are healthy, your brain and kidneys (responsible for filtering the blood and maintaining fluid levels in the body) will manage shifts in water balance to a certain extent. When you are dehydrated, your water levels become more difficult to balance if you have a fever, are exposed to excessive heat for any length of time or have a stomach bug with vomiting or diarrhea. Infants, small children and seniors are more likely to suffer from severe dehydration. When you are properly hydrated, your body produces light-colored urine every 3 to 4 hours.

Dehydration Symptoms

- Dry mouth
- Fatigue
- Rapid heartbeat
- Weakness
- Headache
- Dry, flushed skin
- Muscle cramps and pain
- Thirst
- Dizziness

If dehydration continues, water moves from the space around the cells into the bloodstream, cells begin to shrivel and don't work properly, and body tissues begin to dry out. Brain cells are highly vulnerable to dehydration, leading to confusion and lightheadedness, even fainting. The salts that regulate cell activity (called electrolytes) become unbalanced as well, blood pressure is affected, and eventually the kidneys could shut down. If dehydration continues, toxic waste products can build up and cause severe damage to internal organs and, possibly, death.

Strategies for Preventing and Reversing Dehydration

1. As a rule of thumb, for every 100 pounds (45 kg) of body weight, drink 40 ounces (5 cups/1.125 L) of fluid a day to maintain good health and reduce the risk of headache.

2. When consulting your doctor about dehydration and headache, be prepared to discuss your activity level, your environment and your intake of caffeine (often considered a diuretic).

Eating Habits (Dieting)

The food that you choose for your diet nourishes your growth and development, providing you with the energy you need to stay alive. From cradle to adolescence and from adulthood to your golden years, a balanced, nutrient-rich diet is critical for healthy development and for reducing the risk of chronic disease, including primary headache.

Yo-Yo Diets

How you eat is equally as important as what you eat. Many people eat a yo-yo diet while trying to lose weight. Today they follow the diet program, tomorrow they don't. This pattern of weight loss and weight gain puts you at high risk for heart disease as well as other chronic disease states. The yo-yo habit can also trigger primary headaches. By cutting caloric intake, blood sugar issues go away, but if we return to the poor nutritional habits that got us to the higher weight, the weight quickly comes back. So goes the yo-yo.

There is no one-size-fits-all when it comes to what we look like. Our size and shape depend on our genes and other factors. It is possible to be fat and fit. Health is more dependent on how much belly fat you are carrying and the profile of your blood sugar. We each do have an optimal weight, however. Waist circumference is the true test of your level of obesity. If your goal is to lose weight, start by calculating your caloric balance, which is the number of calories you take in versus the number of calories you burn through exercise. If you burn more calories than you consume on a daily basis, you will lose weight.

Extreme Diets

Extreme diets include fasting or abstaining from certain essential foods, which can result in nutrient deficiencies that trigger primary headache. The popular high-protein, low-carbohydrate diet that focuses on one food group at the expense of others, for example, can increase risk of chronic disease. Research has shown that shifting even a small percentage away from a balanced diet can increase the risk of cardiovascular disease.

Some health dangers come with extreme diets, so it is important to discuss any severe diet change with your doctor. Extreme diets often do not provide the daily nutrition we require and can be life-threatening. And any of these diet patterns can be a factor in chronic primary headache.

Strategies for Improving Your Eating Habits and Avoiding Triggers

Making long-term changes to your eating habits requires considerable effort. Try this three-step process:

1. *Reflect.* Make a list of your current eating habits. Include behaviors that trigger habits you would like to change or improve. Write down behaviors that lead to good eating habits. Use a diary to record everything you eat, when you eat it and why (your mood, level of tiredness, level of stress and how hungry you were). Do you skip breakfast except on weekends? Do you crave sweets in the evenings?

   Examples of habits you might like to change:
   - Eating even if you are not hungry
   - Eating food directly from packages rather than setting out a serving
   - Eating processed food because it is easier to prepare

2. *Replace.* Set out a plan to replace poor eating habits with healthy ones. Select a couple of habits you would like to change — your success rate will be better if you focus on one or two changes rather than take on too much. Recognize your good habits that you don't want to change; build on your successes.

   Examples of good habits:
   - Eating meals on a regular schedule
   - Choosing healthy snacks over treats most of the time

   Determine whether you can avoid the behavior cue that doesn't involve other people:
   - Try not stopping at your usual fast-food place on your way home; instead, try a different route that goes past a take-out restaurant with healthy choices.
   - Leave your change at home so you can't hit up the vending machine at work for a snack, but make sure you take healthy food that you like to work with you.

   For situations you can't avoid, try making decisions for conscious change, such as a shared dinner with several friends where each person brings a healthy dish according to a list you all agree upon.

Exercise new strategies to replace old habits:

- Turn off the news during dinner. Play some quiet music, set the table, and be mindful of each bite of food you put in your mouth to develop an appreciation of healthy, nutritious food and how it makes you feel rather than mindless eating while being distracted.
- Plan shopping trips around a meal plan to be sure that you have whole fresh food available and to prevent the fast-food grab after a busy day.

3. *Reinforce.* Establish conscious strategies that reinforce your healthy eating habits, new and longstanding.

- Understand that it takes time to replace habits.
- Understand that you will fall back into old habits on occasion.
- Ask yourself why you have reverted, to prevent it from happening in the future.
- Every day is a new opportunity to enjoy a healthy, nutritious diet. You will be pleased with the results.

Lifestyle Remedies for Migraine Headaches

One of the issues that people face when they suffer from migraine attacks is a sense of loss of control of their lives. Making lifestyle changes, developing a headache management strategy and creating treatment goals and expectations increases people's level of coping and sense of control. Some of the lifestyle choices that may increase your ability to manage migraine attacks include:

- Using stress management and muscle relaxation techniques (e.g., meditation, yoga, prayer)
- Being active and exercising regularly, pacing yourself as your headaches demand
- Making diet choices based on possible food sensitivities and triggers
- Taking preventive medications (make sure you are aware of any possible side effects or the possibility of medication overuse headaches)

Lifestyle Remedies for Cluster Headaches

If you suffer from cluster headaches, making some changes in your lifestyle may help to manage your headaches. You can improve your quality of life by following some common-sense guidelines that may also enhance your aerobic endurance and flexibility — without triggering cluster headaches or making them worse. Lifestyle factors that can help you manage your cluster headaches include:

- Eating a healthy, nutritious diet
- Following a regular meal schedule (not skipping meals)
- Adopting a regular sleep schedule
- Avoiding caffeine
- Participating in cognitive behavioral therapy to de-stress
- Maintaining routine aerobic exercise

Lifestyle Remedies for Tension Headaches

If you suffer from tension headaches, some practical lifestyle changes may help to manage your headaches. Eat nutritious food at regular mealtimes and follow a regular sleep and exercise schedule. Behavioral therapies (relaxation, biofeedback, cognitive behavioral therapy) have been shown to be effective for managing tension-type headaches.

Chapter 6
The PARR Lifestyle Program

CASE HISTORY
Overwhelmed

Martha is a 40-year-old college professor who is overwhelmed by her migraine headache attacks and how little control she has in her life because it seems she is either having a migraine attack, getting over a migraine attack or worried about having another one. She is very stressed about the impact of the migraines on her job situation, as well as her personal life. With two children aged 7 and 10 and a husband in the military forces, Martha is in charge of chauffeur duties for getting her kids to soccer, swimming and music lessons through the week and on weekends. Her nurse practitioner has scheduled a 2-hour visit to assess Martha's situation and develop a 12-step headache therapy strategy that will include a rescue tool kit.

Primary headaches are complex disorders that require patience and hard work to manage. For some people, management requires many visits to their health-care professionals, specialists, therapists and dietitians and (out of desperation) trying anything else that someone up the street may have suggested. In some cases, everything recommended by the physician (identifying and avoiding trigger factors, making lifestyle changes, trying a number of medications) has been tried — and may fail to control the disabling headaches. Based on the management principles of PARR — prevent, avoid, reduce and rescue — the following 12-step program may offer relief.

PARR

The acronym PARR is a handy tool for identifying the purpose of various treatments for primary headaches. Regardless of the treatment modality, the aim is the same:

Prevent, as much as possible, primary headaches from attacking.
Avoid triggers for primary headaches in all aspects of your life.
Reduce the frequency, severity and length of your primary headaches.
Rescue — use strategies that ensure you are taken care of if you have a headache attack.

Prevent

Accepting that for whatever reason you are a person who has primary headaches is an important first step to good management. Since primary headache is a chronic disorder that currently has no cure, developing a headache prevention plan is critical. Your headache therapy strategy must focus on preventing, avoiding and reducing your headaches. For most people, this can be accomplished through identifying environmental triggers to remove from your life and taking prescribed preventive medication that is proven to prevent headache attacks.

> Since primary headache is a chronic disorder that currently has no cure, developing a headache prevention plan is critical.

Avoid

Once you have determined your specific primary headache triggers, developing a strategy to avoid them is next. Most workplaces are supportive of the need to respect personal health risks, whether that means removing a carpet from your office or requesting that people not wear scents, or even that you don't shake hands upon greeting someone. A thorough assessment of your home and lifestyle, as well as the places you frequent, such as your gym or your children's daycare, will reveal more triggers to avoid.

Reduce

The personalized therapy strategy you develop with your health-care professional will help you recognize lifestyle changes that may successfully reduce headache frequency and severity, supported by possible preventive and acute medication as prescribed by your doctor.

Rescue

One of the critical components of a good therapy strategy is to have a rescue plan for when you feel the onset of a headache attack. Take steps to ensure that you are prepared to take care of yourself when a headache hits. Plan for a quiet, dark room where you can rest, for easy access to nutritious food and drinks that you can stomach, and keep medication within reach. Having a plan to take care of business during a headache is also important, whether that business be work or family-related. Who will pick up your kids, let the dog out, or send off that big project for you? A support network is an essential part of your headache therapy strategy.

Safe Care

Once again, be sure to discuss your headache therapy with your health-care provider. To provide optimum and safe care, all medications, herbal remedies, nutritional supplements, exercise regimens or anything else that may alter homeostasis in your body should be discussed. Follow your doctor's directions for taking any medication prescribed.

---

12 Steps to Prevent, Avoid, Reduce and Rescue

Now let's apply our understanding of the cause and course of primary headaches by condensing the action items on our agenda.

Step 1
Keep a health journal

A good way to figure out what lifestyle choices could be causing your headaches, or making them worse, is to keep a health journal. Knowing what happens in your daily life can help you understand the basis of your headaches. An accumulation of irregular events — missed meals, lack of sleep, going without fluids, stress, wine with dinner — may add up to a major headache a few days later. Keeping track may help you recognize specific or combined triggers and learn to manage your headaches by avoiding or reducing exposure to triggers. It may also improve your quality of life. For the most common triggers, see page 42.

How to Keep a Health Journal

Use a notebook, the journal in your computer or phone app, or just sheets of paper. Consider your habits and choose the vehicle that makes it easiest for you to stay motivated to write in it. Do your best to have at least 6 weeks of diary entries about your headaches before your first appointment with your doctor. Think of it as playing detective — the more information you have for every day, the more helpful your diary will be. With the information you provide, your health-care provider is more likely to be able to provide a headache therapy that works for you.

Episode Information

As soon as possible during or after any headache attack, record:

1. Date and time for beginning and end of any headache.
2. Location and whether it moved.
3. Pain severity and consistency. Typically, primary headache management is described as prevent, avoid, reduce and rescue.
4. Weather conditions, temperature, environmental conditions.
5. Activities at the time that the headache struck.
6. Stage in menstrual cycle.
7. Any signs and symptoms before, during, or after your headache is gone.
8. Exact details about your food intake: what, when, where and how much.
9. If and when you exercised, what kind of exercise, and intensity level.
10. Regular bedtime and when you bounce out of bed in the morning.
11. Stressful events you experienced recently.

General Information

Write or record answers to these questions:

1. Where is the pain typically located (head, neck)?
2. When did you have your first serious headache?
3. Do you have any headache symptoms prior to the attacks?
4. How would you describe the frequency and length of each headache attack?
5. What is the usual timing of your headache attack?
6. Are each of your headache attacks exactly the same? What are the differences, if any?
7. Do your headaches occur at specific times in your menstrual cycle?
8. Describe every single thing you have done to relieve the headache and list the effectiveness of each item.
9. When you are physically active, are your headaches worse?
10. What are the noticeable triggers for your headache attacks?

continued...

After a few weeks, you should be able to see possible relationships between your headaches and your lifestyle patterns from the history of your headaches in your journal. Continue keeping your headache journal even after you start more formal treatments so you can see which treatment is most effective.

Medication Effectiveness

Information about your headache medication:

1. Full drug name.

2. Directions and dosage as given by your doctor.

3. Assign a rating for effectiveness in reducing your headache pain (for example, no difference, better than it was, much improved, pain is gone).

4. How much time passed before you noticed any changes to your headache after taking the drug?

5. How effective was the drug for the entire headache attack?

6. Did you experience any noticeable side effects from this medication?

Always follow your doctor's directions for dosage and time between doses of medications. Rebound headaches may occur from overmedicating. See your doctor to discuss any changes in your medication. Carefully note any symptoms when starting a new medication, and note whether the medication has any impact on your usual activities.

Did You Know?

Smartphone Apps

Several smartphone apps are available to help you manage your headaches. Check them out to see which one best fits your needs.

Step 2
Create a daily schedule

Establish regular meal and snack times to help manage headache frequency. Hunger can be a trigger for headaches. Try to avoid letting mealtimes slip or missing them altogether, as often happens on weekends or busy workdays for many people.

Step 3
De-stress

Talk to a life coach or a cognitive behavioral counselor to reduce stress in your life. Bringing your health diary with you may help give these stress specialists some idea of what your day-to-day life includes, and they may in turn give you tools that make life easier. Many mind-body techniques have been found to be useful for managing stress. These include biofeedback, relaxation methods, meditation, hypnosis, cognitive behavioral training and yoga. For more information on stress management, see page 57.

Step 4
Stay hydrated

Be choosy about what you drink because some beverages (for example, orange or grapefruit juice and some bottled waters) have high levels of histamine or liberate histamine. Avoid diet drinks because aspartame is a known headache trigger. Be aware of your caffeine intake. Coconut water is a natural hydrator that balances your electrolytes and is fat-free. For more information on avoiding dehydration, see page 61.

Step 5
Clean it up

Keep your food preparation area squeaky clean and wash all food carefully to avoid or reduce histamine responses from food. Bacterial microbes found on cutting boards and in the sink increase histamine levels and worsen headache pain. For more information on avoiding high-histamine foods, see page 141.

Step 6
Buy fresh

Vegetables and fruits purchased from local markets or direct from the farmer have lower histamine levels than supermarket produce. Fresh cuts of meat can be purchased from a local butcher to freeze. For more information about food choices to prevent primary headache, see Chapter 13 (page 138).

Step 7
Get some sleep

Sleep — especially regular sleep — restores health. Histamine disrupts sleep, so reducing your histamine levels may improve your sleep patterns. Going to bed at a regular time, sleeping in a dark, quiet space and getting up at the same time every day helps reduce headache risk. Get the *right* amount of sleep for you. Most adults require 6 to 8 hours of shuteye every night. Set a schedule for regular bedtimes and set an alarm to get up at the same time every day. For more information on the value of sleep for preventing primary headache, see page 58.

Sample Journal Page

Headache Diary		
Date	Time headache began	Time headache ended
Medication name and dosage taken	Time medication taken	Time medication became effective (if ever)

Notes		
Weather	Changes in weather	Environment (noise, bright light)
Food eaten	Time food was eaten	Activity when headache started

Level of pain (0 is no pain at all, 10 is the worst pain ever experienced)	Location of pain	If pain moved during the headache, indicate where

Rate effectiveness of medication (0 is no difference, 3 is helped somewhat, 5 is pain totally gone)	Any side effects and time when occurred; use a level to indicate severity (1 is not as bad as 2 is not as bad as 3)	Headache symptoms and time symptom occurred

Stress levels (0 is no stress at all, 10 is the worst stress ever experienced)	Note any possible triggers	Menstrual cycle (note day since start)

If and when you exercised and level of intensity (0 is low, 3 is medium, 5 is high intensity)	When did you go to bed?	When did you get up?

Step 8
Be mindful

Mind-body exercises reduce stress and bring joy to our lives. Find time for activities like tai chi, yoga, massage or stretching. Or take time every day for an activity you enjoy, such as music, theater, sewing, photography, painting, drawing, cooking or walking — you won't regret it as your headaches become less severe. For more information on mind-body strategies for reducing the risk of primary headache, see page 109.

Step 9
Step it up!

Exercising 5 or 6 days a week for half an hour to an hour will help you de-stress. Although research does not conclusively say whether being overweight or obese increases the risk of headache, it may reduce the risk of comorbid conditions. For people who experience migraine after exercise, gentle forms of exercise, such as walking and tai chi, are effective too. Stay aware of your pulse rate to reduce the risk of exercise-associated headache.

Step 10
Be social

Take part in group activities to keep you connected to your community. Volunteering for events is one way to start. Take your time to find an activity that suits your lifestyle and does not add to your stress load. Headaches can isolate you and lead to depression. Reconnect for a better quality of life. For more information on reducing the psychological symptoms of primary headache, see "Mind-Body Treatments," page 109.

Step 11
Make a rescue plan

Accepting that you get headaches that prevent you from fully participating in some areas of your life is the first step to becoming prepared to rescue yourself once a headache starts. When you feel a headache coming on, do your best to find a quiet, darkened room where you can relax. Try

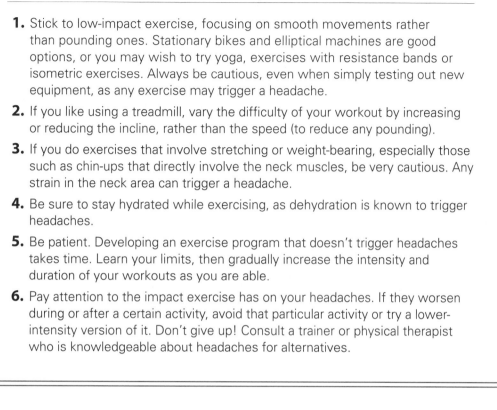

Avoiding Headaches Triggered by Exercise

1. Stick to low-impact exercise, focusing on smooth movements rather than pounding ones. Stationary bikes and elliptical machines are good options, or you may wish to try yoga, exercises with resistance bands or isometric exercises. Always be cautious, even when simply testing out new equipment, as any exercise may trigger a headache.

2. If you like using a treadmill, vary the difficulty of your workout by increasing or reducing the incline, rather than the speed (to reduce any pounding).

3. If you do exercises that involve stretching or weight-bearing, especially those such as chin-ups that directly involve the neck muscles, be very cautious. Any strain in the neck area can trigger a headache.

4. Be sure to stay hydrated while exercising, as dehydration is known to trigger headaches.

5. Be patient. Developing an exercise program that doesn't trigger headaches takes time. Learn your limits, then gradually increase the intensity and duration of your workouts as you are able.

6. Pay attention to the impact exercise has on your headaches. If they worsen during or after a certain activity, avoid that particular activity or try a lower-intensity version of it. Don't give up! Consult a trainer or physical therapist who is knowledgeable about headaches for alternatives.

placing a wrapped ice pack behind your neck, or massage your scalp gently. Practice relaxation techniques such as progressive muscle relaxation, yoga or meditation, all of which are equipment-free. Instruction on these techniques is easily accessible online, on videos and in books, or you may find classes in your area. To promote relaxation in your daily routine, try to set aside a half-hour every day to do something you enjoy and that relaxes you, whether it's enjoying soothing music, soaking in a hot bath, reading, going for a walk or even gardening. For more information on rescue strategies, see pages 76 and 154.

Step 12
Ask for help

Nothing is to be gained by being tough. Take pain-relief medications early in the onset of a headache, if needed. Discuss your rescue plan with your doctor and with your family.

Rescue Tool Box

Be prepared for headache attacks by assembling a rescue tool box.

- If you have nausea, check that you have natural remedies or medication to soothe your stomach. Ginger is a good remedy for nausea and vomiting.
- Keep plenty of fluids beside your bed or wherever you prefer to rest.
- Freeze small servings of low-histamine soups to have on hand when you have a headache.
- Stock fresh young coconut water or milk in your pantry. Coconut is a natural isotonic low-histamine beverage that helps balance electrolytes.
- Prepare a small plastic container to carry with you that contains the following items in case of a headache attack when you're out: a bottle of water; a small snack; typical pain-relief medication used at the onset of a migraine; preventive medication in case you are gone longer than anticipated; emergency or rescue medication in case your pain relief does not work (anti-nausea medication or ginger, plus an anti-inflammatory compress for your head).

Chapter 7
Medications for Primary Headaches

CASE HISTORY
Holistic Medicine

Drew, a 40-year-old building contractor, has had migraines since he was a teenager. He tried some of the over-the-counter and prescription medicines his doctor recommended to treat migraines when he was younger, but they didn't really make it any better, so he quit taking them — he didn't like the side effects either. About 4 years ago, he started having a different kind of headache and found out he had high blood pressure, which his doctor has not yet been able to control. Drew still gets bad migraines, but not as often as before. Usually, the symptoms stop after he takes an ASA and goes to bed for a few hours.

During his last doctor's visit for high blood pressure, he talked to her about newer anti-migraine medication. She explained that the newer medications are much better at reducing the symptoms of migraine headaches. She recommended that he try a medication, such as a beta-blocker or a calcium channel blocker, that would both treat his high blood pressure *and* prevent migraine attacks. With his doctor's support, he plans to make some lifestyle changes too, like losing some weight and following an approved exercise program, along with seeking some counseling to reduce stress.

If your health-care providers diagnose your headache as being migraine, cluster or tension-type in nature, they will work with you to tailor a treatment plan for your condition. The plan will likely include medication therapy, especially if your pain is acute. Some medications are designed to be preventive, reducing the frequency and duration of headache attacks; others are called acute or abortive, helping you to weather the storm of symptoms during the attack.

Medication Actions
Preventive Medications

Taken on a regular basis, preventive drugs reduce the frequency or intensity of your headaches. Preventive medication therapy is recommended if you find that your headaches occur on a regular basis and have significantly affected your quality of life and your work efficiency. Providing your health-care providers with your headache diary will help them to make the right decision about the most effective medication strategy for preventing attacks. If your doctor has prescribed medication that prevents headache, take the medication as directed and be aware of when the prescription needs to be refilled to make sure that you don't run out. Symptoms can return quickly.

Acute, or Abortive, Medications

These drugs are prescribed to stop symptoms of headaches once they have begun. They should be taken only during a headache. Using medication therapy only for headache symptoms is recommended if your headache attacks are not disabling or, if they are, they occur less than 4 days a month.

Warning: Some medications are not recommended for you if you are pregnant or breastfeeding, and in some cases, menstruating or on birth control pills. Some medications are not recommended for children. Please consult your doctors if in doubt.

Safety

Some over-the-counter pain-relief medication may interact with foods you eat or with other medication you may be taking. Your pharmacist and your dietitian can give you the best information about food and medication interactions and contraindications. Talk to your doctor if your over-the-counter medications are not working to relieve your headaches. Your doctor may prescribe a stronger type of medication or a combination of medications for you.

Taking over-the-counter and prescribed medications for headaches may also result in side effects. Side effects can be mild, severe, temporary or permanent. Everyone has different responses to a medication, including side effects. It is standard practice to list all possible side effects on the box for over-the-counter drugs and on a separate page with prescription drugs. If you have a concern about a side effect you are experiencing, contact your doctor or, if serious, visit your hospital emergency room.

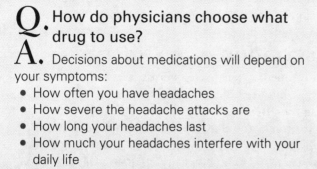

Q. How do physicians choose what drug to use?

A. Decisions about medications will depend on your symptoms:

- How often you have headaches
- How severe the headache attacks are
- How long your headaches last
- How much your headaches interfere with your daily life
- Any other medical conditions you may have

Medications for Migraine Headaches

Some standards and guidelines apply to managing or aborting an acute migraine attack with medications:

1. A headache-specific approach, choosing the initial treatment based on the severity of the attack, is recommended. Migraine-specific drugs include triptans for moderate to severe attacks, and analgesics plus non-steroidal anti-inflammatory drugs (NSAIDs) for mild to moderate attacks.

2. Take the lowest dosage of the most appropriate drug as soon as possible after your headache attack has started.

3. Unless otherwise directed by your physician, medications with one active drug are safest.

4. For best outcomes, it is a good strategy to provide some alternative medications for attacks of different severity.

5. Rescue drugs should be provided in case the first-choice medication fails.

Preventive Medications for Migraine

If you have severe, frequent migraines or migraines with neurological symptoms, your doctor will usually recommend a preventive medication strategy that includes lifestyle and diet changes, daily vitamin supplements and prescription medications. It is interesting to note that many of the medications now known to be effective at preventing migraines were originally developed to treat another medical issue (such as blood pressure, epilepsy or depression).

Prescription Adjustments

Preventive medications have been successful at reducing how often, how intense or how long migraines last. They may also increase the effectiveness of other medications taken during migraine attacks to relieve migraine symptoms. Your doctor may prescribe preventive medications to be taken on a daily basis or when a trigger is known to happen, such as before or during menstruation.

Most of the time, the preventive medication will not totally eliminate your headaches, and some carry a risk of dangerous side effects. If your preventive medications have been effective for 6 months (you have been migraine free), your doctor may recommend reducing the medication slowly until you are no longer taking it — a process called tapering off. If your migraines do not return, you will not need the preventive medication anymore.

Medications for Cluster Headaches

If you have cluster headaches, your doctor will develop a strategy to prevent attacks, reduce the severity of pain and reduce the length of the headache. Over-the-counter pain relievers (aspirin or ibuprophen, Advil, Motrin and others) may not work because your headache attack, although intense, may not last very long. Other treatments for acute pain can be effective in controlling your cluster headaches.

Preventive Medications for Cluster Headaches

Your doctor might prescribe preventive medications to stop cluster headache attacks before they happen. Details about the length and regularity of your cluster headaches will help your doctor decide which preventive therapy is best for you. Any drugs prescribed can be tapered off once the episode is over.

Medications for Tension-Type Headaches

If you have frequent tension headaches, please visit your doctor to discuss a medication therapy strategy. A wide selection of over-the-counter and prescription drugs are available to stop or relieve tension headache pain, but if you treat your headaches with over-the-counter pain relievers for a long period, you could cause what are called overuse headaches.

Tolerance

Pain relievers take away the pain on a temporary basis. Taken over a long period, painkillers and other medications may stop being effective against your headaches. You may also develop new headaches from the medication itself. To prevent medication overuse headaches, keep your use of over-the-counter drugs below 9 days per month. Continue to discuss any medication you take on a regular basis with your doctor, even if it is over-the-counter. All medications have some kind of side effect in the short or long term. Discussing with your doctor possible causes for your headaches, such as stressors, is part of a patient-centered treatment plan to reduce the use of medication and improve your quality of life.

Preventive Medications for Tension Headaches

If you have frequent or severe headaches or both, some medications could reduce your suffering. Your doctor may prescribe one of the preventive medications in the chart on pages 82–85 if you suffer from frequent headaches or those that don't get better from pain-relief medication or mind-body therapies, such as stress management or yoga. If your headaches cause you pain that disables you or causes you to take more pain-relief medication than is recommended, or if other medical issues prevent you from taking pain medications, your doctor may recommend preventive medication.

As well, your doctor may prescribe an antidepressant to prevent tension headache. If you have chronic headache, antidepressants may help, because antidepressants stabilize levels of brain chemicals such as serotonin, which can be a cause of headache pain. These drugs are effective for headache prevention even if you don't have depression.

Summary of Preventive Medications and Therapies for Treating Primary Headaches

Warning:

- The information about medication for primary headaches is intended as a guide for discussion with your health-care professional only.
- The information does not cover all possible uses, directions, precautions, interactions with other conditions or other medications, or possible side effects of what may or may not occur in actual clinical care or treatment.
- Always consult your physician before beginning any treatment therapy or altering treatment regimens.

Medication or Therapy	Common Name	Migraine	Cluster	Tension
Acupuncture therapy (up to 10 sessions of acupuncture over a 5–8 week period)		✓		✓
Anti-epileptic	Topiramate	✓	✓	✓
Anti-nausea medication	Domperidone	✓		
Anti-nausea medication	Metoclopramide (Reglan)	✓		
Anti-nausea medication	Prochlorperazine (Compro)	✓		

- Be aware that medication overuse headache is a risk if you use acute medications as therapy for your headaches. Keeping track of how often you have headache, how often you take medication and how effective that medication is for your headache is necessary to identify this condition.
- When a health-care provider recommends over-the-counter or prescription medication for an individual who suffers from primary headaches, personal preferences, other medical conditions, and possible side effects are all considered.

Action	Possible Side Effects	Cautions
Prevention or reduction of headache symptoms	Side effects are rare (complications have resulted from inadequate sterilization of needles and from improper treatment delivery; new disposable needles from a sealed package offer reduced risk)	Serious side effects may occur if therapy is not delivered properly. Acupuncture therapy should be administered by qualified practitioners only.
Controls certain types of seizures: partial seizures, tonic-clonic seizures, or Lennox-Gastaut syndrome	Vision problems, dizziness, drowsiness, burning or tingling, menstrual changes, confusion, nervousness, concentration problems, fatigue	May cause fetal malformation during pregnancy or reduce effectiveness of hormonal contraceptives. Discuss all possible side effects with your health-care provider and pharmacist. Call your physician or seek medical help immediately if you have concerns about possible side effects from medications you have been prescribed.
Controls vomiting; can be combined with other medications	Breast pain, breast milk flowing from the nipple, dry mouth, headache, hot flashes	Contact your doctor right away if you experience any of the following: burning, difficult, or painful urination; fast, irregular, pounding, or racing heartbeat or pulse; loss of balance or muscle control; redness of the eye; or sores inside the mouth.
Controls vomiting; can be combined with other medications	Drowsiness, excessive tiredness, weakness, headache, dizziness, diarrhea, vomiting, breast enlargement or discharge, missed menstrual period, decreased sexual ability, frequent or uncontrolled urination	Discuss all possible side effects with your health-care provider and pharmacist. Call your physician or seek medical help immediately if you have concerns about possible side effects from medications you have been prescribed.
Controls vomiting; can be combined with other medications	Changes in menstrual period, constipation (mild), decreased sexual ability, dizziness, drowsiness, dry mouth, fatigue,headache, nasal congestion, nausea, sweating, swelling or pain in breasts, trouble sleeping, watering of mouth, weight gain (unusual)	Discuss all possible side effects with your health-care provider and pharmacist. Call your physician or seek medical help immediately if you have concerns about possible side effects from medications you have been prescribed.

Medication or Therapy	Common Name	Migraine	Cluster	Tension
Beta-blocker	Propranolol	✓		
Calcium channel blocker (L-type)	Verapamil (Isoptin, Verelan, Verelan PM, Calan, Bosoptin, Covera-HS)	✓	✓	✓
Corticosteroid	Dexamethasone	✓	✓	
Triptans (available by prescription and over-the-counter, depending on country and specific drug)	Sumatriptan (Imitrex) Rizatriptan (Maxalt) Almotriptan (Axert) Naratriptan (Amerge) Zolmitriptan* (Zomig) Frovatriptan* (Frova) Eletriptan (Relpax)	✓	✓	✓
Vitamin Therapy: riboflavin (400 mg once daily)		✓		

Action	Possible Side Effects	Cautions
Lowers portal vein pressure, inhibits norepinephrine	Tiredness, dizziness; increases risk of type 2 diabetes; possible sleep disturbance	Use with caution if you have any of the following conditions: diabetes mellitus, hyperthyroidism, peripheral vascular disease, phaeochromocytoma, hypertension, myasthenia gravis, or if you take drugs with bradycardic effects.
Vasodilator; controls ventricular rate	Headaches, facial flushing, dizziness, lightheadedness, swelling, increased urination, fatigue, nausea, constipation	Discuss all possible side effects with your health-care provider and pharmacist. Call your physician or seek medical help immediately if you have concerns about possible side effects from medications you have been prescribed.
Reduces pain, anti-inflammatory artificial steroid; may be prescribed in combination with other pain-relieving medication	Constipation, darkening or lightening of the skin color, diarrhea, difficulty sleeping, dizziness or lightheadedness, flushing of face or cheeks, hiccups, increased or decreased appetite, increased sweating, indigestion and nausea, nervousness or restlessness, vomiting, redness, swelling, or pain at the place of injection	Discuss all possible side effects with your health-care provider and pharmacist. Call your physician or seek medical help immediately if you have concerns about possible side effects from medications you have been prescribed.
Reduces pain, nausea, light sensitivity, sound sensitivity *Recommended for women (and girls) with predictable menstrual hormone-related migraine that is not responding to usual acute treatment	Nausea, dizziness, muscle weakness	Triptans should not be taken if you have any of the following conditions: uncontrolled high blood pressure, coronary artery disease, history of ischemic stroke, peripheral artery disease, pregnancy and lactation, or if you are over 65 years old. Some triptans may interfere with birth control medication.
Will reduce frequency and intensity of migraine for some people; three months of riboflavin therapy may be necessary before results are seen	May cause urine to turn yellow-orange color; in high doses, may cause diarrhea, increase urine production	Recommended amounts of riboflavin during pregnancy or lactation are 1.4 mg per day. May interact with medications given for depression. May interact with phenobarbital (Luminal) to increase speed of breakdown of riboflavin. May interact with probenecid (Benemid) by increasing the amount of riboflavin in the body.

Summary of Acute Medications for Treating Primary Headaches

Medication or Therapy	Common Name	Migraine	Cluster	Tension
Analgesic	Acetaminophen (Paracetamol, Anacin, Atasol, Tylenol, Panadol)	✓		✓
Anti-epileptic	Gabapentin	✓		
Anti-nausea medication	Domperidone	✓		
Anti-nausea medication	Metoclopramide (Reglan)	✓		
Anti-nausea medication	Prochlorperazine (Compro)	✓		
Calcium channel blocker (L-type)	Verapamil (Isoptin, Verelan, Verelan PM, Calan, Bosoptin, Covera-HS)	✓		✓
Combination	Acetaminophen, aspirin and caffeine (Excedrin Migraine)	✓		✓

Warning: Consult with your family physician before taking any new medication or changing your medication therapy. This table is for information purposes only.

Action	Possible Side Effects	Cautions
Pain relief for mild to moderate headaches	Possible liver damage from overdose; people with liver disease should not use analgesics	Stop taking acetaminophen products immediately if you experience rash; hives; itching; swelling of the face, throat, tongue, lips, eyes, hands, feet, ankles, or lower legs; hoarseness; difficulty breathing or swallowing.
	Dizziness, sleepiness, possible infection	Call your physician or seek medical help immediately if you have concerns about possible side effects, such as rash, itching, swelling (face, throat, tongue, lips, eyes), hoarseness, difficulty swallowing/breathing, seizures or others.
Controls vomiting; can be combined with other medications	Breast pain, breast milk flowing from the nipple, dry mouth, headache, hot flashes	Contact your doctor right away if you experience any of the following: burning, difficult, or painful urination; fast, irregular, pounding, or racing heartbeat or pulse; loss of balance or muscle control; redness of the eye; sores inside the mouth.
Controls vomiting; can be combined with other medications	Drowsiness, excessive tiredness, weakness, headache, dizziness, diarrhea, vomiting, breast enlargement or discharge, missed menstrual period, decreased sexual ability, frequent or uncontrolled urination	Discuss all possible side effects with your health-care provider and pharmacist. Call your physician or seek medical help immediately if you have concerns about possible side effects from medications you have been prescribed.
Controls vomiting; can be combined with other medications	Changes in menstrual period, constipation (mild), decreased sexual ability, dizziness, drowsiness, dry mouth, fatigue, headache, nasal congestion, nausea, sweating, swelling or pain in breasts, trouble sleeping, watering of mouth, weight gain (unusual)	Discuss all possible side effects with your health-care provider and pharmacist. Call your physician or seek medical help immediately if you have concerns about possible side effects from medications you have been prescribed.
Vasodilator, controls ventricular rate	Headaches, facial flushing, dizziness, lightheadedness, swelling, increased urination, fatigue, nausea, constipation	Discuss all possible side effects with your health-care provider and pharmacist. Call your physician or seek medical help immediately if you have concerns about possible side effects from medications you have been prescribed.
To reduce mild to moderate pain	Ulcers, gastrointestinal bleeding, rebound headaches	Risk of possibly fatal liver disease due to acetaminophen. Alcohol consumption increases risk. Do not give aspirin to people <16 years old, due to possible Reye's syndrome.

Medication or Therapy	Common Name	Migraine	Cluster	Tension
Combination	Ergots and caffeine (Migergot, Cafergot)	✓		
Combination	Sumatriptan and naproxen sodium (Treximet)	✓	✓	✓
Combination	Triptan plus NSAIDs	✓		
Corticosteroid	Dexamethasone	✓	✓	
Ergot derivative (available as nasal spray and injection)	Dihydroergotamine (D.H.E. 45) (Migranal)	✓		
NSAID	Acetylsalicylic acid (ASA) (Aspirin)	✓		✓
NSAID	Naproxen sodium, over-the-counter or prescription (Aleve, Anaprox, Antalgin, Apranax, Nalgesin, Naposin, Proxen, Synflex)	✓		✓

Action	Possible Side Effects	Cautions
Effective for migraines that last >48 hours and for throbbing headaches; not considered as effective as triptans	Nausea, dizziness, anxiety	Can cause severe rebound headaches if taken on a frequent basis. Not recommended if you have hypertension or cardiac risk factors. Do not take ergots if you are pregnant or may become pregnant (may cause uterine contractions leading to abortion and could restrict blood flow to the fetus).
More effective migraine relief than either medication alone	Nausea, dizziness, muscle weakness	Discuss all possible side effects with your health-care provider and pharmacist. Call your physician or seek medical help immediately if you have concerns about possible side effects from medications you have been prescribed.
	See side effects for each medication.	Discuss all possible side effects with your health-care provider and pharmacist. Call your physician or seek medical help immediately if you have concerns about possible side effects from medications you have been prescribed.
Reduces pain, anti-inflammatory artificial steroid; may be prescribed in combination with other pain-relieving medication	Constipation, darkening or lightening of the skin color, diarrhea, difficulty sleeping, dizziness or lightheadedness, flushing of face or cheeks, hiccups, increased or decreased appetite, increased sweating, indigestion and nausea, nervousness or restlessness, vomiting, redness, swelling, or pain at the place of injection	Discuss all possible side effects with your health-care provider and pharmacist. Call your physician or seek medical help immediately if you have concerns about possible side effects from medications you have been prescribed.
Effective for migraines that last >48 hours and for throbbing headaches; more effective than ergots	Nausea, abdominal cramps, dizziness, dry mouth	Too much of this drug may cause rebound headaches. Frequent use can lead to physical dependence. When prescribed, ergot derivatives should be taken no more than twice weekly. Short-term therapy only. Cannot be taken in combination with triptans.
Pain relief and anti-inflammatory for mild to moderate headaches	Possible stomach bleeding, heartburn, gastrointestinal ulcers, tinnitus at higher doses	NSAIDs used more than 15 days a month could increase the risk of increased migraine attack. Do not give Aspirin to people <16 years old, due to possible Reye's syndrome.
Pain relief and anti-inflammatory for mild to moderate headaches	Heartburn, constipation, diarrhea, ulcers, stomach bleeding	Increases risk of cardiovascular disease and stroke.

Medication or Therapy	Common Name	Migraine	Cluster	Tension
NSAID	Ibuprofen (oral and gel/topical) Ibuprofen lysine (oral and intravenous use) (Motrin, Nurofen, Advil, Nuprin)	✓		✓
NSAID	Diclofenac sodium (oral, rectal, intramuscular, intravenous, topical) (Voltaren, Aclonac, Arthrotec [misoprostol added for gastric protection], Dyloject)	✓		✓
NSAID	Ketorolac (Toradol)	✓		✓
NSAID	Indomethacin	✓		✓
Opiates (barbiturate-containing analgesic compounds — narcotics)	Codeine	✓	✓	Not recommended for tension headaches
Oxygen			✓	
Triptans (available by prescription and over-the-counter, depending on country and specific drug) (Oral, nasal or subcutaneous preparations)	Sumatriptan (Imitrex) Rizatriptan (Maxalt) Almotriptan (Axert) Naratriptan (Amerge) Zolmitriptan* (Zomig) Frovatriptan* (Frova) Eletriptan (Relpax)	✓	✓	✓

Action	Possible Side Effects	Cautions
Pain relief and anti-inflammatory for mild to moderate headaches	Nausea, dyspepsia, gastrointestinal ulcers, diarrhea, constipation, dizziness, priapism, rash, salt and fluid retention, hypertension, headache	Regular use may lead to hearing loss. Increases risk of cardiovascular disease and stroke. Increases risk of kidney cancer. Interacts with alcohol consumption to increase risk of stomach bleeding. Dangerous for people with asthma.
For more severe headache pain	Peptic ulcer, nausea, dyspepsia, gastrointestinal ulcers, diarrhea, constipation	Increases risk of cardiovascular disease and stroke. Possible hepatitis. Possible kidney damage.
For moderate to severe pain relief, short-term use only	Edema, hypertension, palpitation, fainting, rash, dizziness, headache, sweating, peptic ulcer, nausea, dyspepsia, gastrointestinal ulcers, diarrhea, constipation	Possible kidney failure. Possible hemorrhage. Hypersensitivity reactions. Increases risk of cardiovascular disease and stroke.
For mild to moderately severe pain; reduces pain and inflammation and relieves upset stomach	Headache, dizziness, vomiting, diarrhea, constipation, irritation of the rectum, constant feeling of the need to empty bowels, ringing in the ears	Discuss all possible side effects with your health-care provider and pharmacist before taking any medication. Call your physician or seek medical help immediately if you have concerns about possible side effects from medications you have been prescribed.
Controls pain	Constipation, dizziness, lightheadedness, feeling faint, drowsiness, dry mouth, headache, lack of energy or tiredness, nausea or vomiting, sweating; dependence is an issue	Discuss all possible side effects with your health-care provider and pharmacist. Call your physician or seek medical help immediately if you have concerns about possible side effects from medications you have been prescribed.
Relieves cluster headache pain		Dangerous to use oxygen around open flame. May interact with chemotherapy.
Reduces pain, nausea, light sensitivity, sound sensitivity; used in combination with either NSAID or paracetamol; nasal or subcutaneous triptans recommended for cluster headaches *Recommended for women (and girls) with predictable menstrual hormone-related migraine that is not responding to usual acute treatment.	Nausea, dizziness, muscle weakness	Triptans should not be taken if you have any of the following conditions: uncontrolled high blood pressure, coronary artery disease, history of ischemic stroke, peripheral artery disease, pregnancy and lactation, or if you are over 65 years old. Some triptans may interfere with birth control medication.

Patience

Be patient. Preventive medications can take several weeks before you start to notice any change in your headaches. In addition, one of the side effects of taking painkillers or overusing caffeine is that your preventive medication might be less effective. Using acute pain-relief medication only as a last resort will make the combination of painkillers and preventive medications most effective with the fewest side effects. Regular visits with your doctor to monitor your overall treatment strategy are important. If your preventive medication has effectively reduced the frequency of your headaches, your doctor may recommend gradually decreasing the dosage.

Emergency Care for Primary Headaches

If you have any of the following symptoms, see your doctor right away or go to a hospital emergency room for medical treatment.

Emergency Care for Migraines

If you experience the following symptoms during a migraine attack, they might indicate a more serious condition that needs to be looked at immediately:

- Speech problems, vision changes, poor or no balance, unable to move arms or legs
- Changes in your headache intensity, or the typical pattern is different
- Your headache is much worse if you lie down
- You have never had such a bad headache before

Emergency Medications for Migraine (Acute)

There are several medications that have been proven effective for emergency situations.

Non-steroidal anti-inflammatory drugs (NSAIDs) other than aspirin are the most widely preferred drugs. Paracetamol and aspirin follow. Metoclopramide is the preferred anti-emetic drug for acute episodic migraine in most countries.

Emergency Care for Cluster Headache (Acute)

Cluster headache onset is sudden and the pain level is severe. Over-the-counter pain relief medication may not be effective here.

Emergency Medications for Cluster Headache

- 100% oxygen at a minimum flow rate of 12 quarts (12 L) per minute using a non-rebreathing mask and a reservoir bag
- Nasal or tablet form of a triptan (zolmitriptan) medication: Zomig
- A local anesthetic may numb cluster headache pain: lidocaine (Xylocaine)

Emergency Care for Tension-Type Headache (Acute)

It is rare that tension headaches require emergency treatment. People who have cluster headaches and migraine attacks are more often seen in the emergency setting. Seek medical attention if your headache changes in some way, if you have a "new" headache, or if medication that has previously worked to relieve headache pain is no longer effective.

Medication Cautions

Cardiovascular disease: If you have already been diagnosed with cardiovascular disease, it is important to avoid ergotamines, triptans and COX-2 inhibitors when you are trying to stop a migraine. Migraine with aura is known to increase the risk of cardiovascular disease. If you experience this type of migraine, it is crucial to strictly control other risk factors for cardiovascular disease, such as high blood pressure, smoking and oral contraceptive use.

Antidepressants: Although tricyclic antidepressants (TCAs) increase the risk of abnormal heart conduction, if you have been diagnosed with both migraine and depression, TCAs and selective norepinephrine reuptake inhibitors (SNRIs) may help prevent headaches. Flunarizine (commonly prescribed in Europe and Asia) and beta-blockers are not good choices, as they may make depression worse, especially if you are elderly. If you have both migraine and restless leg syndrome, avoid neuroleptics, selective serotonin reuptake inhibitors (SSRIs), SNRIs, mirtazapine and flunarizine.

Note: The medications described in this chapter are based on Carville S, Padhi S, Reason T, Underwood M. Guideline Development Group. Diagnosis and management of headaches in young people and adults: Summary of NICE guidance. BMJ, 2012 Sep 19;345:e5765; the side effects listed are derived from Health Canada drugs and health products information monographs, accessed January 2013 at http://webprod5.hc-sc.gc.ca/dpd-bdpp/info.do?code=73377&lang=eng, and Body and Health.Canada.com, accessed January 2013 at http://bodyandhealth.canada.com/drug_info_details.asp?channel_id=0&brand_name_id=4082&page_no=2#AdverseEffects.

Chapter 8
Physiotherapy for Primary Headaches

CASE HISTORY
Attention

As a personal coach, Stephen spends a great deal of time at the computer doing research and setting up exercise routines for clients. His business is just getting off the ground, and he often works late into the night, updating his website and Facebook page. More and more often, Stephen is getting intensely painful headaches that feel like someone is tightening steel pinchers around his head. The headaches are lasting a few hours and happening almost every day. Stretching his neck and shoulders helped for a while, and taking over-the-counter pain-relief medications stopped the headache for a day or so before it came back. His family doctor diagnosed Stephen's headaches as being tension headaches, prescribed a mild NSAID to take when Stephen felt a headache coming on, and set up an appointment with a physiotherapist to help him assess his working lifestyle to see if they could reduce the frequency and intensity of his tension headaches. Stephen needs to spend more time and effort coaching himself.

Physiotherapy is a health-care profession that evaluates your physical function while providing treatment and exercises to restore and maintain your normal level of physical function. As participants in a holistic treatment team committed to PARR, physiotherapists work to restore movement and reduce pain in patients with primary headaches.

Physiotherapy Options

Your doctor might recommend physical therapy as part of your management strategy, especially if you are having frequent tension headaches. A physical treatment plan will be most effective if it combines training in appropriate ergonomics for the workplace and home with exercise and stretching.

Manual Therapies for Migraine

Manual therapies, such as relaxation therapy, massage therapy, chiropractic care or physiotherapy, may enhance the effectiveness of your migraine management strategy. Massage therapists use their hands, forearms, elbows and feet to work on the skin and muscles of the body. There are many different kinds of massage therapy; some are gentle and some are "deep tissue" and intense.

Manual Therapies for Cluster Headaches

The periodic nature of cluster headaches makes it more difficult to seek manual therapies on a regular basis. If you suffer from cluster headaches, you may need to see your physiotherapist on short notice.

Manual Therapies for Tension-Type Headaches

Some tension headaches can be caused by dysfunction in the musculoskeletal ecosystem of the neck region. As an example, a disorder of the neck joints or connecting muscles between the base of your skull and your neck may send pain signals to your head.

Your headaches might be caused by neck problems if

- No other possible causes have turned up in discussions with your doctor and resulting tests
- Pressure at the base of your skull relieves headache pain
- Your headache pain is worsened by neck movement or by holding your neck in one position (for example, working at a computer monitor)
- Your headache is not always relieved by medication

A physiotherapist might use the following treatments for your tension-type headaches:

- Mobilization of stiff joints
- Stretching exercises
- Heat treatments
- Acupuncture or dry needling
- Trigger point therapy to release tight muscles

Chiropractic Care

Chiropractic care is an alternative therapy based on the idea that some health problems can be successfully treated with spinal manipulation. Although it doesn't work for everyone, chiropractic treatment could bring as much relief from your tension headaches as short-term prescription medications.

Chiropractors focus on health problems with the musculoskeletal and nervous systems and the effects of these on general health and daily life (back pain, neck pain, arm or leg joint pain and headaches). Chiropractic care is a drug-free, hands-on approach with strong diagnostic skills, and chiropractors are trained to recommend therapeutic and rehabilitation-based exercises and to counsel patients on nutrition, diet and lifestyle. Chiropractors also refer patients to other health-care providers as needed.

Caution: Stroke Risk

Although manipulation of the cervical spine (neck) can provide benefits in certain situations, there is some evidence that this therapy may increase the risk of stroke or transient ischemic attack. Be cautious when considering this treatment and discuss your concerns with your chiropractor or doctor.

Did You Know?

Multimodal Therapy

Researchers say that physical therapy can reduce headache frequency, intensity and duration for people who have chronic tension headaches. Overall, these physical treatments are most beneficial when integrated into a multimodal treatment plan that includes exercise and stretching, as well as training in how your environment affects your physical and mental health in both the home and the workplace (ergonomics). Exercise and stretching exercises are more effective than massage or heat or cold application.

Trigger Point Treatments

Muscle usually accounts for nearly 50% of the body's weight. We each have about 400 muscles (there are variations from one person to another), and any one of these muscles can develop trigger points and cause pain that is felt in another part of the body (called referred pain) and dysfunction. Symptoms can range from intolerable, described as agonizing pain, to an almost painless restriction of movement and distortion of posture. Trigger points are tender when pressed and may feel like a small lump, but healthy muscles don't have trigger points and are not tender when pressed.

Trigger Point Injection

Trigger points are known to cause irritation to the surrounding nerves (referred pain). Injection into trigger points (called TPI) is a therapy used to treat painful trigger points or knots of muscle in tense muscle areas and may be an option if your headache pain is muscle-related. A health-care professional will insert a small needle that contains a local anesthetic, sometimes including a corticosteroid, into your trigger point. A brief course of TPI usually deactivates the point, reducing or eliminating the pain, and is effective for some time. TPI therapy is a quick process that takes place at your family physician's clinic, and several trigger points can be treated in a visit. TPI is effective for reducing pain in the neck, lower back, arms and legs; for relieving tension headaches; and for treating fibromyalgia.

Bite Equilibrium

Your bite equilibrium describes the mechanics of how your teeth fit together when you close your mouth and how your jaw bones align. Temporomandibular joint (TMJ) disorders indicate that something is not working properly in how these joints work together and is usually considered a factor in secondary rather than primary headache, but could also be the cause of your tension headaches. Factors that affect the likelihood that TMJ is causing your headaches include age, specific symptoms, susceptibility and pain threshold.

TMJ Therapy

See your doctor and your dentist for a thorough examination to determine whether a temporomandibular joint (TMJ) issue is causing headaches for you. Physiotherapy, orthodontic appliances and surgery are possible solutions to discuss with your doctor. Other therapies may include:

- Jaw exercises to strengthen muscles and improve flexibility and range of motion
- Heat therapy for blood circulation in the jaw
- Ice therapy to reduce swelling and relieve pain
- Massage to relieve overall muscle tension
- Training to improve posture and correct jaw alignment

Did You Know?

Wisdom Teeth

Impacted wisdom teeth may be a cause of headaches, but would generally fall under the secondary headache rule, since once the teeth are removed or break through the gums, the headaches should end. If your wisdom teeth have not yet emerged, and you have swollen gums and related pain along with headaches, make an appointment with your dentist to have a look at your wisdom teeth. Getting checked to see if you are grinding your teeth at night could also reduce chronic headaches.

TMJ Treatments

A physiotherapist uses many techniques to relax, stretch and release tight muscles and scar tissue. Movement of the temporomandibular joint releases scar tissue that has been preventing normal muscle use, thereby improving the patient's range of motion. The use of high-frequency sound waves (ultrasound therapy) directed to the temporomandibular joint reduces pain and swelling and improves circulation.

Transcutaneous Electrical Nerve Stimulation (TENS)

In this therapy, a mild electrical current is applied to the skin around the jaw joint, which is believed to interrupt the pain signals arising from the joint. Some people gain headache relief from TENS therapy, and may also experience more relaxed muscles and improved blood flow.

Posture

Learning to be aware of your posture may help prevent headaches. Tension in your neck area, shoulders and upper back muscles can be the result of how you sit at your computer or the way you walk.

Guidelines for Improving Your Posture and Preventing Headaches

- Keep your back in a neutral position (not arched, not slumped forward).
- Sit straight up in your chair.
- Be sure that your lower back is supported.
- Stretch your neck, arms and back muscles every hour when you're sitting at a computer.
- Ensure that the top of your computer monitor is level with your eyes so you are looking slightly down at the computer. A document holder helps keep papers at the same eye level.
- Never prop the telephone headset between your ear and your shoulder. A headset or speakerphone is better for frequent telephone use.
- Don't reach up and down in your work space. Adjust your work surface to a comfortable level.
- If you are standing for any length of time, use a small stool to support one foot.
- Lift items with your legs rather than with your neck or back. Keep your body square to the item you're lifting rather than twisting to pick something up.
- Be aware of exercises that hyperextend the neck (such as racing bicycles).

Chapter 9
Surgery for Primary Headaches

CASE HISTORY
Out of Options

Peter felt a stabbing pain in his eyes when his wife turned on the bedroom lights. He groaned as he quickly covered his head with the blankets. She apologized quietly, turned out the light, found her way to the closet for her sweater and left, closing the door softly. Now 43 years old, Peter has been struggling with migraines since he was in his early 20s. He would start seeing the odd jangly aura that gave him some warning of the headache to come, and then the pain of the migraine would take over, sometimes for a few hours, but more often for more than a day — when he couldn't bear any light, when sounds brought tears of pain, and he would barely be able to eat anything. Although he had a wonderful family physician who worked with him tirelessly to discuss possible lifestyle changes and to find the right medication mix that would give him back his life, nothing seemed to keep the headaches away for any length of time. Peter's doctor suggested that he consider surgery.

Surgery for Migraine Headaches

If you have migraine headaches (with or without aura) and do not get any relief from lifestyle changes, medication therapy or physiotherapy strategies, your doctor may discuss migraine surgery with you.

Peripheral Nerve Stimulation for Migraine

This therapy is used to treat chronic migraine patients who have not found medication effective in relieving their pain. Mild electrical impulses are used to stimulate the two occipital nerves (greater and lesser) of the brain. These two nerves are located at the back of the head and are part of the peripheral nervous system involved in migraine attacks. Small metal electrodes are implanted below the skin at the back of the head, with the leads attached to a device called a neurostimulator that can be implanted below the clavicle or shoulder blade, or in the chest, lower abdomen or buttock.

Botox

Produced by the bacterium *Clostridium botulinum*, botulinum toxin type A (Botox) is a protein molecule that acts on the nervous system (a neurotoxin). Botox has the ability to block or reduce nerve messages to muscles and, by doing so, stops the muscle from contracting.

Botox was first used for cosmetic purposes to reduce facial wrinkles, but research was conducted to assess the effectiveness of Botox for people suffering from migraines. After much testing, Botox has been approved for treatment of chronic migraine headaches in adults. To treat migraine, Botox is injected into specific forehead and neck muscles (not for cosmetic purposes, however). For this treatment to be effective, it must be repeated every 12 weeks.

Nerve Decompression Plastic Surgery for Migraine

For some people, migraine attacks are triggered by irritation or overstimulation of the trigeminal nerve, which is a large cranial nerve in the face and neck. Either irritation or overstimulation of the nerve can set off a cascade of events that leads to a migraine attack. Different migraine symptoms require different nerve decompression surgery. A piece of the irritated nerve might be removed; muscle around the irritated nerve may be removed; other nerves or muscles in the face may be removed or reduced; or septoplasty, repair of a deviated septum, could be done for nasal trigger points.

Caution: Infection and bleeding are risks of this surgery. On rare occasions, people have lost a minimal amount of hair around the surgery incision line. Some numbness may occur to the area where the surgery is done. For some people, the numbness lasts for a long time or can be permanent.

Surgery for Cluster Headaches

If you have cluster headaches and get no relief from medication or any other therapy, your doctor may recommend surgical treatment. However, the surgery could cause side effects that are worse than the cluster headache.

Radiofrequency Thermocoagulation

This is the most common surgical technique for severe cluster headaches because it interrupts pain signals by heating up small areas of nerve tissue. The radiofrequency needles are accurately placed using fluoroscopic X-rays. The doctor will confirm that the needle has been inserted in the cluster headache nerve trigger by having the patient confirm when he or she feels a tingling sensation. Pain signals are blocked for a prolonged period, but nerve pathways may grow back after some time has passed.

Side effects: Bruising, bleeding, headaches, moderate to severe facial numbness, loss of feeling in the cornea and anesthesia dolorosa, which is severe pain in the area where the anesthesia has been given.

Caution: Intracranial hemorrhage, stroke, infection and motor weakness that typically resolves in 1 to 6 months; even death is possible.

> **Did You Know?**
>
> **Deep Brain (Hypothalamus) Stimulation**
> A stimulator placed in the hypothalamus can stop cluster headaches from occurring. For some patients, cluster headache pain stops immediately, but for others, pain continues for another 4 months. No side effects have been seen. Still an experimental procedure, hypothalamic stimulation requires further studies to confirm its safety and effectiveness.

Glycerol Trigeminal Rhizotomy

Used as an alternative to radiofrequency thermocoagulation, glycerol trigeminal rhizotomy is a surgical intervention that uses sterile glycerol to cut off the nerve supply by injecting the glycerol into the sensory ganglion (a mass of nerve cell bodies) of the trigeminal nerve (gasserian ganglion). Although this intervention has a higher rate of recurring cluster headache than radiofrequency thermocoagulation, side effects also occur less frequently.

Trigeminal Nerve Root Section

This is an effective treatment known for a better surgical outcome. The trigeminal nerve is cut (or lesioned) at the root entry zone.

Microvascular Decompression

In this procedure, the trigeminal nerve is destroyed by a radiation beam from the gamma knife. This outpatient procedure usually takes a few hours. Few medical institutions have gamma knife capabilities, however, and high relapse rates are associated with this procedure. More research is required.

Chapter 10
Complementary and Alternative Medicine

CASE HISTORY
Alternative Care

Susan put away her hockey gear for the last time. She had been playing recreational hockey with the same group of women for several years, but on the advice of a neurologist, she was giving up the game because of the cluster headaches she suffered after many games. People would stare at her in the change room as her face flushed a dangerous purple. Over-the-counter pain-relief medication was not much help. Most of the time, Susan would awaken around 3:00 a.m. with her head pounding fiercely, and unable to stay in one place, she would begin pacing. She would be exhausted when the headache finally let go, feeling bruised in her face and head. Family physicians had not been able to help with the headaches, and the neurologist had simply advised that she stop playing hockey.

Susan turned to a new family doctor trained in Western and Chinese medicine. He was highly skilled in acupuncture, with considerable success treating other patients with classic migraine. Susan received acupuncture treatments several times a week for the first few weeks, then once every 2 weeks. Susan found that the headaches were less severe, and although she still had the occasional headache — mostly when she played tennis — they were not as intense or prolonged. Acupuncture once every 6 weeks seemed to be sufficient for keeping the headaches at bay. It was a relief to not be reliant on medication and to be able to participate more fully in social events than she had been able to for some time.

Around the world, people suffering from primary headache use complementary and alternative medicine (CAM), often at the suggestion of a friend or relative. Common CAM therapies for headaches include acupuncture, traditional medicines, homeopathy, breathing exercises, yoga and therapeutic touch. When employed with caution, these alternatives can help patients improve management of their headaches by reducing their frequency, intensity and duration.

Traditional Chinese Medicine

According to the principles of traditional Chinese medicine, migraine headaches, tension-type headaches and cluster headaches share the same cause, or etiology: a blockage in the body resulting in insufficient flow of *qi* in the liver and/or gallbladder meridian. The concept of *qi* refers to the life energy that normally flows through the main organs (the *zang* and *fu* organs), their 12 main meridians and 356 classical pressure points. Various illnesses and disorders of the human body are described in terms of too little or too much *qi* in particular organs or areas of the body, resulting from insufficient flow or blockages in the flow of blood and *qi*.

Migraine headache can sometimes correspond to the TCM syndromes called liver yang rising and gallbladder heat or a combination of both. The liver is known as the organ that maintains a smooth flow of *qi* through the body. The gallbladder is a subsidiary organ closely related to the liver. When *qi* becomes congested in the liver and gallbladder, the yang energies of the liver travel up to the head, which results in headache syndromes.

Traditional Chinese Herbs

Certain dried flowers and herbs are prescribed to help with headaches. As with Western medicine, a proper diagnosis is only possible from a trained TCM practitioner, based on receiving a detailed history, palpating the pulse points and looking at the tongue. Sometimes a tea made from 10 to 12 dried rosebuds helps soothe an attack of migraine, cluster or tension-type headache.

Did You Know?

Popularity

Acupuncture is becoming more popular in the Western world, thanks in part to an increase in practitioners trained in TCM-based acupuncture, and in part to word-of-mouth from friends and relatives who have experienced improved quality of life after acupuncture. In the United States, 2.13 million people are currently being treated by an acupuncturist, and 4.1% will visit one at some point in their lives.

Acupuncture

A pillar of traditional Chinese medicine and CAM, acupuncture is used to treat myriad medical conditions and to combat addictions. It often targets conditions that involve pain, including osteoarthritis, menstrual cramps, fibromyalgia, lower back pain and carpal tunnel syndrome — and, of course, headaches. One out of 10 people who visit an acupuncturist is seeking relief from headache pain.

By inserting needles at specific acupuncture points, acupuncturists try to restore balance in the body, clearing blockages that prevent the flow of *qi* to the areas of the body affected by a particular condition. Recent studies have successfully explained the effectiveness of acupuncture in terms of conventional neurophysiology, which may make it more accepted in the Western world, and some acupuncturists now explain it to their patients in those terms.

The take-home message from research and case studies is that acupuncture is a reliable, cost-effective alternative for people suffering from migraine headaches. In particular, it is a good option for those who cannot tolerate medications or for whom traditional therapies have been ineffective. Acupuncture may also be of some benefit to people with chronic or frequent episodic tension-type headaches, though the research evidence to support this is not as strong.

Analgesic Effect

At this time, researchers do not fully understand how acupuncture relieves pain. One theory suggests that certain structures in the nervous system that are known to control pain perception are activated by acupuncture therapy. Another hypothesizes that acupuncture influences connections within the brain and between the brain and the spinal cord. Acupuncture's proven anti-inflammatory effect could also play a role in its success in the treatment of pain.

Naturopathic Medicine

Naturopathic medicine is an eclectic practice including acupuncture, lifestyle counseling, clinical nutrition, botanical medicine, hydrotherapy, mind-body therapies and homeopathic medicine. The aim in treating primary headache is to remove impediments to healing before interceding. This involves removing headache triggers and maintaining adequate hydration and nutrition, reducing stress, eliminating food allergies and avoiding vasoactive and amine foods.

Elimination Diet

Naturopathic physicians and other CAM practitioners often use an elimination diet to investigate headache triggers. One by one, they eliminate potential allergens from the diet, and after a period of 1 to 2 weeks, or until symptoms improve (indicating the offending food has been eliminated), they slowly reintroduce one possible symptom-causing food group every 2 days to see if symptoms return. For people who have migraines once or twice monthly, it may be important to reintroduce foods more gradually. If a migraine occurs after all foods have been reintroduced, it becomes a more lengthy process to see if a combination of food and environment, or a total load of vasoactive and amine foods, has tipped the balance toward a migraine. A laboratory test called ELISA (enzyme-linked immunosorbent assay) can be used to identify the antibodies that signal food allergies (IgE and IgG) and offer information that is more precise without requiring an elimination diet.

Homeopathic Medicine

Homeopathy is a holistic practice of medicine that aims to treat the whole person, mind and body, not just the complaint. Homeopathic medicine is designed to trigger our natural internal healing system and works on a law known as "similars," also called "like cures like." This involves giving the minimum dose possible (called minute) of a substance (called a remedy) that when given at full strength to a healthy person is known to cause the symptoms (called rubrics) experienced by the patient. The principle behind the minute dose is that the effectiveness of the medication is related to the size of the dose — the lower the better. Many homeopathic remedies are diluted so many times that no measurement of the original substance is possible.

Remedies are made from plants, minerals or animals — mountain herbs (such as arnica), crushed whole bees, belladonna (deadly nightshade) and white arsenic, to name a few. The remedies can be provided as gels, drops, creams, ointments, tablets or sugar pellets that melt under your tongue. Your homeopath will individualize your remedy to suit your medical situation. Even though side effects from remedies are rare, if you are taking homeopathic remedies for your headaches, please tell your doctor what you are taking, because interactions are possible between remedies and any medications you may be taking.

Homeopathic Remedies for Primary Headaches

Remedy	Rubrics
Strychnos nux-vomica	For headaches from stimulant abuse or a migraine that is triggered by anger, overwork or coffee
Spigelia	For headaches on the left side with pain radiating from the back of the head (called the occiput) into the eye
Sanguinaria	For right-sided headache radiating from the occiput to the eye, accompanied by vomiting
Iris versicolor	For headache with vomiting and burning sensation in gastrointestinal tract

Ayurvedic Medicine

The goal of Ayurvedic medicine is to balance and integrate mind, body and spirit to promote wellness and prevent illness. Current Ayurvedic migraine treatment includes four herbo-mineral formulations, three meals and three snacks in a day, with 8 hours of sleep at night, while avoiding tea, coffee and carbonated drinks, as well as reheated, deep-fried and canned food. Research has shown that this treatment reduces the frequency, intensity and associated symptoms in migraine patients. Because the herbs are given together, it is difficult to assign side effects to any one.

Safety Concerns

Although Ayurvedic medicine has been practiced in India for centuries, there remains some concern about the possible toxicity and interactions with other therapies, and the lack of scientific evidence for therapies. Please check your government health website for required certification for Ayurvedic medicine practitioners and request to see the credentials of any Ayurvedic therapist you may visit. If you are taking herbs or following a specialized diet based on Ayurvedic therapy, please tell your doctor. Sharing any information with your doctor about complementary and alternative practices you follow will ensure that you receive coordinated, integrated care.

Mind-Body Treatments

These treatments are considered an excellent choice when stress is identified as a headache trigger, as well as for muscle tension, insomnia and mood disorders considered difficult to resolve. Biofeedback techniques, guided imagery, cognitive behavioral therapy, meditation, music therapy, relaxation training and stress management have been proven to be safe and effective for headache. The use of these therapies with medication has shown a synergistic improvement, where all therapies work together for a better outcome than each alone, reducing anxiety and depression in particular, and increasing the sense of self-control in improving headache symptoms.

Bodywork

Exercise, stretching, massage, manual therapy, manipulation and craniosacral therapy have been most effective when combined with biofeedback, relaxation training and exercise. An educational and physical program including simple relaxation exercises and stretching reduced headache frequency, neck and shoulder pain, and medication use after 6 months. Yoga has been especially effective for migraine without aura.

Therapeutic Touch

Therapeutic touch (TT) involves holding the hands a short distance from the body (no physical contact) first to identify, then to correct the patient's energy field imbalances. Sessions can be as brief as 5 minutes or go as long as 30 minutes. Healing touch also focuses on helping patients to realize their strengths, encouraging commitment to self-care and establishing a beneficial relationship between patient and practitioner. Therapeutic touch has been used for pain, stress (anxiety), headache, well-being and depression but should not be used in place of therapies with proven effectiveness for severe conditions.

Four-Step Therapeutic Touch Protocol

1. *Centering:* Focus attention on the patient and calm her or his mind.

2. *Assessing:* Evaluate the patient's energy flow for imbalances.

3. *Intervening:* Facilitate a symmetrical flow throughout the patient's energy field.

4. *Evaluating/closure:* Verify the impact of the intervention and complete the therapy session.

Meditation

Meditation is a complementary mind-body therapy used in the treatment of many health-related problems, including all forms of primary headaches. All the various means of meditation address "the breath" in some way.

Five Kinds of Meditation

1. **Mantra meditation** involves repeating a word, sound or symbol within a group practice. Examples include transcendental meditation, relaxation response meditation and clinically standardized meditation.

2. **Mindfulness meditation** is meant to build nonjudgmental awareness, acceptance and the ability to stay "in the moment." Examples include Vipassana meditation, Zen Buddhist meditation, mindfulness-based stress reduction and mindfulness-based cognitive therapy.

3. **Yoga** includes physical postures (asanas), breath techniques (pranayama), eye positions, mantras and meditation. Hatha yoga and kundalini yoga are two examples out of many.

4. **Qi gong** combines self-regulation through breathing patterns with postures, movements and meditation.

5. **Tai chi**, also called moving meditation, is a collection of slow exercises for mental concentration, relaxation, improved posture, flexibility and well-being.

Chapter 11
Nutritional and Botanical Supplements

CASE HISTORY
Taking Care of Yourself

Angela gathered up the piles of student nurse assignments she still had to mark when she got home from her clinical nursing class. She held her head briefly, then checked her backpack for the preventive medication she normally took whenever a headache started. Feeling a little faint, she took a moment before filing the papers into a folder marked DUE TOMORROW. Her trendy water bottle was empty again, but she still had coffee, so she chased the medication with the cold beverage before heading out to her car. Between taking her son to his dentist's appointment and preparing her students' assignment, Angela hadn't had a chance for lunch, even though she had prepared her favorite grilled vegetable wrap with almonds, a pear and some tapioca for snacks. It was still in the car where she'd left it. Her family physician was concerned about her general state of health and her iron-deficient blood. As he prescribed an iron supplement for her anemia, he warned Angela that her headaches would only get better when she started taking better care of herself.

Poor nutrition and nutritional deficiencies can trigger primary headaches, so it makes sense to eat nutrient-rich food to prevent them. At times, however, the deficiency is so extreme and the food sources so poor that individual nutrients are needed to supplement your food supply. Recently, nutrients have been shown to be not just preventive of headache but also therapeutic when taken in large doses. Medical practitioners, especially specialists in clinical nutrition, have begun to prescribe nutrients as therapy, often instead of pharmaceutical medications.

Therapeutic Nutrients

- Vitamins
- Minerals
- Essential fatty acids
- Amino acids

Nutrient Supplementation

Traditionally, plants have been used as medicine for many illnesses, including headache. Botanical, or herbal, medicines have been shown to be effective and safe, when used with caution, in many credible scientific trials. It is important to discuss supplements with your doctor to rule out interactions with any other conditions you have or medications that you may be taking.

Causes of Nutrient Deficiencies

- Reduced or inadequate intake
- Decreased absorption: Inability of the body to break down foods and absorb the nutrition
- Decreased utilization: An inability of the body to make use of nutrients absorbed due to some breakdown in the metabolic process, such as blocking an enzyme function
- Increased destruction of nutrients: Exposure to medications in the diet may break down nutrients
- Increased wastage: Diarrhea, vomiting, excess menstrual bleeding, or lactation, to name a few
- Increased nutrient requirement: Growth, pregnancy, menopause

Aims of Nutritional Supplementation

- Provide the nutrients required to prevent disease conditions
- Overcome metabolic deficiencies that prevent nutrient absorption
- Compensate for lifestyle (smoking, alcohol consumption), nutrient depletion in soil where crops are grown, or medication
- Compensate for nutrient dependency when an error in genetic makeup prevents normal metabolic pathways for specific nutrients
- Treat specific conditions (such as magnesium to reduce risk of migraine attack)

Selected Nutrient Supplementation for Headaches

Nutrient	Action	Possible Side Effects
Magnesium	Some migraine sufferers have lower levels of magnesium in their brain and body during migraine as well as at other times. Magnesium prevents vasospasms, stabilizes cell membranes (reducing inflammation) and inhibits platelet aggregation. Including magnesium-rich foods or adding magnesium supplements may reduce your risk of migraine headaches.	Diarrhea, stomach upset, nausea, vomiting. Large doses of magnesium may build up in the body, causing confusion, low blood pressure, slowed breathing, irregular heartbeat, coma and even death. Do not take high doses of magnesium if you have a heart blockage, and don't take it at all if you have a kidney disorder. Magnesium may interact with antibiotics or some medications.
Riboflavin (vitamin B_2)	Riboflavin (vitamin B_2) is part of the chain of activity that leads to the production of oxygen for energy use in our bodies. For some people with migraine, if a metabolic dysfunction is a trigger, then supplementing with riboflavin may prevent and reduce migraine symptoms, frequency, intensity and duration of attacks. Riboflavin may reduce the need for acute medication use. Daily doses of riboflavin may improve mitochondrial function by increasing the stores of brain mitochondrial energy, with minimal side effects.	In high doses, may cause diarrhea, increase urine production and have other possible side effects. May interact with some medications. Dosage of 0.08–100 mg per day is safe for pregnant or breastfeeding women.
Coenzyme Q10	Improves metabolic efficiency and protects mitochondria (site of oxygen/energy production) from free-radical damage. Reduces activation of trigeminal nerve in central nervous system.	May cause stomach upset, loss of appetite, nausea, vomiting, diarrhea, allergic skin rashes, and possibly lower blood pressure. May interact with some medications or during surgery.
Vitamin B_{12}	Vitamin B_{12} has been seen to reduce migraine frequency by 50%. The use of NSAIDs for pain control can lead to reduced B_{12} levels, so taking B_{12} can protect from NSAID side effects. (More research is necessary on the use of B_{12} as therapy for migraine attacks.)	Vitamin B_{12} supplementation can lead to itchiness, blood clots, diarrhea and severe allergic reactions in some people, and should not be taken by individuals with Leber hereditary optic neuropathy or allergies/sensitivities to cobalamin or cobalt. Vitamin B_{12} may interact with some medications.

continued...

Nutrient	Action	Possible Side Effects
Niacin (vitamin B3)	Niacin causes flushing that could abort migraine symptoms by vasodilating intracranial blood vessels. This is known to be the case for peripheral blood vessels, but more study is required to understand whether niacin also affects central blood vessels.	For some people, niacin may raise histamine levels and possibly cause headache.

Botanical Medicine

Botanical, or herbal, medicine is a traditional medical practice that uses plant-based medicines to preserve good health and to prevent and treat illness, both physical and mental. The use of herbal medicines is long established and considered safe and effective, with some cautions. Botanical medicine practitioners recommend or make remedies that use herbs and herbal materials, herbal preparations and finished herbal products. Active ingredients from plant parts, other plant materials or combinations of the above are also included. During preparation of remedies, active ingredients should be standardized for safety.

Components of Herbal Remedies

Dried herbs	Leaves, stems, wood, roots, bark, fruit, seeds, flowers, rhizomes and other parts of the plant. The parts may be used whole, crumbled or ground.
Herbal materials	In addition to herbs, these may contain fresh juices, fixed oils, gums, resins, essential oils and/or dry powders. Processing may include roasting, steaming or baking with liquor, honey or other ingredients.
Herbal preparations	Comminuted (very diluted) or powdered herbal materials, extracts and tinctures, along with fatty oils of herbal materials. Production of the material may include extraction, fractionation, purification, concentration or other physical or biological processes (steeping or heating herbal materials in alcoholic beverages, honey and others).
Finished herbal products	Herbal preparations that are made up of one or more herbs (called a mixture herbal product when more than one). May also contain a vehicle or medium (called excipients) or synthetic ingredients along with active ingredients. When synthetic or chemically defined active substances have been added, the product is no longer considered to be herbal.

Standardization

Like drugs, herbal products can be dangerous if taken without direction from an experienced practitioner. Herbal products can increase your risk for medical conditions or interact with Western medications you may be taking for other medical conditions. Unless the product is standardized so that you know exactly what a dose contains and it is produced in a regulated and safe way, you may be at risk of ingesting toxic materials along with the herbs. Government websites provide lists of approved herbal products that are proven to be standardized and safe when taken as directed.

Traditional Herbal Remedies

The herbs listed in this table have been used historically for relief from headaches. Although other herbs are also recommended for primary headaches, information was not available from a reliable source about possible side effects or safety, so they have not been included here. Before using any herbs, discuss your situation and all medications, supplements and herbs you are taking with your doctor, pharmacist and dietitian, if possible, for the optimal and lowest-risk integrated strategy for managing your headaches.

Herbal Remedies for Primary Headache		
Botanical	**Action**	**Possible Side Effects**
Tanacetum parthenium (feverfew)	Migraine prevention, may work by inhibiting serotonin release, helping to prevent initial vasoconstriction that could begin an attack	Open sores in mouth, upset stomach. Not recommended for pregnant or breastfeeding women.
Petasites hybridus (butterbur)	Reduces headache frequency	Upset stomach for some. Look for butterbur products labeled or certified as PA-free (pyrrolizidine alkaloids are potentially harmful chemicals). Not recommended for pregnant or breastfeeding women.
Salix alba, Salix nigra (white willow, black willow) Source for salicylic acid (aspirin)	Reduces pain, anti-inflammatory	Some people experience stomach upset, mild nausea, ulcers and stomach bleeding with white willow. Avoid if you are prone to stomach upset or have stomach or intestinal ulcers.
Zingiber officiale (ginger) Ginger tea: Steep 1 slice of gingerroot in 1 cup (250 mL) hot water.	Pain relief, anti-inflammatory, relieves stomach upset	Few side effects noted from small doses. Possible side effects most often associated with powdered ginger include gas, bloating, heartburn and nausea.

Chapter 12
Dietary Therapy

CASE HISTORY
Sick and Tired

Conrad was sick and tired of losing his life to migraines. He had tried many medications, with some success, but he didn't like the side effects, so he would often skip the preventive medications intended to stop the migraines before they started. He was ready to make a major change. This time, he decided to explore dietary therapy.

On the advice of his physician and dietitian, Conrad began keeping a health journal so he could see if his food choices affected the onset, duration and severity of his headaches. At his next visit, they asked Conrad to shift his diet to gluten-free to see if that helped. Conrad rolled his eyes, but he had signed an agreement with his wife and children to see this through. He thought it would be impossible to shop for and live on gluten-free food, but he was pleasantly surprised to find many gluten-free foods available in his grocery store. Conrad had a new skip in his step on his next visit with his doctor and dietitian. He'd had four headache-free days in a row, something he hadn't experienced since he'd been a young teenager, he had found it much easier to focus on his research projects, and he wasn't as irritable.

Conrad had also experimented with caffeine in this month, going without coffee for 2 of 4 weeks and returning to it for the final 2 weeks, and discovered he is one of the people for whom caffeine is not a trigger for headaches. He found no difference whatsoever between the coffee and coffee-free times. Conrad's next challenge was to try following a low-histamine diet, but his previous successes using food as therapy gave him the courage to make this more radical change in his diet. His family was also eager to help him. They like the new Conrad better than the old, irritable husband and father.

Does the food you eat affect your headaches? It seems like every week we hear about another new superfood that will cure headaches — or about foods that will make headaches worse. While these claims are not always substantiated, they do indicate that food choices and primary headache are connected. And while doctors have known for many years that foods such as chocolate, red wine, sausage and rich cheeses seem to cause bad headaches, ongoing evidence-based research in agriculture, diet and nutrition provides us with a better understanding of how we can achieve our optimal health with the foods we prepare for ourselves and our family.

Developing a Dietary Plan

Learning more about how to choose foods that build a healthy and nutritious diet will help you manage your headaches. Understanding basic nutrition will also arm you with the knowledge you need to make your way through the minefields of advertising and decipher exactly what those nutrition information boxes on food packages really mean!

More and more people are using dietary therapy to manage their headache symptoms. Developing a plan with your doctor and dietitian may help you manage yours. Keeping a health diary will also help you recognize how certain foods may affect headache symptoms over time.

Modern vs. Primitive Diets

The modern Western diet has become nutritionally poor because of soil exhaustion and food processing. In one of the great ironies of modern food nutrition, vitamins B_1, B_2 and B_3 are stripped from whole-grain wheat in the process of making white flour for bread products, but white bread is now fortified or enriched with these same three vitamins. But left alone in its primitive, unprocessed state, whole-grain wheat is more nutritious than processed white flour even with the native vitamins added back. In his landmark book, *Hoffer's Laws of Natural Nutrition* (reissued as *Healing with Clinical Nutrition*), Dr. Abram Hoffer worked out a diet dialectic to show the differences between the modern and primitive diets.

Modern diet	Primitive diet
Artificial	Whole
Dead	Alive
Stale	Fresh
Monotonous	Varied
Toxic	Non-toxic
Abundant	Scarce
Exogenous	Endogenous
Often artificially flavored	Naturally flavored
Complex	Simple

Some research indicates that the modern diet is conducive to primary headaches, while the primitive diet is preventive and, if the headaches are chronic, therapeutic.

Food Facts and Guides

Dietitians typically divide food into two nutrient groups: macronutrients and micronutrients. Macronutrients provide us with the energy, or calories, that keep us alive, and include carbohydrates, proteins and fats. Micronutrients include vitamins, minerals, essential fatty acids and amino acids that support the digestion, absorption and dissemination of macronutrients in the body. These digestive functions are enabled by enzymes, which are biological catalysts for chemical reactions in the body. Neurotransmitters and hormones enable communication between the gut and the brain, signaling the feeling of satiety, for example, so you do not overeat and become overweight. And our immune system protects us from the pathogens that may enter the body by many means — including through food. Improperly cleaned or stored foods may carry bacteria or spoil, adding or increasing food-borne pathogens.

Food Guides and Food Groups

The United States Department of Agriculture (USDA) and Health Canada have categorized foods in different groups based on their nutrients. In the USDA food guide, known as MyPlate, foods that share similar nutritional values are organized into six groups:

- Fruits
- Vegetables
- Grains
- Protein products
- Dairy
- Oils

In addition, these food guides recommend the size of a serving of food in each group. This nutritional analysis is the basis of the nutrition facts printed on food labels.

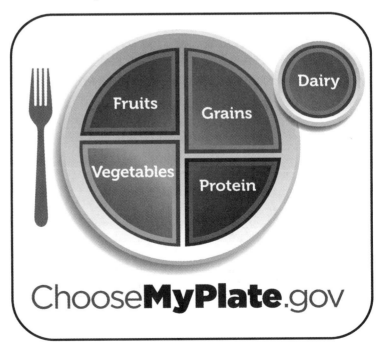

How to Read a Food Label

The Nutrition Facts label that is required on food labels in Canada and the United States is a valuable guide to help manage your shopping, planning and cooking, compare products or determine nutrient value.

Understanding Food Nutrition Facts Labels

1. Check serving size and total number of servings.
  - A single serving is used to calculate information.
  - How many servings are in a package.
  - When comparing products, check serving size first.

2. The % daily value (% DV) indicates what percentage of the recommended daily intake of a nutrient is supplied by one serving of the food.
  - Choose foods that are high or low in a nutrient (5%=low; 20%=high)
  - The % DV is based on a 2,000-calorie/day diet and is meant as a general guide to adjust according to your needs.

Nutrition Facts	
① Per ½ cup (125 mL)	②
Amount	**% Daily Value**
③ **Calories** 70	
④ **Fat** 0.5 g	1%
Saturated 0 g + Trans 0 g	0%
Cholesterol 0 mg	
⑤ **Sodium** 250 mg	10%
Carbohydrate 13 g	4%
⑥ Fibre 2 g	8%
Sugars 6 g	
⑦ **Protein** 2 g	
⑧ Vitamin A 2%	Vitamin C 2%
Calcium 0%	Iron 4%

3. Pay attention to calories per serving.
  - Check calories per serving and compare to fat per serving.
  - Sometimes low fat has as many calories as the full-fat version.

4. Learn which fats you are eating.
  - Comparing labels and learning to choose foods that have less saturated fat, trans fat and cholesterol will reduce your risk of heart disease. The % DV for total fat includes all fats shown.

5. Limit your intake of sodium to lower your risk of developing high blood pressure.

6 Fiber and sugars are healthy sources of carbohydrates.
  - Compare sugars in foods to limit those with added sugars, such as sucrose, glucose, fructose, or corn syrup.
  - Beware of foods that have added sugars as item 1, 2 or 3 in the ingredient list.

7. When choosing proteins, lean, lower-fat or fat-free are the best options.

8. Look for nutrient-rich foods.
  - Comparing food nutrition labels will help you to choose foods that are higher in valuable nutrients.
  - Compare brands to get higher nutrient value with fewer calories.

Source: Adapted from Health Canada. Interactive nutrition label. Get the facts. The nutrition facts table. Accessed April 2013 from http://fwww.hc-sc.gc.ca/fn-anAabel-etiquet/nutrition/consflnl_main-eng.php#a.

Eating Well with Canada's Food Guide

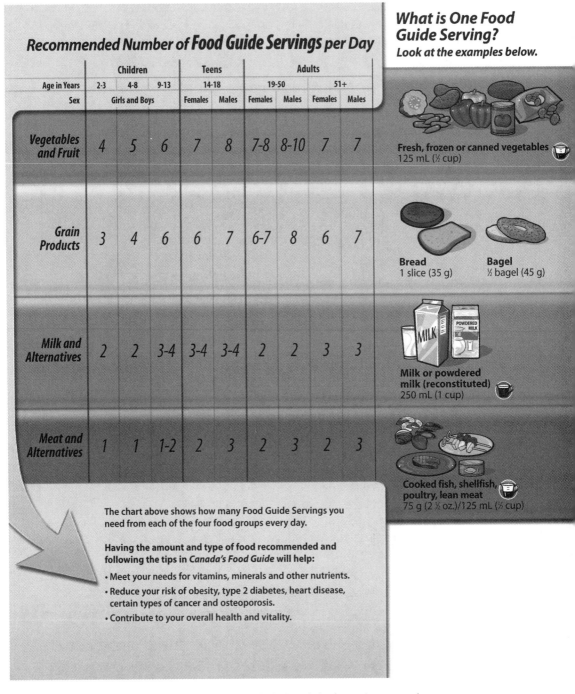

Recommended Number of *Food Guide Servings* per Day

	Children			Teens		Adults			
Age in Years	2-3	4-8	9-13	14-18		19-50		51+	
Sex	Girls and Boys			Females	Males	Females	Males	Females	Males
Vegetables and Fruit	4	5	6	7	8	7-8	8-10	7	7
Grain Products	3	4	6	6	7	6-7	8	6	7
Milk and Alternatives	2	2	3-4	3-4	3-4	2	2	3	3
Meat and Alternatives	1	1	1-2	2	3	2	3	2	3

What is One Food Guide Serving?
Look at the examples below.

Fresh, frozen or canned vegetables
125 mL (½ cup)

Bread
1 slice (35 g)

Bagel
½ bagel (45 g)

Milk or powdered milk (reconstituted)
250 mL (1 cup)

Cooked fish, shellfish, poultry, lean meat
75 g (2 ½ oz.)/125 mL (½ cup)

The chart above shows how many Food Guide Servings you need from each of the four food groups every day.

Having the amount and type of food recommended and following the tips in *Canada's Food Guide* will help:

• Meet your needs for vitamins, minerals and other nutrients.
• Reduce your risk of obesity, type 2 diabetes, heart disease, certain types of cancer and osteoporosis.
• Contribute to your overall health and vitality.

For the full guide, please contact Health Canada or visit their website (www.hc-sc.gc.ca).

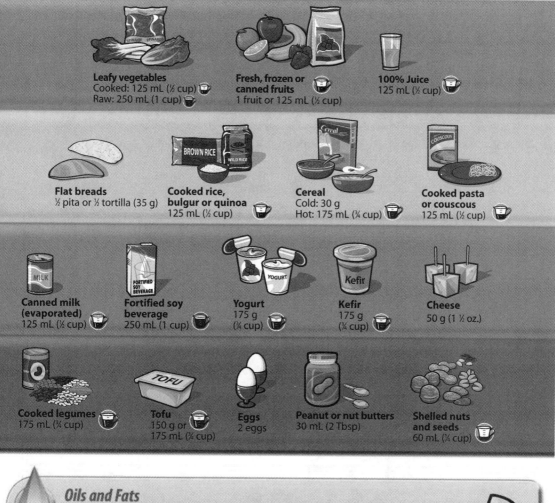

Leafy vegetables
Cooked: 125 mL (½ cup)
Raw: 250 mL (1 cup)

Fresh, frozen or canned fruits
1 fruit or 125 mL (½ cup)

100% Juice
125 mL (½ cup)

Flat breads
½ pita or ½ tortilla (35 g)

Cooked rice, bulgur or quinoa
125 mL (½ cup)

Cereal
Cold: 30 g
Hot: 175 mL (¾ cup)

Cooked pasta or couscous
125 mL (½ cup)

Canned milk (evaporated)
125 mL (½ cup)

Fortified soy beverage
250 mL (1 cup)

Yogurt
175 g
(¾ cup)

Kefir
175 g
(¾ cup)

Cheese
50 g (1 ½ oz.)

Cooked legumes
175 mL (¾ cup)

Tofu
150 g or
175 mL (¾ cup)

Eggs
2 eggs

Peanut or nut butters
30 mL (2 Tbsp)

Shelled nuts and seeds
60 mL (¼ cup)

Oils and Fats

- Include a small amount – 30 to 45 mL (2 to 3 Tbsp) – of unsaturated fat each day. This includes oil used for cooking, salad dressings, margarine and mayonnaise.
- Use vegetable oils such as canola, olive and soybean.
- Choose soft margarines that are low in saturated and trans fats.
- Limit butter, hard margarine, lard and shortening.

Macronutrient-Balanced Diet

Nutrition agencies like the USDA and Health Canada recommend a balanced, or proportioned, diet of macronutrients. Here is the case for an average adult, 19 years or older:

- 45% to 65% carbohydrates
- 10% to 35% protein
- 20% to 35% fats

The food guides give good explanations of which foods fall in each category (such as vegetables, fruit, grain products, milk and alternatives, meat and alternatives) and give more detailed recommendations of servings per day for children, teens and adult females and males. If you follow the recommendations of the national food guides, you will be less likely to suffer from nutrient deficiencies and weight issues, and you should be able to maintain good health. The focus of food guides is on achieving optimal health through nutritional therapy.

Dietary Aims

Achieving these aims should improve your general health and help fend off primary headaches.

1. Learn to evaluate the variety and quality of the carbohydrates, fats and proteins in your diet.
2. Get plenty of fiber by choosing the right carbohydrates, including fruit, vegetables and whole grains.
3. Avoid eating highly processed "white" carbohydrates (breads or baked goods made from white flour; white rice; white-flour pasta; and products with added sugars, such as high-fructose corn syrup).
4. Eat good fats, such as olive oil and omega-3 oils from fish and some plants, such as flax seeds.
5. Avoid high-dose saturated fats (animal sources) and trans fats (commercial baked goods, some vegetable oils and dressings, fried foods).
6. Choose lean animal and plant protein.
7. Avoid grain-fed, hormone-supplemented commercial beef (which contains saturated fat plus excessive omega-6 fatty acids).
8. Because of its heart-friendly properties, eating dark chocolate in small amounts is acceptable even though it contains saturated fats.

Guide to Food Groups and Primary Headaches

Items from some food groups seem to trigger primary headaches, while other items tend to prevent them. Take the time to make a list of problematic foods to avoid and have the foods that help prevent your headaches at hand in your pantry or refrigerator.

Carbohydrate Sources

Fruits, vegetables and grains are the prime sources of carbohydrates. These foods "fire" your body with the energy needed to live and act. These food groups also include fiber, which is used by your body to digest food and expel body waste.

Fruits and Vegetables

Fruits and vegetables provide the essential vitamins, minerals and fiber to build good health and fight off disease. Fruits and vegetables are low in unhealthy fats, have few calories and are filling. Eating vegetables of different colors — making a rainbow on your plate — provides the widest range of nutrients, from vitamin A to zinc. At first glance, it may not seem possible to eat as many servings of fruits and vegetables as recommended by the guidelines, but the suggested serving sizes are relatively small.

Grains and Grain Products

Grains are a good source of fiber and several of the B vitamins (thiamin, riboflavin, niacin and folate). Aim to eat whole grains because they contain the kernel (bran, germ and endosperm). Refined grains have gone through the milling process, which removes the bran and germ from the kernel. Milling improves shelf life and gives grain a finer texture but removes dietary fiber and many of the B vitamins.

Breads, rice, pasta and cereals made from mostly processed or refined white flours with refined sugars or corn syrup (used in most cakes, cookies and candies) can cause poor digestion in your gut, disrupt your body's balance and lead to disease. Increase the nutritional value of your food by switching to whole grains whenever possible. Include barley in vegetable soups, or grains in casserole dishes or stir-fries.

Whole grains are also sources of magnesium and selenium. Selenium protects your cells from oxidation (being broken down in the same way that metal rusts when exposed to air) and supports your immune system.

Did You Know?

Disease Protection

Fruits and vegetables protect us by reducing the risk of cancer and other chronic disease states, including primary headaches, but many people do not eat enough fruit and vegetables for optimal health. A diet with insufficient quantities of these foods may lead to nutrient deficiencies that could increase headache risk.

Did You Know?

Fiber Foundation

Dietary fiber is known to reduce blood cholesterol levels and your risk of heart disease, obesity and type 2 diabetes. Fiber helps to maintain healthy bowel function and reduces constipation and diverticulosis (a form of small bowel disease). Including fiber in your diet is also valuable in maintaining a slower release of sugars into your bloodstream — valuable for people who suffer from primary headaches, because low blood sugar is one of the possible headache triggers.

Q. What is gluten?

A. Gluten is a protein found in grains, such as wheat, rye, barley and other products (durum flour, farina, graham flour, semolina). Oats or other grains can be contaminated during processing, so reading labels carefully and looking for items that are gluten-free is important. Gluten in your diet may damage hair-like structures called villi in the inner wall of the small intestine. Villi absorb nutrients from the food that you eat, so damage may cause digestive upset and other symptoms. Recurring migraines are one of the many symptoms of celiac disease (diagnosed through testing) or gluten sensitivity (usually identified by removing foods containing gluten from the diet and observing symptoms over time). A gluten-free diet may be right for you. Discuss your symptoms with your health-care provider and dietitian.

B Vitamins

B vitamins are essential in your diet to support your nervous system. If the neurovascular system is impaired by a deficiency of the key B vitamins (vitamins B_2, B_6 and B_{12}), you are more susceptible to headache attacks. B vitamins are also involved in your body's metabolism because they help release energy from the protein, fat and carbohydrates you eat. B vitamins from the protein food group help you release energy from the proteins you eat, are actively involved in the nervous system, help to form red blood cells and help to build tissues.

Protein Sources

Your age, sex and level of physical activity determine your need for protein. The foods in the protein food group provide protein, B vitamins, vitamin E, iron, zinc and magnesium. The proteins you eat are building blocks for your bones, muscles, cartilage, skin and blood; enzymes, hormones and vitamins are built (metabolized) from proteins; and proteins provide the calories required by your body for fuel. Lean cuts of meat, fish and seafood, nuts and seeds, legumes (beans and peas — also part of the vegetable group), eggs, processed soy and cheese are all sources of protein. A healthy diet includes at least 8 ounces (250 g) of fish or seafood a week unless you are vegetarian or vegan.

Fat Sources

Fat is the major source of energy stored in your body and helps insulate your body organs and absorb some essential vitamins. Dietary fat has 9 calories per gram, twice as many as either carbohydrates or protein, so too much fat in your diet can be harmful to your health and increase the risk of obesity, high blood cholesterol and heart disease. However, some fats are essential for your body to function at its best. Fats also maintain healthy skin and hair.

Common Foods Rich in Magnesium

Food	Serving	Magnesium (mg)
Oat bran	½ cup (125 mL), uncooked	96.0
100% bran cereal	½ cup (125 mL)	93.1
Brown rice	1 cup (250 mL), cooked	86.0
Almonds	1 ounce (30 g), about 23 almonds	78.0
Swiss chard	½ cup (125 mL), chopped, cooked	75.0
Molasses, blackstrap	1 tbsp (15 mL)	48.0
Okra	½ cup (125 mL), cooked	47.0
Hazelnuts	1 ounce (30 g), about 21 nuts	46.0
Milk 1% fat	1 cup (250 mL)	34.0

Did You Know?

Zinc Support

Zinc is essential for biochemical reactions in your body and supports the immune system. In addition, normal levels of zinc in the blood inhibit the release of histamines from the body's mast cells. Zinc deficiency is related to chemical sensitivity.

Meat Safety

- Keep raw, cooked and ready-to-eat foods in separate containers.
- Store raw meats in containers that will not drip onto other foods.
- Do not wash or rinse your meat or poultry.
- Wash all cutting surfaces with warm, soapy water after preparing each food item.
- To destroy microorganisms, cook foods to the recommended temperature using a meat thermometer that will display the safe internal temperature for each kind of meat.
- Never defrost foods on the counter.
- Avoid raw or undercooked meats and eggs.
- Be aware of mercury content in some fish, especially for pregnant or nursing women and for children.

Kinds of Fat
Cholesterol

A fat-like substance found in all cells of your body, cholesterol is necessary to make hormones, vitamin D and some of the substances that help digest your food. Your liver produces sufficient cholesterol for your needs, but it is also present

Q. What is fat?

A. In nature, carbon, hydrogen and oxygen are the essential chemical units that come together to form molecules. Saturated, polyunsaturated, monounsaturated and trans fats are all forms of fatty acids — chains of hydrogen and carbon that form the basic chemical units for fats — whose composition, or structure (determined by the length of the carbon chain), controls how the fat looks, whether it is solid or liquid at room temperature and how it affects the cholesterol levels in your bloodstream. When you look under the "Fat" heading in food labels, you will see the total fat and then the types of fats in the product, broken down into saturated and trans fats, in grams but also the percentage of the total fat in the product.

in foods. Lipoproteins, so called because they are made up of fats — lipids — and an outer shell of proteins, package cholesterol to travel through the bloodstream. High levels of low-density lipoproteins (LDLs, or "bad" cholesterol) can lead to a cholesterol buildup, increasing the risk of coronary or artery disease. On the other hand, increased levels of high-density lipoprotein (HDLs, or "good" cholesterol) in your arteries may reduce the risk of heart disease. Your diet can have an impact on the levels of both kinds of lipoproteins in your bloodstream.

Saturated Fats

This kind of fat is found in animal products (meat and butter) and plant products (cocoa butter, coconut and palm oils). Overall, your optimal diet should include no more than 10% saturated fats in your daily calorie intake. In your body, your liver manufactures cholesterol from saturated fats. Saturated fats are known to raise blood cholesterol levels (in particular low-density lipoprotein, or LDL — the unhealthy cholesterol) and increase risk of heart disease and stroke.

Trans Fats

Trans fats are manufactured to improve the shelf life and texture of polyunsaturated fatty acids. For example, margarine is made solid at room temperature by saturating it with hydrogen (called hydrogenization). The product of this reaction is called a partially hydrogenated vegetable oil (PHVO) and is the main ingredient of vegetable shortening and margarine. Trans fats are found in snack foods, commercially made cookies and cakes, and other products. Trans fats, like saturated fats, may increase LDL and decrease HDL cholesterol blood levels. Read labels carefully to avoid trans fats whenever possible.

Polyunsaturated Fats

There are two kinds of unsaturated fats: polyunsaturated and monounsaturated. Polyunsaturated fats (PUFAs) are found in plant-based oils (safflower, vegetable, sunflower, soybean and corn oils) and are not known to raise blood cholesterol levels. PUFAs are also known to reduce the risk of type 2 diabetes.

Monounsaturated Fats

Monounsaturated fats (MUFAs) are found in olive and canola oils. These fats may raise high-density lipoprotein (HDL — the healthy cholesterol), which has been associated with a reduced risk of heart disease and diabetes.

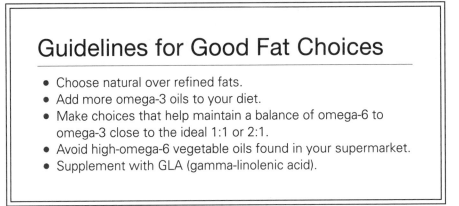

Guidelines for Good Fat Choices

- Choose natural over refined fats.
- Add more omega-3 oils to your diet.
- Make choices that help maintain a balance of omega-6 to omega-3 close to the ideal 1:1 or 2:1.
- Avoid high-omega-6 vegetable oils found in your supermarket.
- Supplement with GLA (gamma-linolenic acid).

Fat Facts

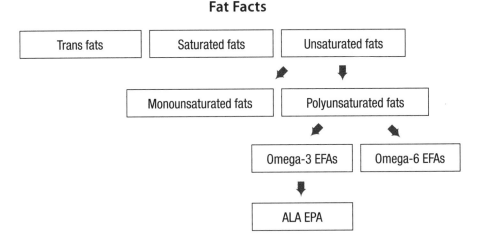

| Trans fats | Saturated fats | Unsaturated fats |

| Monounsaturated fats | Polyunsaturated fats |

| Omega-3 EFAs | Omega-6 EFAs |

| ALA EPA |

Essential Fatty Acids

There are two kinds of essential fatty acids (EFAs): alpha-linolenic acid (ALA), which is a type of omega-3 acid, and linoleic acid (LA), an omega-6 fatty acid. ALA and LA are essential oils — "essential" because they must be included in your diet; your body cannot synthesize them — required for good health. Once digested, ALA is converted in your body to eicosapentaenoic acid (EPA) and docosahexaenoic acid (DHA).

Essential fatty acids are involved in responding to injury, infection, stress and certain disease states. They are also involved in cell division and growth, blood clotting, muscle activities, secretion of digestive juices, hormone production and the movement of calcium and other substances through the bloodstream. EPA produces molecules (eiconsanoids) that protect against potential strokes and heart attacks, as well as inflammation-based conditions, such as arthritis, lupus and asthma. EPA also reduces cytokines — the molecules that increase inflammation.

Omega-3 fatty acid DHA is the major fat found in our brains and is important for its development and how it functions. For example, DHA is responsible for the signal transmission along neurons, and also for the inflammation response in the brain.

Dairy Products and Alternatives

Dairy foods are hard to categorize because they contain fat, protein and carbohydrates, but including dairy products in your diet can increase bone health and reduce your risk of osteoporosis. Dairy products have also been linked with reduced risk of cardiovascular disease and type 2 diabetes and are known to lower blood pressure in adults.

Dairy foods contain calcium — and are the primary source of calcium in some populations — used for building and maintaining bone mass, including your teeth. Yogurt, milk and soy milk (soy beverage) also provide potassium, which could help you maintain healthy blood pressure. In addition, dairy products that are fortified with vitamin D help to build and maintain bones and teeth by protecting the calcium and phosphorous levels.

A high intake of dairy products may add to the level of saturated fats and so contribute to higher risk of a range of diseases, but low-fat or fat-free forms of dairy foods will add little or no fat to the diet.

Sources of Good Oils

Some foods that are high in good oils include nuts, olives, avocados and some fish. Mayonnaise, some salad dressings and soft margarine (with no trans fats) are oil-based foods that are included in most diets.

- Canola oil
- Cottonseed oil
- Corn oil
- Soy oil
- Sunflower oil
- Olive oil
- Avocado oil
- Walnut oil
- Small amounts of coconut oil

Anti-Fatty Food Preparation

Some fats are made unhealthy by the way we use them in the kitchen.

- Put your frying pan away; instead, broil, grill, poach or boil your meat, poultry and fish.
- Reduce the amount of meat-related fat you consume by draining off any fat from your meat before serving.
- Use herbs, spices and ground nuts for breading. Pat the mixture onto the meat's surface instead of rolling, so you use less.
- Choose recipes that don't include sauces and gravies; use fresh or dried herbs for flavoring instead.
- Choose beans, which provide a lower-fat alternative to meats.
- Use nuts for snacks, in salads and in main dishes.
- Replace meat or poultry in recipes with nuts.

Dairy Alternatives

The most common alternatives to dairy products include beverages, cheese, yogurt and ice cream products made from soy, rice, almond or coconut. Soy may cause allergies and headaches for some, and fermented soy (some soy sauce, tofu products and tempeh) may cause histamine reactions as well. Soy is known for having an estrogen-like effect, so it may affect women who have hormone-related migraine attacks.

Rice milk may contain canola oil, which is known to cause headaches for some people, especially those with rice allergies or sensitivities. Although it is lactose-free, rice milk is higher in carbohydrates than cow's milk and may have added sugar.

Almond milk may be a healthy milk alternative for some, but caution is advised for those with thyroid problems because it may lead to a goiter. Some people may also be sensitive to almonds or to chemicals used during processing that could lead to headaches.

For any new foods added to your diet, keeping your diary up to date on any positive or negative changes in headache symptoms will help you choose the best dairy alternative.

Sweeteners

Sugar, natural or processed, is a simple carbohydrate that your body uses for fuel. Food sources of carbohydrates, such as fruits, vegetables and dairy foods, all contain sugars. On labels, "added sugars" refers to the sugars or syrups added during processing to increase the appeal of processed foods. Sugar helps preserve foods (jellies, jams), bulks up foods (baked

Dairy Product Safety

- Avoid unpasteurized (raw) milk or products that have been made from raw milk.
- Put any dairy foods in the fridge right away.
- Do not defrost frozen foods on the counter.
- Put any leftover food from meals that contain dairy products in the fridge immediately after food has been served.
- If dairy products are left on the counter for 2 or more hours, throw them away.

goods, ice cream), balances acidity of foods that contain vinegar and tomatoes, gives baked foods texture and color, and adds flavor to processed foods.

Reading Sugar Content

Reading nutrition labels for sugar content can be confusing. Sugar has many names based on what it is made from and the refining process. If you look at the list of ingredients, names that end in "ose" are chemical names for many sugars (fructose, glucose, maltose, dextrose). Other sugars include honey, molasses, fruit juice concentrate, fruit nectars, cane syrup, cane juice, corn sweeteners, high-fructose corn syrup and malt syrup. When you look at the list, the placement of the ingredient's name — first, second or third — shows how much of that ingredient is in the product compared to the other ingredients.

Q. What is lactose intolerance?

A. Some people are unable to digest dairy products because they may not have sufficient amounts of the enzyme that breaks down lactose (called lactase) into glucose and galactose. Symptoms of lactose intolerance include cramps, abdominal bloating, nausea, flatulence, diarrhea, rumbling stomach (called borborygmi) and vomiting. Lactase deficiencies can be genetic in origin, caused by injuries to the small intestine or, more rarely, there is a complete lack of lactase. Lactose-free dairy alternatives are available if you are lactose intolerant. You should also supplement your diet with calcium from food sources, such as canned fish, soy products, leafy greens (collard, turnip greens, kale, bok choy) and calcium-fortified juices, cereals, breads, milk and almond milk.

Sugar Problems

- Tooth decay from bacterial growth around teeth combined with poor oral hygiene.
- Possible weight gain from empty calories.
- Increased triglycerides.
- Replacing healthy food choices, which leads to poor nutrition.

Artificial Sweeteners

Sugar substitutes or artificial sweeteners are carefully assessed by government food regulatory bodies before they are permitted for public use. Often, artificial sweeteners are labeled as GRAS (generally recognized as safe). The maximum amount that is considered safe for each artificial sweetener is set by regulatory bodies as an acceptable daily intake (ADI) and is set much lower than the maximum amount that could contribute to health problems.

Artificial sweeteners are popular because they have no calories and don't contribute to tooth decay or cavities. People with diabetes also use artificial sweeteners because they don't raise blood sugar levels. Even though these products are widely used, some health concerns exist, so we recommend limited use. If you have health issues and are considering the use of artificial sweeteners, discuss the possible adverse effects with your health-care provider or dietitian.

How to Reduce Your Sugar Intake

Choose water rather than sugary drinks or flavored coffee beverages. When juice is your beverage of choice, 100% fruit juice is a healthier choice than fruit drinks. From a nutritional point of view, whole fruit is always better than fruit juice.

Choose:
- Sugar-free, whole-grain cereals rather than the sugary versions
- Fruit and vegetables; low-fat cheese; low-fat, low-calorie yogurt; and whole-grain crackers for snacks
- Syrups, jams, jellies and preserves that have few ingredients and reduced sugar (not replaced with artificial sugars)
- Water-packed canned fruit

Approved Artificial Sweeteners

- Acesulfame potassium (acesulfame K)
- Aspartame
- Neotame
- Polydextrose
- Sucralose
- Thaumatin
- The sugar alcohols (called polyols) sorbitol, isomalt, lactitol, maltitol, mannitol, xylitol
- Steviol glycosides (a sweetener based on the stevia plant)

Artificial sweeteners, along with other sugar substitutes, are common ingredients in foods:

- Ice cream
- Yogurt
- Fruit drinks
- Baked goods
- Jellies
- Soft drinks
- Chewing gum
- Candy

Chemical Additives and Preservatives

Food additives are designed to help make food flavorful, nutritious, safe, convenient, colorful and affordable. Preservatives slow the food spoilage that is caused by mold, air, bacteria, fungi and yeast. They also help to control contaminants that cause foodborne illness (botulism, for one). Antioxidants help prevent fats and oils from becoming rancid or from going "off." They are also responsible for preventing foods like apples from turning brown. However, these additives have been shown to affect headaches and other disease conditions adversely. Avoid them or reduce their intake when possible.

Beverages

In every cell of our bodies, water is essential for maintaining good health every day. Some of our water needs are satisfied through the foods we eat, such as celery, tomatoes, oranges, melons (foods that are 85% to 95% water) or prepared foods, such as soups and casseroles. Drink when you are thirsty.

Did You Know?

Avoiding Additives
Some food additives (MSG, benzoate, sulphites, nitrites, glutamate and food dyes, for example) are known to cause headaches and other symptoms, such as hyperactivity. Please read food labels carefully and record any symptoms as they occur to be able to track possible relationships between foods and headache symptoms.

How to Stay Hydrated

If you wait until your lips are dry and you are really thirsty, your body is already in a state of dehydration. Manage your fluid intake with these tips:

- Carry a water bottle with you.
- Freeze some water in a container that will not break down in the freezer (stainless steel or freezer-safe plastic). The water will stay cold throughout your day.
- When you are having meals in restaurants, choose water rather than other beverages. Juices, sports drinks and pop have added sugar and calories, and diet drinks have artificial sugars.
- Make your water more appealing by adding a squeeze of your favorite fruit juice — you might drink more water than you would otherwise.
- Be aware of how many cups of coffee or tea you drink during the day. Both coffee and tea increase your urine output (called the diuretic effect), which may lead to dehydration. Caffeine may also have an impact on your sleeping patterns.

Quick Guide to Dietary Therapy for Primary Headache

Food Group	Diet Trigger	Diet Therapy
Carbohydrates Fruits and vegetables	Folate may increase histamine levels. Vegetables high in folate include black-eyed peas, spinach, great northern beans and asparagus.	Eat a wide variety of fruits and vegetables to reduce the risk of ingesting too much of any one substance.
	Some fruits and vegetables are histamine-rich and may trigger headaches. Strawberries, bananas, tomatoes and asparagus are all examples of histamine-rich foods.	Follow the low-histamine meal plan, choose low-histamine foods more often and eat histamine-rich foods in small amounts.
	Being deficient in magnesium may trigger headaches.	Include magnesium-rich foods in your diet and consider magnesium supplements. Swiss chard and okra are foods that are naturally high in magnesium.

Food Group	Diet Trigger	Diet Therapy
Carbohydrates Grains and grain products	Gluten may be a trigger for headaches for some people. Gluten is found in wheat, rye and barley. Other foods, such as oats, may be contaminated with gluten during processing.	Gluten-free versions of foods are readily available. Read labels carefully for gluten in food. Many restaurants also now offer gluten-free dishes.
Carbohydrates Sweeteners	Poor food choices, such as soft drinks or commercial snacks and desserts, may lead to too many empty calories from sugars and cause obesity or increase the risk of heart attack.	Reduce sugar intake by eating whole fresh foods whenever possible. Replace sugary drinks and caffeinated beverages with water.
Protein Meats, fish, legumes, nuts	Meat with nitrites, fermented or aged meats, fish skin or meats left to defrost on a counter or in a refrigerator may have a higher level of histamine.	Choose cuts of meat from the low-histamine list. Choose fresh meat from the meat counter. When buying ground meat, have it ground at the time of purchase and use immediately.
	Iron deficiency may lead to anemia.	Protein is often a good source of iron. Eat a variety of protein sources every day.
	Some legumes are histamine-rich.	Follow the low-histamine meal plan, choose low-histamine foods more often and eat histamine-rich foods in small amounts.
	Some nuts are histamine-rich.	Some nuts (such as almonds and hazelnuts) are high in magnesium. Include small amounts of low-histamine nuts, instead of meats, with meals.
	Too much fat in your diet can lead to obesity, which may trigger headaches for some people and could increase risk of heart disease.	Choose leaner cuts of meat to reduce risk of heart disease. Include less meat in your diet — and when you do include meat, eat smaller portions.
Omega-3 Fats	Omega-3 fats reduce stress, aid in digestion and reduce inflammation. Low-fat diets may be a headache trigger for some people.	To increase your intake of omega-3 and lower your intake of omega-6 EFAs, eat less meat at a sitting, use more olive and nut oils than safflower or corn oils, eat fish more often and eat more leafy vegetables on a daily basis. Fats in moderation are necessary for a healthy, nutritious diet.

Food Group	Diet Trigger	Diet Therapy
Dairy Products	Some dairy products are histamine-rich.	Choose lower-fat milk products, such as 1% or 2% milk or alternatives. Choose fresh, unfermented cheeses for less histamine. 1% milk is a good source of magnesium.
Additives and Preservatives	Some food additives (MSG, benzoate, sulphites, nitrites, glutamate and food dyes, for example) are known to cause headaches and other symptoms, such as hyperactivity.	Read labels carefully to avoid additives. Using fresh leafy herbs to flavor your meals may reduce headache frequency.
Sodium	A high-sodium diet may trigger headaches as well as increase risk of heart disease or stroke.	Reading food labels will help you identify how much sodium is in your diet. Choosing fresh whole foods over processed foods will reduce your sodium intake. Be aware that restaurant meals may be high in hidden sodium.
Beverages	Dehydration may be a trigger for headache for some people.	Choose whole fresh foods that have a higher water content (pears, apples, fresh leafy vegetables). Carry water bottles with you to ensure you stay hydrated.
	Caffeine is a headache trigger for some; for others, it may be a pain reliever.	Read food and beverage and medication labels to be aware of how much caffeine you ingest on a daily basis. Record caffeine intake to be able to assess any association with headache.

Part 3

Low-Histamine Diet Program

Chapter 13
Low-Histamine Diet Principles and Practices

CASE HISTORY
An Education in Histamines

During his freshman year at university, Joe began to suffer from serious headaches. Here's how he described his symptoms when he visited the campus health clinic: "Not only did I start to have severe headaches, I also started getting hives. Some mornings, my eyes are very swollen and my body itches from head to toe. I've been having scary heart palpitations, even when I'm just reading or sitting in class."

Although he had never had allergies and was typically healthy, it appeared that Joe was having some kind of allergic response, but no allergies were found through testing. Meeting as a team, his dietitian and family physician discussed Joe's secondary symptoms — hives, swelling, heart palpitations — and wondered if histamine intolerance or sensitivity was a factor, since no other cause had been found. As well as being given medication for relief from his headaches, Joe was referred to the university's school of dietitians, where his diet was assessed for high levels of histamines. Because some evidence indicates that headaches and other symptoms like Joe's may be related to histamine intolerance, a low-histamine diet was suggested for possible relief. Joe left his assessment with a list of high-histamine foods to avoid, a set of meal plans to follow for 14 days, and corresponding recipes.

Joe was initially reluctant to change his diet, thinking that the low-histamine foods would be difficult to find or cook. He did miss the high-nitrite sausage he had become somewhat addicted to but was less reluctant to give up fermented foods, such as sauerkraut. He found that being careful to not eat too much high-histamine food in one day was more important than avoiding it altogether. He also found that gluten-free food was easy to find and that many restaurants offered gluten-free versions of his favorite foods.

After 2 weeks of a mostly low-histamine diet, the hives had faded and Joe was no longer itchy. Joe recorded one headache during that period, and that happened after a stressful exam when he had been up late studying and was definitely dehydrated. He also recorded that the panicky feeling from the heart palpitations was not happening anymore. Joe continues to keep a health journal to ensure a healthier and happier university career.

A well-proportioned, or balanced, diet built on the foundation of authoritative food guides will improve your general health and prepare you for doing battle with your headaches. In addition to this armory, there is a dietary strategy that may prevent or reduce headaches for some people. Choosing low-histamine, antihistamine and histamine-blocking foods could remove a significant trigger for your headaches. Recent research has shown that for some people, a diet that reduces the intake of histamine may prevent, reduce, or even eliminate the symptoms experienced with primary headaches.

Histamine Theory

Histamine is a biogenic amine formed in our bodies by normal cellular metabolism. Biogenic amines are also commonly found in fermented meat, some beverages, dairy products, sauerkraut and spoiled fish, to name a few sources. There are several forms of biogenic amines in food (histamine, tyramine, cadaverine, putrescine, spermidine, and spermine), but tyramine and especially histamine are most commonly associated with food reactions.

Histamine Reaction

Histamine serves to regulate bodily functions in three ways: as a messenger, a neurotransmitter and a mediator. It is involved with the wake/sleep cycle (circadian rhythm), bowel movements and immune system function. The normal cell lifecycle for histamine is as follows: it is produced in our bodies, stored in certain types of cells, and, when required, acts as a messenger. All stored histamine is released at one time. Then histamine is either ingested by immune system scavengers or broken down by one of the two enzymes able to do so — diamine oxidase (DAO) or histamine N-methyltransferase (HNMT). Of the two enzymes, diamine oxidase, which is active in the intestine, is thought to be the likely cause of histamine intolerance. When the histamine rises to a "tipping point" in the body, histamine attached to receptors in some of the body systems described above may cause symptoms that mimic allergy. However, typical tests for food allergies will not be positive because the immune system is not involved.

Histamine Intolerance (HIT)

Many factors can influence histamine levels in our bodies. Histamine is found in the foods you eat, and if levels of histamine have increased to the point that your enzymes are unable to break it down, histamine toxicity may be the result.

For some people, eating foods high in histamine leads to symptoms similar to those experienced as a result of an allergy or food poisoning. Some experience common cold symptoms as a result of high histamine levels. Because HIT can be episodic for some people or chronic for other people, it is not easy to relate symptoms directly to diet. This food sensitivity or intolerance is recognized as a metabolic disorder because of the inability of the enzymes to break down the ingested histamine.

Histamine Intolerance Symptoms

Histamine intolerance symptoms differ from person to person. Possible histamine intolerance symptoms include:

- Flushing, headache, migraine, dizziness
- Nausea, vomiting
- Sleep disturbances, general fatigue
- Breakouts of sweating or hot flashes, changes in temperature sensation (you feel like the room is freezing but everyone else is just fine)
- Sneezing, runny nose, coughing up mucus or phlegm, an irritated throat, swollen nasal passages, or even trouble breathing
- Possible digestive problems include abdominal pain, heartburn, gas or diarrhea
- Drop in blood pressure, heart palpitations, tachycardia
- Swelling and water retention (swollen fingers or eyelids)
- Menstrual symptoms
- Increase in eczema symptoms
- For people who experience severe allergic responses (anaphylactic), histamine intolerance may also affect their condition

This disorder is also called biogenic amines intolerance. While a few people are born with HIT, it is seen most often in women aged 40 and over.

Range of HIT Severity

The spectrum of HIT symptom severity ranges from not affected at all to extremely affected. Every person is affected by histamine levels above a threshold called a limit of tolerance. Infused histamine is one of the molecules that has been used in clinical research to successfully trigger headache and non-aura migraine. For some people, some histamine intolerance symptoms, such as flushing or severe headache, may occur only after a meal that includes several foods high in histamine (tomatoes, strawberries, aged cheese, and red wine, to name a few), and for others, small amounts of any foods containing histamine may result in severe HIT symptoms.

How Foods Affect Body Histamine Levels

The low-histamine diet may provide a dietary structure by which you could reduce frequency, intensity or duration of primary headaches. Keeping a life diary, reducing stress wherever possible, practicing mind-body therapies, taking preventive medications as directed by your health-care provider and maintaining a meal and sleep schedule to the best of your ability may give you the tools to improve your quality of life. Learning the foods or combinations of foods that may trigger headaches will help you to recognize the symptoms of food-related histamine toxicity with or without other exposure to headache triggers.

High-Histamine Foods

The amino acid histidine is a precursor of histamine in food. One of the essential 20 amino acids, histidine is part of any protein and can be converted to histamine by histidine decarboxylase, which is produced by some of the bacteria that live in our large bowel. The resulting histamine is moved from the digestive system elsewhere in the body.

The same histidine decarboxylase is present in the gut of fish. When the fish dies, histidine is released as part of the breakdown of tissues, resulting in a massive increase of

<aside>
Did You Know?

Stress Trigger
Stress is another factor known to raise histamine levels in the body, making it difficult to assess histamine response on diet alone. Diamine oxidase and HNMT enzyme levels, as well as histamine blood or urine levels, may be useful in a diagnosis of HIT but are not reliable as a response indicator, so testing of this nature is rarely conducted.
</aside>

<aside>
Did You Know?

Back to Basics
Excessive carbohydrates in your diet can promote bacterial growth and fermentation in your large bowel, possibly leading to increased production of histamine. Maintaining a balanced or proportioned diet as recommended in food guides may be one of the easiest methods of reducing possible headache triggers related to foods.
</aside>

Did You Know?

Overall Good Nutrition

In one major study, patients followed a histamine-free diet for 2 weeks and showed reductions in severity of all histamine-related symptoms. An important factor to the success of this study was improving nutrition overall — ingesting a balanced diet, such as recommended by Canada's Food Guide and the U.S. MyPlate Program.

histamine as time goes by. Since shellfish are not gutted as part of processing, gut histidine continues to produce histamine until it is cooked. Food sources that are naturally high in histamine (such as some fish, shellfish and fermented foods) should be avoided altogether or eaten in limited amounts if you are histamine intolerant. Some fruits and vegetables have consistently high levels of histamine (strawberry, grapefruit, eggplant and tomatoes, among others). It is thought that higher levels of histamine are produced as fruits and vegetables ripen, so they should be eaten as soon as possible.

Foods That Release or Liberate Histamine

Ingestion of some foods has been found to cause histamine release in the body through a non-allergy-related physiological process even though the specific foods are not high in histamine (such as sunflower seeds, wheat germ, egg white and organ meats). Avoiding these foods may reduce or eliminate headache triggers, since some people seem to be more sensitive to histamine-liberator foods than to high-histamine foods.

Food Storage

Bacterial growth from improper storage of food can result in increased histamine levels in all food groups.

Principles of the Low-Histamine Diet

Based on the functions of histamine in the body and the pathophysiology of primary headaches, the low-histamine diet

1. Includes low-histamine foods and limits histamine-containing foods

2. Avoids or eliminates foods that liberate histamine from mast cells

3. Reduces the external introduction and development of histamine through

   - Informed food buying
   - Safe food storage
   - Clean food preparation

A diet based on reducing the intake of histamine from food and the production of histamine in food preparation may prevent, reduce or eliminate the symptoms you experience from primary headaches. The meal plans and recipes in this book will provide you with a healthy and nutritious diet that will prevent high levels of histamine from accumulating in your body.

Low-Histamine Diet Goals

Setting goals is necessary for making changes in your diet. Being realistic about your diet goals can be the difference between success and failure. Setting a few goals at a time and practicing these goals for a month or so is a realistic approach. Keep track of your progress. Knowing that the goals you meet are making a difference may keep you motivated.

Did You Know?

Antihistamines

Fresh or frozen leafy herbs have natural antihistamine action, while over-the-counter antihistamines are used for relieving nasal congestion and the effects of histamine-bearing insect stings.

Did You Know?

Keep on Keeping Your Diary

For your first few weeks on the low-histamine diet, maintain your health journal so you can determine if reducing your histamine intake is successful for managing your headaches.

Sample Monthly Goals

For this month, I will shop more often to ensure that fruits and vegetables are fresh. I will buy fresh meat from the local butcher to prevent histamine buildup.

OR

For this month, I will eat a gluten-free diet and monitor any changes to see if it helps.

OR

For this month, I will follow the low-histamine meal plan.

Low-Histamine Diet Guidelines

Before selecting foods to purchase and prepare on the low-histamine diet, quickly review these 10 practical guidelines for implementing and maintaining this diet:

1. **Balanced food groups**

   Start by reviewing the USDA MyPlate (page 118) and Canada's Food Guide (page 120) to ensure you develop a balanced diet by using the food groups as guidelines when you're shopping. Prepare your vegetables and fruit with little to no added fat, sugar or salt. Consume whole vegetables or fruit more often than juice. Prepare whole grains rather than processed grains and grain products; they are lower in fat, sugar and salt and higher in nutrients.

2. **Low-fat foods**

   Include milk or an acceptable alternative beverage in your diet every day, selecting lower-fat, calcium-rich alternatives. Choose leaner meats with little or no added fat or salt, as well as protein alternatives. Be aware of how much sodium you are including in your diet. Eat at least 2 servings of fresh fish per week, but beware of eating more, because fish can be high in histamine content. Eating large or frequent servings of a particular food may also lead to an accumulation of histamine.

3. **Fresh foods**

   Buy fresh food. Histamine levels in fruit, vegetables and meat increase as the foods ripen or age. Shop more often for fruit, vegetables and meat to keep fresh food on your plate.

4. **Clean kitchen**

   Wash your fruit and vegetables and clean your refrigerator, food preparation areas and sink area often to prevent bacterial growth that may increase the histamine levels of your food.

5. **Safe storage**

   Maintain high standards for food storage and preparation to prevent increased histamine levels in your food. Buy meat fresh from your local butcher and freeze or use it immediately.

6. Well-prepared food

When preparing food, take it out of the refrigerator or freezer at the last minute, defrost it in the microwave, if necessary, then wash, prepare and serve it immediately. Leaving food on the counter for any length of time increases histamine levels.

7. Safe defrosting

Defrost meat in your microwave, not on the counter. After your meal is prepared, plate the food, separate out extra servings before the meal and freeze them immediately to provide healthy meals for times when you have a headache attack.

8. Low-histamine foods

Select foods that are naturally low in histamine, such as cottage cheese, mozzarella, farmer's cheese, fresh beef, chicken, almonds, olive oil, green beans, apples, blackberries, coconut, grapes, mango and more. Including a variety of these foods at every meal reduces the risk of accumulated histamine.

9. Histamine-liberating foods

Avoid foods that are histamine liberators. These foods release body histamine from the mast cells where it is stored and may result in an overabundance of histamine in your body. Some histamine liberators include egg whites, seafood, shellfish, a variety of nuts, avocado, lentils and watermelon.

10. Histamine blockers

Avoid foods that block diamine oxidase (DAO), one of the two enzymes that break down histamine. Some DAO blockers include beer, wine, green tea, mate tea and energy drinks. Include histamine blockers in your meals. Leafy herbs, such as basil and parsley, block histamine from being released from mast cells. Keeping a window box of herbs close to your kitchen makes it easier to include them in your meals. When adding herbs to cooked dishes, add dried herbs when you start cooking but fresh herbs at the end. If you are using dried herbs, buy small quantities on a more frequent basis (date your spice containers). When buying fresh herbs, you will know if your herbs are fresh from the fragrant smell, bright color and crispness of the stalks.

Egg White Risk

Egg whites have high levels of histamine, plus they are histamine liberators, although the yolk has no histamine. Using whole eggs on occasion will not cause symptoms of headache.

Histamine Food Lists

No definitive list of histamine values in specific foods is included in the pages that follow because histamine levels shift depending on the food's freshness, storage conditions and cleanliness during preparation. Helping you understand the value of purchasing fresh food, of storing food properly and of maintaining clean preparation standards gives you the ability to evaluate the likelihood of higher histamine levels in your diet on a day-to-day basis. Try to include foods that are low in histamine

1. Foods to Avoid, with High Levels of Histamine

These foods can lead to intense headache symptoms after a normal serving.

Vegetables

Avocado • Eggplant • Pickled cucumber, any vegetable pickled in vinegar • Porcini mushrooms, morel mushrooms, different types of mushrooms (except white button mushrooms) • Sauerkraut, pickled cabbage • Spinach • Tomatoes

Fruits

Bananas • Grapefruit • Guava • Kiwifruit • Oranges • Papaya • Pineapple • Raspberries • Strawberries

Grains

Buckwheat • Wheat germ

Meat Products

Dried meats (any kind) • Ground meat (bought premade from butcher or prepackaged) • Ham (cured, dried) • Innards and entrails • Salami • Sausages (all kinds) • Smoked meat

Fish and Seafood

Seafood • Shellfish (mussels, oysters, clams) • Tuna • Fish (anything that isn't fresh or fresh frozen) • Fish skin

Legumes

Lentils • Peas • Red beans • Soybeans • White beans

Nuts and Seeds

Sunflower seeds • Walnuts

Dairy Products

All mature (old) cheeses • Cheddar cheese • Fontina • Parmesan • Raw milk cheese • Ready-made cheese for melting • Ready-made cheese products with other ingredients • Roquefort

Fats and Oils

Hydrolyzed lecithin • Walnut oil

Spices and Seasonings

Bouillon cubes (because of additives) • Cayenne pepper • Chili powder • Curry • Meat extract • Mustard, mustard seeds, mustard powder • Paprika • Rose hips, dog rose • Soy sauce • Stinging nettle • Red wine vinegar, white wine vinegar, balsamic vinegar • Yeast, yeast extract as much as possible, but remember that no diet is totally histamine free. Only ranges, not absolute values of histamine, can be given for specific foods listed here.

1. Foods to avoid, with high levels of histamine
2. Foods to limit, with a small amount of histamine
3. Foods to eliminate that liberate histamine
4. Foods to eliminate that block diamine oxidase (DAO)
5. Foods to include that block histamine
6. Foods to enjoy, with no histamine

Alcoholic Beverages

Alcohol, pure (ethanol) • Alcoholic beverages • Beer • Brandy • Champagne • Liquor: schnapps, spirits, clear (colorless) • Wine

Beverages

Black tea • Drinks containing cocoa, hot chocolate, chocolate drinks, malted drinks • Energy drinks • Mate (*Ilex paraguariensis*) tea • Orange juice • Tomato juice • Soy milk

Sweeteners

Licorice root • Malt extract

Additives

Sulfer dioxides • Sulfites

Food Coloring

Amaranth • Azorubine, carmoisine • Carmine, cochineal, crimson lake • Curcumin • Erythrosine • Ponceau 4R, cochineal red A • Quinoline yellow • Red 2G, acid red 1, azogeranine • Sunset yellow FCF, orange yellow 5 • Tartrazine

Preservatives

Benzoic acid and salts • Orthophenyl phenol, 2-hydroxybiphenyl • PHB-ester (parabens), para-hydroxy-benzoic acid (PHB) • Salicylic acid • Sodium orthophenyl phenol, sodium • Sorbic acid and salts, sodium, potassium, calcium sorbate • Sulfites, sulfur dioxide

Flavor Enhancers

Glutamates, glutamic acid

Thickeners

Carob, carob bean hum, carubin

Flavorings

Quinine (in bitter lemon or tonic water)

Vitamins

Folic acid

Stimulants

Theobromine (xantheose) (found in chocolate, tea, acai)

Preparations and Mixtures

Chocolate • Licorice • Mustard • Tofu

2. Foods to Limit, with a Small Amount of Histamine

You may find that foods from this list do not cause symptoms, especially if your diet is already mostly low-histamine foods. Exposure to other headache triggers along with eating these foods may cause symptoms, however, so keeping your journal up-to-date will help you recognize when it is safe to have foods from this list.

Vegetables

Brussels sprouts • Kohlrabi (German turnip) • Leeks • Onions • Peas • White button mushrooms

Fruits

Figs • Plums • Watermelon*

Grains

Barley • Bread, baked goods • Cereals in general • Malt • Rye • Sago, pearl sago • Sweet corn, canned • Wheat

Dairy Products

Buttermilk • Cream with no additives • Feta cheese • Lactose-free milk • Milk powder • Products made from unprocessed milk • Raw milk • UHT (ultra-high-temperature) milk • Yogurt

Nuts and Seeds

Cashews • Hazelnuts • Sesame seeds

Fats and Oils

Sunflower oil

Spices and Seasonings

Ginger • Nutmeg • Poppy seeds • Turmeric • Vanilla pod, vanilla powder, vanilla sugar, vanilla extract • Cider vinegar

Alcoholic Beverages

Low-histamine wine (<0.1 mg/L)

Beverages

Carbonated spring water with lots of sulfur, fluorine and iodine; mineral water; sparkling bottled water • Coffee • Green tea • Herbal teas (several ingredient mixtures) • Oat drink, oat milk • Stinging nettle (*Urtica dioica*) tea • Rice milk, rice drink • Soft drinks

Food Coloring

Flavin mononucleotide • Indigo carmine, indigotine (E132) • Patent blue V, sulphan blue

Thickeners

Carrageenan, processed eucheuma seaweed • Guar gum

Leavening Agents

Baking powder

Caution: Since watermelon is also a histamine liberator (releasing histamine from mast cells in the body), keep track of whether you get a headache after eating it to determine if it is a trigger for you.

3. Foods to Eliminate That Liberate Histamine

Foods that release histamine from mast cells may cause a headache reaction, depending on how much of the food you eat, whether you are eating other histamine foods, and whether you have environmental or internal histamine exposures.

Egg Whites

Vegetables

Avocado • Peas • Tomatoes

Fruits

Grapefruit • Kiwifruit • Oranges • Papaya • Pineapple • Plums • Prunes • Strawberries • Watermelon

Grains

Wheat germ

Meat Products

Innards and entrails • Pork (possibly) • Salami (possibly) • Smoked meat (possibly)

Fish

Seafood • Shellfish (mussels, oysters, crab, lobster, shrimp)

Legumes

Lentils • Red beans • Soybeans • White beans

Nuts and Seeds

Cashews • Hazelnuts • Sunflower seeds • Walnuts

Alcoholic Beverages

Pure alcohol (ethanol) • Beer • Brandy • Champagne • Histamine-free wine (<0.1mg/L) • Liquor: schnapps, spirits, clear (colorless) • Rum • Wine

Beverages

Mineral water, bottled sparkling water • Orange juice • Tomato juice

Additives and Flavorings

Cocoa, cocoa powder • Folic acid • Licorice • Mustard, mustard seeds, mustard powder • Potassium iodide (e.g., as additive in iodized salt) • Rose hips, dog rose • Yeast, yeast extract

4. Foods to Eliminate That Block Diamine Oxidase (DAO)

These foods can block DAO enzymes and thereby prevent histamine breakdown. Foods from this list may trigger headaches for you because the levels of histamine in your body may rise and cause toxic symptoms. If possible, eliminate these foods and substances from your diet.

Alcohol

Beer • Black tea • Energy drinks • Green tea • Mate tea • Theobromine (xantheose) • Wine

5. Foods to Include That Block Histamine

Fresh or frozen leafy herbs:

Basil, chives, parley, sage, savory

6. Foods to Enjoy, with No Histamine Response

Include these foods in your diet at any time. Consider using them therapeutically when you know you are going to be in a stressful situation or will be exposed to histamine triggers, such as bad weather.

Vegetables

Beets • Bell peppers (not hot chiles) • Cabbage • Carrots • Celery • Cucumbers • Fennel • Garlic • Gourds, squashes • Green beans • Lettuce, both head and leaf lettuces • Napa cabbage, celery cabbage, Chinese cabbage • Parsnips • Red radishes • White radishes • Zucchini

Fruits

Apples • Black currants • Blackberries • Blueberries • Coconut, shredded or flaked • Dates, fresh or dried • Grapes • Lingonberries, cowberries • Mangos • Melons (except watermelon) • Pears • Persimmons, kaki, Sharon fruit • Raisins • Red currants • Rhubarb • Sallow thorn, common sea-buckthorn

Herbs

Basil • Chives • Parsley • Sage • Savory

Grains

Corn flakes cereal (if no additives) • Dried sweet corn, cornmeal, corn flour • Millet • Oats • Quinoa • Rice, rice cakes, rice crackers, crisp rice cereal • Spelt • Sweet corn, corn on the cob, fresh or frozen

Meat and Poultry Products

Beef, veal (fresh) • Chicken • Ground meat, if eaten immediately after being minced

Fish

Fish (freshly caught or fresh frozen)

Nuts and Seeds

Almonds • Chestnuts, sweet chestnuts • Hemp (*Cannabis sativa*) seeds

Dairy Products

Brick cheese • Butter • Cottage cheese • Cream cheese • Cream with no additives • Egg yolks • Gouda cheese (young) • Mascarpone cheese • Mozzarella cheese • Ricotta cheese • Pasteurized milk • Quark, curd cheese, farmer's cheese

Fats and Oils

Canola oil • Margarine • Olive oil • Peanut oil • Safflower oil • Sunflower oil

Spices and Seasonings

Bouillon powder and cubes (with no additives) • Plain caramel (E150a), caramel (E150)

Beverages

Elderflower cordial • Mango nectar • Still mineral water • Tap water

Miscellaneous

Gelatin

Sweeteners

Caramel (browned sugar) • Fructose (fruit sugar) • Honey • Lactose (milk sugar) • Maltose, malt sugar (pure) • Maltodextrin • Maple syrup • Stevia (leaves, liquid, powder) • Sugar, sucrose (beet sugar, cane sugar)

Histamine Food lists amended with permission from Swiss Interest Group Histamine Intolerance (SIGHI), www.histaminintoleranz.ch/en/therapy_dietarychange.html.

Compliance and Complications

Making changes to your established eating habits and developing new habits requires an acceptance of the need for the dietary changes and an ability to motivate family members to participate to some extent. Understanding that the food you eat can affect your state of health is a powerful first step. Considering food as fuel for your brain and body makes it easier to build and follow a meal plan and diet that meet your specific needs. Barriers to changing diet for better health include low desire, little interest and lack of knowledge.

Goal Setting

Figuring out the strategy that works best for your lifestyle and making a list of goals to follow that suit your personality (all at once or one step at a time) can make all the difference to maintaining your healthy diet plan.

Meeting with your doctor and dietitian to discuss dietary changes is also important for goal setting. Making diet part of your overall therapy strategy will help to maintain motivation. Talking to your family or the group of people you eat most meals with is important for the success of your dietary changes. You will need to enlist the help of your family, friends and maybe people at work to help with the changes needed for buying, storing and preparing food for the low-histamine diet.

Stay Informed and Motivated

Every time you visit your health-care providers, take along a list of questions about your diet:

- Can I commit to making dietary changes to help my headaches?
- What steps do I need to take to shop, store and prepare food for the low-histamine diet?
- What do I need to do to put together an emergency food rescue kit after a headache has started?
- How many servings of fruit and vegetables can I eat now?
- Can I add to that list?
- How much white bread, pasta and desserts can I eat now?
- How do I feel about not eating some of those foods?
- How many servings of beans and less common vegetables, such as bok choy, should I eat?
- How do I feel about not eating shellfish?
- Am I eating too much of one food group?

Chapter 14

Low-Histamine Diet Program Cooking Tips

Making changes to your cooking habits may reduce your headache risk, and a few kitchen and shopping tricks will help you prepare for these challenges.

Preparing Your Kitchen
Quick Tips

1. Keep your cooking area very clean.
2. Check your pantry supplies for high-histamine items. Mark them clearly so that you don't use them by mistake.
3. Prepare and cook meals just before mealtime, because having food sit on counters or in the fridge may raise histamine levels.
4. Avoid slow cooker recipes, because this form of cooking raises histamine levels.
5. Keep your recipe items in the fridge until you are ready to prepare that item; this will avoid raising histamine levels.

Kitchen Design

> Design your kitchen area with the express purpose of reducing your risk of headache.

1. Design your kitchen area with the express purpose of reducing your risk of headache.
2. If you have tension headaches, keep your tools and dishes within easy reach. Aggravating the muscles in your neck and the back of your head by reaching and looking upward into high kitchen cupboards may trigger headaches for you.
3. Consider the weight of your pots and pans. Could you find smaller, lighter versions that might reduce your risk of headaches?
4. Be aware of the lighting in your kitchen; some lights may be more likely to trigger headaches than others.

5. Try installing soft lighting under the cabinets or counters to reduce the risk of headache.

6. Think about using racks for plates, pots and pans to reduce any banging and crashing that may trigger a headache.

Grocery Shopping

Planning your grocery shopping will help you meet your low-histamine diet goals. Knowing your headache triggers and planning your shopping expeditions around them will help you manage your headaches.

1. Prepare a shopping list based on the low-histamine meal plan and recipes.

2. Bring along your lists of low-histamine, high-histamine, histamine liberators and DAO blockers when you shop.

3. Shop in a store where you are familiar with the layout and the goods that are carried there. If you are not familiar with the store's layout, take a walk through (when you're not hungry is best) with a piece of paper and draw a plan showing where items are located, marking low-histamine items with a star and marking items you need to avoid with an X. Then plan your list based on the store's design.

4. Shop around the outside of the grocery store, where the produce, meat, and dairy products are located. Avoid the aisles with processed food products.

> Shop around the outside of the grocery store.

5. Shop often for fresh vegetables and fruits. If you have a busy schedule, consider ordering from a local farm or butcher. Some farms will deliver a selection of fresh fruits and vegetables, and some butcher shops will deliver a wide range of fresh cuts.

6. Shop after a meal; you will be less tempted by baked goods and snacks.

7. Be aware of your list of triggers. If your headaches are triggered by chemicals and perfumes, avoid the aisle with detergents and ask for help in getting the products you need from that aisle. Or you may find that ordering your groceries online or by phone, to be delivered, may reduce your risk of headaches.

8. The lights in grocery stores may trigger headaches for you. If this is the case, order online or find a smaller grocery store that has friendlier lighting.

9. Some grocery stores play music all day. If you find that your headaches are triggered by noise, you may want to choose a quieter grocery store.

Headache Rescue Kit

1. Prepare an easily accessible drawer or cupboard as your rescue cupboard when you have a headache. Although it is important to keep your medications in a safe place, out of reach of children, be sure that the medications you use to stop headache pain are within reach.

2. Have medications, teas or foods (such as ginger) that help reduce stomach upset within reach.

3. Keep coconut water, known to balance electrolytes, available in the fridge as part of your rescue kit.

4. Keep nutrient-dense foods, like figs, in your pantry or vegetable crisper for those moments when you need energy. Keep small servings of frozen soups and broth at hand for defrosting to keep energy levels up when a headache starts.

5. Tell family members where to find your headache rescue kit or keep a list on the inside of a cupboard door.

6. When traveling, prepare two rescue kits that each contain pain-relief and headache prevention medication as well as anything you take for stomach upset; eye drops to reduce eye strain; ear plugs to protect from bus, plane, or car noise; and protein bars to keep blood sugar even for times when food is not available, etc. One kit should be kept with you at all times and the second packed in your luggage. Keep a copy of any medication prescriptions in your carry-on luggage in case you are asked for it at any point during your trip or if you need more. Whenever possible, drink bottled water to maintain your hydration level.

6. Ask for help. School-aged children are often able to help with meals and household chores if given instruction when you don't have a headache.

> Have medications, teas or foods (such as ginger) that help reduce stomach upset within reach.

When All Else Fails...

When you have a headache and don't want to cook, what are your options for a quick and nutritious dinner? Following the low-histamine diet at a restaurant can be challenging. Salads, vegetable plates and many meat dishes are acceptable, as long as sauces are requested on the side.

But it is possible to eat a healthy, nutritious meal with very little cooking. Here are some strategies (recognizing that some are not practical for all of us):

1. Check local health food stores for healthy, gluten-free frozen meals for emergencies.

2. Purchase precut and trimmed foods from grocery stores for a quick vegetable stir-fry. Have the meat department grind beef or poultry to be cooked as soon as you are home.

3. Hire a personal chef. Many local chefs will come to your home or prepare a week's worth of frozen meals to your specifications. Hiring a housekeeper who will keep house and make meals may also work for you.

4. Become a regular at a local restaurant. They may be willing to prepare a meal to your specifications.

5. Make large batches of food and freeze meal-sized portions.

6. Create a low-histamine dinner club. A group of people can meet on a regular basis, with each member cooking batches of a meal and freezing meal-sized portions to share, allowing each member to come away with a variety of dishes that follow the low-histamine diet plan.

7. Start a community kitchen. This very old concept embraces the idea of people coming together as a community to procure and prepare food for meals. Working together as a group to prepare low-histamine meals can provide support for anyone with a headache.

Meeting your needs for a healthy, nourishing diet is a priority for managing your headaches. Get creative with and within your community for solutions that meet your individual circumstances. Ask your doctor and dietitian for information about existing services that will support your needs.

Chapter 15
Low-Histamine Diet Menu Plans

CASE HISTORY
Full Support

Bill, a 45-year-old father of two boys, started the low-histamine diet 2 weeks ago and now faces several challenges.

Once he understood the principles of how histamine could be affecting his body, Bill had put his hand to his cheek, thinking of how often he would be flushed before the headache started its relentless pounding. He had also thought about the many rashes he'd had while growing up and wondered if they were related to the food he'd been eating. He'd been willing to give a low-histamine diet a try.

Bill posted three lists of foods — low-histamine, some histamine and high-histamine — inside his cupboard doors. His oldest son, Steve, carefully keyed the lists into his smartphone so he would have the information with him when he shopped for groceries. With the dietitian's advice about organizing his kitchen, Bill was finding it less stressful to cook, and he found he had fewer headaches after preparing a meal. The recipes included on the meal plan turned out to be tasty and added some new flavors and foods to the family's usual diet.

There were days when Bill slipped up and ate foods from the high-histamine list, but he was finding that if he had been eating low-histamine foods for the rest of the day, and if his other triggers were low or absent, his headaches were much, much better. In the final week of his program, Bill checked his journal to find that he'd had one headache in the previous week and that the headache had lasted for 2 hours; taking over-the-counter medication had been enough to quiet his head. Bill continued on with the diet. At the end of 3 months, he found that while he'd had occasional slip-ups, if he was careful to stay on a scheduled meal plan and drink lots of fluids, having some high-histamine foods didn't always mean headaches. A lot of other histamine intolerance symptoms were also better. Although the 3 months had been hard work, and many days he had been grumpy, it was worth it. What was more, his family had stuck through it with him and hadn't minded the little changes to favorite family recipes he had made. Bill knew he would need the support of his family to stick with this new lifestyle.

M eal planning can be addictive, and looking for new low-histamine recipes or sharing recipes with friends and family that have worked for you can be satisfying — and even fun. Before preparing the delicious and nutritious recipes provided in Part 4 of this book, work up to the following 28-day menu plan. These daily plans ensure your meals will have a solid nutritional foundation, meet food guide standards for good health and provide low-histamine foods. After you become more accustomed to the foods that have low levels of histamine, you can make up your own menus and adapt your shopping list accordingly.

Plan Ahead

It will help if you keep several menus with simple, easy-to-prepare recipes posted on your pantry or refrigerator door. Have all needed ingredients close at hand in the pantry or freezer for a quick option for you or someone else (if you are out of commission with a headache). When you have headache-free days, cook extra food and freeze it right away. Then if you have a headache or headache hangover day, you will have nutritious food ready to go. In addition, if you do as much food preparation as you can on a headache-free day, you will have a head start and reduce your stress load.

Good Nutrition

Each menu has been designed to meet the energy requirements for women (1800 calories) and men (2300 calories). They were chosen to help women and men maintain their current weight. Consult a dietitian if you are interested in losing weight. Calculating how to reduce calories without sacrificing nutrition is a job for a professional.

These meal plans feature low-histamine food recipes. Some recipes are included to help you learn how to adapt family favorites to low-histamine options. Snacks are included for every day. Remember to make a schedule you can live with. The value of keeping regular mealtimes can't be stressed enough.

Good Cheer

The recipes chosen for the meal plans help us remember that choosing the foods we eat and preparing them for ourselves and for those we love fuels our bodies but also feeds our souls. Shopping for and preparing food, as well as the sights and smells from cooking meals, should be an ongoing source of pleasure.

Be proud of your ability to make nourishing yourself a priority!

4-Week Menu Plan

Calories per day for women: 1800
Calories per day for men: 2300
For recipes from the book, the typical serving size is 1 serving for women and 2 servings for men, unless otherwise noted.

Meal	Menu Plan for Women	Menu Plan for Men
Day 1: Monday		
Breakfast	1 Quinoa Crêpe (page 185) with 1 tbsp (15 mL) honey or maple syrup 1 serving of fresh fruit or $\frac{1}{2}$ cup (125 mL) 100% juice 1 cup (250 mL) milk or milk alternative Herbal tea or decaf coffee	2 Quinoa Crêpes (page 185) with 2 tbsp (30 mL) honey or maple syrup 1 serving of fresh fruit or $\frac{1}{2}$ cup (125 mL) 100% juice $\frac{1}{2}$ cup (125 mL) milk or milk alternative Herbal tea or decaf coffee
Morning Snack	1 Honey Whole Wheat Muffin (page 201) with 1 tsp (5 mL) butter or 1 tbsp (15 mL) jam	2 Honey Whole Wheat Muffins (page 201) with 2 tsp (10 mL) butter or 2 tbsp (30 mL) jam
Lunch	Red and Yellow Bell Pepper Soup (page 225) $2\frac{1}{2}$ oz (75 g) mild cheese 2 gluten-free crackers 1 cup (250 mL) milk or milk alternative	Red and Yellow Bell Pepper Soup (page 225) $2\frac{1}{2}$ oz (75 g) mild cheese 4 gluten-free crackers 1 cup (250 mL) milk or milk alternative
Afternoon Snack	$\frac{1}{2}$ cup (125 mL) yogurt with $\frac{1}{2}$ cup (125 mL) grapes	1 cup (250 mL) yogurt with 1 cup (250 mL) grapes
Dinner	Veal Meatloaf (page 284) Cool Cucumber Salad (page 240) $\frac{1}{2}$ cup (125 mL) cooked brown rice $\frac{1}{2}$ cup (125 mL) mashed baked butternut squash 1 cup (250 mL) milk or milk alternative	Veal Meatloaf (page 284) Cool Cucumber Salad (page 240) 1 cup (250 mL) cooked brown rice 1 cup (250 mL) mashed baked butternut squash 1 cup (250 mL) milk or milk alternative
Evening Snack	$\frac{1}{2}$ cup (125 mL) sliced cantaloupe	1 cup (250 mL) sliced cantaloupe
Day 2: Tuesday		
Breakfast	1 slice Old-Fashioned Cornbread (page 196) 1 boiled egg 1 serving of fresh fruit or $\frac{1}{2}$ cup (125 mL) 100% juice 1 cup (250 mL) milk or milk alternative Herbal tea or decaf coffee	2 slices Old-Fashioned Cornbread (page 196) 1 boiled egg 1 serving of fresh fruit or $\frac{1}{2}$ cup (125 mL) 100% juice $\frac{1}{2}$ cup (125 mL) milk or milk alternative Herbal tea or decaf coffee
Morning Snack	1 medium apple	1 medium apple
Lunch	1 roast beef sandwich made with 2 slices Brown Sandwich Bread (page 190), $2\frac{1}{2}$ oz (75 g) roast beef and 1 tbsp (15 mL) butter $\frac{1}{2}$ cup (125 mL) zucchini and carrot spears $\frac{1}{2}$ cup (125 mL) apple juice	1 roast beef sandwich made with 2 slices Brown Sandwich Bread (page 190), $2\frac{1}{2}$ oz (75 g) roast beef and 1 tbsp (15 mL) butter 1 cup (250 mL) zucchini and carrot spears $\frac{1}{2}$ cup (125 mL) apple juice
Afternoon Snack	5 rice crackers 1 cup (250 mL) low-fat cottage cheese	10 rice crackers 1 cup (250 mL) low-fat cottage cheese
Dinner	Fish Fillets with Corn and Red Pepper Salsa (page 253) Greens and Grains Gratin (page 266) $\frac{1}{2}$ cup (125 mL) steamed green beans 1 cup (250 mL) milk or milk alternative	Fish Fillets with Corn and Red Pepper Salsa (page 253) Greens and Grains Gratin (page 266) 1 cup (250 mL) steamed green beans 1 cup (250 mL) milk or milk alternative

Meal	Menu Plan for Women	Menu Plan for Men
Evening Snack	1 Oatmeal Raisin Cookie (page 310)	2 Oatmeal Raisin Cookies (page 310)
Day 3: Wednesday		
Breakfast	1 poached egg 1 slice toasted Multigrain Sandwich Bread (page 191) with 1 tsp (5 mL) butter and 1 tbsp (15 mL) jam or honey 1 serving of fresh fruit or ½ cup (125 mL) 100% juice ½ cup (125 mL) milk or milk alternative Herbal tea or decaf coffee	1 poached egg 2 slices toasted Multigrain Sandwich Bread (page 191) with 2 tsp (10 mL) butter and 2 tbsp (30 mL) jam or honey 1 serving of fresh fruit or ½ cup (125 mL) 100% juice ½ cup (125 mL) milk or milk alternative Herbal tea or decaf coffee
Morning Snack	¼ cup (60 mL) yogurt cheese 2 gluten-free crackers	¼ cup (60 mL) yogurt cheese 4 gluten-free crackers
Lunch	1 Crêpe (page 184) with ½ cup (125 mL) sliced mango and 1 tbsp (15 mL) cream cheese Cabbage and Carrot Slaw (page 238) ½ cup (125 mL) pear juice 1 cup (250 mL) milk or milk alternative	2 Crêpes (page 184) with 1 cup (250 mL) sliced mango and 2 tbsp (30 mL) cream cheese Cabbage and Carrot Slaw (page 238) ½ cup (125 mL) pear juice 1 cup (250 mL) milk or milk alternative
Afternoon Snack	1 medium apple	1 medium apple
Dinner	Oven-Baked Beef Stew (page 281) 1 Quinoa Popover (page 199) with 1 tsp (5 mL) butter Quick Sautéed Kale (page 292) 1 cup (250 mL) milk or milk alternative	Oven-Baked Beef Stew (page 281) 2 Quinoa Popovers (page 199) with 2 tsp (10 mL) butter Quick Sautéed Kale (page 292) 1 cup (250 mL) milk or milk alternative
Evening Snack	½ cup (125 mL) yogurt with ½ cup (125 mL) blueberries	1 cup (250 mL) yogurt with 1 cup (250 mL) blueberries
Day 4: Thursday		
Breakfast	Not Your Same Old Oats (page 177) 1 slice toasted Multigrain Sandwich Bread (page 191) with 1 tsp (5 mL) butter 1 serving of fresh fruit or ½ cup (125 mL) 100% juice ½ cup (125 mL) low-fat cottage cheese Herbal tea or decaf coffee	Not Your Same Old Oats (page 177) 2 slices toasted Multigrain Sandwich Bread (page 191) with 2 tsp (10 mL) butter 1 serving of fresh fruit or ½ cup (125 mL) 100% juice 1 cup (250 mL) low-fat cottage cheese Herbal tea or decaf coffee
Morning Snack	1 Chewy Coconut Quinoa Bar (page 210)	2 Chewy Coconut Quinoa Bars (page 210)
Lunch	Pasta with Roasted Vegetables and Goat Cheese (page 267) ½ cup (125 mL) salad greens tossed with 1 tbsp (15 mL) Lemon Vinaigrette (page 249) ½ cup (125 mL) apple juice 1 cup (250 mL) milk or milk alternative	Pasta with Roasted Vegetables and Goat Cheese (page 267) 1 cup (250 mL) salad greens tossed with 2 tbsp (30 mL) Lemon Vinaigrette (page 249) ½ cup (125 mL) apple juice 1 cup (250 mL) milk or milk alternative
Afternoon Snack	Sweet Potato Chips (page 211)	Sweet Potato Chips (page 211)
Dinner	Just-for-Kids Honey Lemon Chicken (page 274) 5 spears steamed asparagus* ½ cup (125 mL) steamed sliced beets 1 cup (250 mL) milk or milk alternative	Just-for-Kids Honey Lemon Chicken (page 274) 10 spears steamed asparagus* 1 cup (250 mL) steamed sliced beets 1 cup (250 mL) milk or milk alternative
Evening Snack	Rhubarb Bread Pudding (page 318)	Rhubarb Bread Pudding (page 318)

*Warning: Asparagus is high in folate, which can increase histamine levels. Include asparagus in small amounts on days when your other headache triggers are low.

Meal	Menu Plan for Women	Menu Plan for Men
Day 5: Friday		
Breakfast	Toasted Quinoa Porridge (page 178) with 1 tbsp (15 mL) honey or maple syrup or 1 tsp (5 mL) butter 1 serving of fresh fruit or ½ cup (125 mL) 100% juice 1 cup (250 mL) milk or milk alternative Herbal tea or decaf coffee	Toasted Quinoa Porridge (page 178) with 1 tbsp (15 mL) honey or maple syrup or 1 tsp (5 mL) butter 1 serving of fresh fruit or ½ cup (125 mL) 100% juice 1 cup (250 mL) milk or milk alternative Herbal tea or decaf coffee
Morning Snack	1 medium pear	1 medium pear
Lunch	Sweet Potato Omelet (page 181) ½ cup (125 mL) celery sticks ½ cup (125 mL) apple juice	Sweet Potato Omelet (page 181) 1 cup (250 mL) celery sticks ½ cup (125 mL) apple juice
Afternoon Snack	1 Scottish Oat Cake (page 200)	1 Scottish Oat Cake (page 200)
Dinner	Broiled Rosemary Thighs (page 278) Quinoa Spaghetti with Kale (page 269) Braised Baby Bok Choy (page 286) ½ cup (125 mL) raw baby carrots 1 cup (250 mL) milk or milk alternative	Broiled Rosemary Thighs (page 278) Quinoa Spaghetti with Kale (page 269) Braised Baby Bok Choy (page 286) 1 cup (250 mL) raw baby carrots 1 cup (250 mL) milk or milk alternative
Evening Snack	5 rice crackers 2 tbsp (30 mL) cream cheese	10 rice crackers 3 tbsp (45 mL) cream cheese
Day 6: Saturday		
Breakfast	1 poached egg 1 slice toasted Multigrain Sandwich Bread (page 191) with 1 tsp (5 mL) butter and 1 tbsp (15 mL) jam or honey 1 serving of fresh fruit or ½ cup (125 mL) 100% juice 1 cup (250 mL) milk or milk alternative Herbal tea or decaf coffee	1 poached egg 2 slices toasted Multigrain Sandwich Bread (page 191) with 2 tsp (10 mL) butter and 1 tbsp (15 mL) jam or honey 1 serving of fresh fruit or ½ cup (125 mL) 100% juice 1 cup (250 mL) milk or milk alternative Herbal tea or decaf coffee
Morning Snack	½ cup (125 mL) cooked chopped rhubarb with 1 tbsp (15 mL) maple syrup	1 cup (250 mL) cooked chopped rhubarb with 1 tbsp (15 mL) maple syrup
Lunch	1 grilled cheese sandwich made with 2 slices Brown Sandwich Bread (page 190) and 2½ oz (75 g) mozzarella cheese Braised Green Beans and Fennel (page 291) ½ cup (125 mL) mango juice	1 grilled cheese sandwich made with 2 slices Brown Sandwich Bread (page 190) and 2½ oz (75 g) mozzarella cheese Braised Green Beans and Fennel (page 291) ½ cup (125 mL) mango juice
Afternoon Snack	Quinoa Crunch (page 176) ½ cup (125 mL) milk or milk alternative	Quinoa Crunch (page 176) 1 cup (250 mL) milk or milk alternative
Dinner	Spanish Vegetable Paella (page 264) ½ cup (125 mL) salad greens tossed with 1 tbsp Lemon Vinaigrette (page 249) 1 cup (250 mL) milk or milk alternative	Spanish Vegetable Paella (page 264) 1 cup (250 mL) salad greens tossed with 2 tbsp Lemon Vinaigrette (page 249) ½ cup (125 mL) milk or milk alternative
Evening Snack	½ cup (125 mL) gluten-free ice cream	1 cup (250 mL) gluten-free ice cream
Day 7: Sunday		
Breakfast	2 Oatmeal Pancakes (page 186) with 1 tbsp (15 mL) honey or maple syrup 1 serving of fresh fruit or ½ cup (125 mL) 100% juice ½ cup (125 mL) milk or milk alternative Herbal tea or decaf coffee	3 Oatmeal Pancakes (page 186) with 2 tbsp (30 mL) honey or maple syrup 1 serving of fresh fruit or ½ cup (125 mL) 100% juice ½ cup (125 mL) milk or milk alternative Herbal tea or decaf coffee

Meal	Menu Plan for Women	Menu Plan for Men
Morning Snack	1 Sweet Potato Muffin (page 204) with 1 tsp (5 mL) butter	1 Sweet Potato Muffin (page 204) with 1 tsp (5 mL) butter
Lunch	Chilled Melon Soup with Ginger and Lime (page 219) 1 Traditional Tea Biscuit (page 197) 1/2 cup (125 mL) hummus 1/2 cup (125 mL) raw vegetable cubes or spears 1 cup (250 mL) milk or milk alternative	Chilled Melon Soup with Ginger and Lime (page 219) 2 Traditional Tea Biscuits (page 197) 1 cup (250 mL) hummus 1 cup (250 mL) raw vegetable cubes or spears 1 cup (250 mL) milk or milk alternative
Afternoon Snack	1/2 cup (125 mL) cubed cantaloupe	1 cup (250 mL) cubed cantaloupe
Dinner	Bistecca alla Florentine (page 282) Southwestern Sweet Potato Salad (page 243) 1/2 cup (125 mL) braised chopped celery 1/2 cup (125 mL) steamed sliced beets 1 cup (250 mL) milk or milk alternative	Bistecca alla Florentine (page 282) Southwestern Sweet Potato Salad (page 243) 1 cup (250 mL) braised chopped celery 1 cup (250 mL) steamed sliced beets 1 cup (250 mL) milk or milk alternative
Evening Snack	Mint Yogurt Dip (page 207) 2 gluten-free crackers	Mint Yogurt Dip (page 207) 4 gluten-free crackers
Day 8: Monday		
Breakfast	1 Crispy Brown Rice Treat (page 309) 1 slice toasted Multigrain Sandwich Bread (page 191) with 1 tbsp (15 mL) jam 1 serving of fresh fruit or 1/2 cup (125 mL) 100% juice 1/2 cup (125 mL) milk or milk alternative Herbal tea or decaf coffee	1 Crispy Brown Rice Treat (page 309) 2 slices toasted Multigrain Sandwich Bread (page 191) with 2 tbsp (30 mL) jam 1 serving of fresh fruit or 1/2 cup (125 mL) 100% juice 1/2 cup (125 mL) milk or milk alternative Herbal tea or decaf coffee
Morning Snack	1/2 cup (125 mL) cottage cheese with 1/2 cup (125 mL) pear slices	1 cup (250 mL) cottage cheese with 1/2 cup (125 mL) pear slices
Lunch	1 wrap made with 1 Quinoa Tortilla (page 193), Zucchini and Chickpea Salad (page 244) and 1/4 cup (60 mL) chopped lettuce Sweet Potato Chips (page 211) 1 medium apple, sliced 1 cup (250 mL) milk or milk alternative	2 wraps made with 2 Quinoa Tortillas (page 193), Zucchini and Chickpea Salad (page 244) and 1/2 cup (125 mL) chopped lettuce Sweet Potato Chips (page 211) 1 medium apple, sliced 1 cup (250 mL) milk or milk alternative
Afternoon Snack	1/2 cup (125 mL) cubed cantaloupe	1 cup (250 mL) cubed cantaloupe
Dinner	Salmon with Roasted Vegetables (page 257) Rice, Black Bean and Red Pepper Salad (page 245) 1/2 cup (125 mL) cooked corn kernels 1/2 cup (125 mL) celery sticks 1 cup (250 mL) milk or milk alternative	Salmon with Roasted Vegetables (page 257) Rice, Black Bean and Red Pepper Salad (page 245) 1 cup (250 mL) cooked corn kernels 1 cup (250 mL) celery sticks 1 cup (250 mL) milk or milk alternative
Evening Snack	Eat Your Greens Smoothie (page 216)	Eat Your Greens Smoothie (page 216)
Day 9: Tuesday		
Breakfast	1 poached egg 1 slice toasted Multigrain Sandwich Bread (page 191) with 1 tsp (5 mL) butter 1 serving of fresh fruit or 1/2 cup (125 mL) 100% juice 1/2 cup (125 mL) milk or milk alternative Herbal tea or decaf coffee	1 poached egg 2 slices toasted Multigrain Sandwich Bread (page 191) with 2 tsp (10 mL) butter 1 serving of fresh fruit or 1/2 cup (125 mL) 100% juice 1/2 cup (125 mL) milk or milk alternative Herbal tea or decaf coffee

Meal	Menu Plan for Women	Menu Plan for Men
Morning Snack	1 medium apple	1 medium apple
Lunch	Roasted Cauliflower Soup (page 223) 2 Crêpes (page 184) with 3 tbsp (45 mL) cream cheese 1/2 cup (125 mL) carrot sticks 1 cup (250 mL) milk or milk alternative	Roasted Cauliflower Soup (page 223) 3 Crêpes (page 184) with 3 tbsp (45 mL) cream cheese 1 cup (250 mL) carrot sticks 1 cup (250 mL) milk or milk alternative
Afternoon Snack	1/2 cup (125 mL) mango juice	1/2 cup (125 mL) mango juice
Dinner	Pasta with Roasted Vegetables and Goat Cheese (page 267) Braised Baby Bok Choy (page 286) 1 cup (250 mL) milk or milk alternative	Pasta with Roasted Vegetables and Goat Cheese (page 267) Braised Baby Bok Choy (page 286) 1 cup (250 mL) milk or milk alternative
Evening Snack	1 slice Old-Fashioned Cornbread (page 196)	1 slice Old-Fashioned Cornbread (page 196)
Day 10: Wednesday		
Breakfast	Crustless Zucchini Quiche (page 182) 1 slice toasted Multigrain Sandwich Bread (page 191) with 1 tsp (5 mL) butter 1 serving of fresh fruit or 1/2 cup (125 mL) 100% juice 1/2 cup (125 mL) milk or milk alternative Herbal tea or decaf coffee	Crustless Zucchini Quiche (page 182) 2 slices toasted Multigrain Sandwich Bread (page 191) with 2 tsp (10 mL) butter 1 serving of fresh fruit or 1/2 cup (125 mL) 100% juice 1/2 cup (125 mL) milk or milk alternative Herbal tea or decaf coffee
Morning Snack	5 rice crackers	10 rice crackers
Lunch	Quinoa Salad (page 247) 1/2 cup (125 mL) steamed green beans 1/2 cup (125 mL) apple juice 1 cup (250 mL) milk or milk alternative	Quinoa Salad (page 247) 1 cup (250 mL) steamed green beans 1/2 cup (125 mL) apple juice 1 cup (250 mL) milk or milk alternative
Afternoon Snack	Apple Berry Muesli (page 174)	Apple Berry Muesli (page 174)
Dinner	Rosemary Chicken Breasts with Sweet Potatoes and Onions (page 276) Shaved Beet Salad with Pistachios and Goat Cheese (page 238) 1 cup (250 mL) milk or milk alternative	Rosemary Chicken Breasts with Sweet Potatoes and Onions (page 276) Shaved Beet Salad with Pistachios and Goat Cheese (page 238) 1 cup (250 mL) milk or milk alternative
Evening Snack	1/2 cup (125 mL) yogurt with 1/2 cup (125 mL) blueberries	1 cup (250 mL) yogurt with 1 cup (250 mL) blueberries
Day 11: Thursday		
Breakfast	1 Oatmeal Pancake (page 186) with 1 tbsp (15 mL) maple syrup 2 tbsp (30 mL) ricotta cheese 1 serving of fresh fruit or 1/2 cup (125 mL) 100% juice 1 cup (250 mL) milk or milk alternative Herbal tea or decaf coffee	2 Oatmeal Pancakes (page 186) with 2 tbsp (30 mL) maple syrup 3 tbsp (45 mL) ricotta cheese 1 serving of fresh fruit or 1/2 cup (125 mL) 100% juice 1 cup (250 mL) milk or milk alternative Herbal tea or decaf coffee
Morning Snack	1/4 cup (60 mL) hummus with raw vegetable spears	1/2 cup (125 mL) hummus with raw vegetable spears
Lunch	Oven-Baked Beef Stew (page 281) 1 Traditional Tea Biscuit (page 197) 1/2 cup (125 mL) mango juice 1 cup (250 mL) milk or milk alternative	Oven-Baked Beef Stew (page 281) 1 Traditional Tea Biscuit (page 197) 1 cup (250 mL) mango juice 1 cup (250 mL) milk or milk alternative

Meal	Menu Plan for Women	Menu Plan for Men
Afternoon Snack	1/2 cup (125 mL) yogurt (optional: add 1 tsp/5 mL honey or maple syrup)	1 cup (250 mL) yogurt (optional: add 1 tsp/5 mL honey or maple syrup)
Dinner	Fish Fillets with Corn and Red Pepper Salsa (page 253) Baked Parsnip Fries (page 299) 1/2 cup (125 mL) salad greens tossed with 1 tbsp (15 mL) Cilantro Oil (page 249) 1 cup (250 mL) milk or milk alternative	Fish Fillets with Corn and Red Pepper Salsa (page 253) Baked Parsnip Fries (page 299) 1 cup (250 mL) salad greens tossed with 2 tbsp (30 mL) Cilantro Oil (page 249) 1 cup (250 mL) milk or milk alternative
Evening Snack	2 tbsp (30 mL) raw almonds	3 tbsp (45 mL) raw almonds

Day 12: Friday

Meal	Menu Plan for Women	Menu Plan for Men
Breakfast	1 poached egg 1 slice toasted Multigrain Sandwich Bread (page 191) with 1 tsp (5 mL) butter 1 serving of fresh fruit or 1/2 cup (125 mL) 100% juice 1/2 cup (125 mL) milk or milk alternative Herbal tea or decaf coffee	1 poached egg 2 slices toasted Multigrain Sandwich Bread (page 191) with 2 tsp (10 mL) butter 1 serving of fresh fruit or 1/2 cup (125 mL) 100% juice 1/2 cup (125 mL) milk or milk alternative Herbal tea or decaf coffee
Morning Snack	1 Berry Cheesecake Bar (page 308)	2 Berry Cheesecake Bars (page 308)
Lunch	Dill Carrot Soup (page 221) 1 chicken sandwich made with 2 slices Brown Sandwich Bread (page 190), 2 1/2 oz (75 g) sliced roasted chicken breast and 1/2 cup (125 mL) sliced mango 4 cucumber spears 1 cup (250 mL) milk or milk alternative	Dill Carrot Soup (page 221) 1 chicken sandwich made with 2 slices Brown Sandwich Bread (page 190), 2 1/2 oz (75 g) sliced roasted chicken breast and 1/2 cup (125 mL) sliced mango 6 cucumber spears 1 cup (250 mL) milk or milk alternative
Afternoon Snack	1 Chewy Coconut Quinoa Bar (page 210)	2 Chewy Coconut Quinoa Bars (page 210)
Dinner	Veal Meatloaf (page 284) Garlicky Cauliflower Purée (page 289) Herbed Parsnips (page 294) 1 cup (250 mL) milk or milk alternative	Veal Meatloaf (page 284) Garlicky Cauliflower Purée (page 289) Herbed Parsnips (page 294) 1 cup (250 mL) milk or milk alternative
Evening Snack	1 cup (250 mL) air-popped popcorn with 2 tbsp (30 mL) butter or preferred oil and a pinch of salt (optional: add a pinch of ground turmeric)	2 cups (500 mL) air-popped popcorn with 3 tbsp (45 mL) butter or preferred oil and a pinch of salt (optional: add a pinch of ground turmeric)

Day 13: Saturday

Meal	Menu Plan for Women	Menu Plan for Men
Breakfast	Toasted Quinoa Porridge (page 178) 2 slices toasted Multigrain Sandwich Bread (page 191) with 1 tsp (5 mL) butter 1 serving of fresh fruit or 1/2 cup (125 mL) 100% juice 1 cup (250 mL) milk or milk alternative Herbal tea or decaf coffee	Toasted Quinoa Porridge (page 178) 2 slices toasted Multigrain Sandwich Bread (page 191) with 2 tsp (10 mL) butter 1 serving of fresh fruit or 1/2 cup (125 mL) 100% juice 1 cup (250 mL) milk or milk alternative Herbal tea or decaf coffee
Morning Snack	1 Blueberry Yogurt Pop (page 321)	1 Blueberry Yogurt Pop (page 321)
Lunch	Zucchini Frittata (page 262) 1/2 cup (125 mL) salad greens tossed with 1 tbsp (15 mL) Lemon Vinaigrette (page 249) 1/2 cup (125 mL) apple juice 1 cup (250 mL) milk or milk alternative	Zucchini Frittata (page 262) 1 cup (250 mL) salad greens tossed with 2 tbsp (30 mL) Lemon Vinaigrette (page 249) 1/2 cup (125 mL) apple juice 1 cup (250 mL) milk or milk alternative
Afternoon Snack	1/2 cup (125 mL) cubed mango	1 cup (250 mL) cubed mango

Meal	Menu Plan for Women	Menu Plan for Men
Dinner	Simple Grilled Fish (page 252) Winter Squash Quinoa Bisque (page 228) $\frac{1}{2}$ cup (125 mL) steamed green beans $\frac{1}{2}$ cup (125 mL) milk or milk alternative	Simple Grilled Fish (page 252) Winter Squash Quinoa Bisque (page 228) 1 cup (250 mL) steamed green beans $\frac{1}{2}$ cup (125 mL) milk or milk alternative
Evening Snack	1 Baked Granola Apple (page 312)	1 Baked Granola Apple (page 312) 2 tbsp (30 mL) cream cheese
Day 14: Sunday		
Breakfast	Best-Ever Scrambled Eggs (page 179) 1 Summer Corn and Quinoa Griddle Cake (page 209) 1 serving of fresh fruit or $\frac{1}{2}$ cup (125 mL) 100% juice Herbal tea or decaf coffee	Best-Ever Scrambled Eggs (page 179) 2 Summer Corn and Quinoa Griddle Cakes (page 209) 1 serving of fresh fruit or $\frac{1}{2}$ cup (125 mL) 100% juice Herbal tea or decaf coffee
Morning Snack	$\frac{1}{2}$ cup (125 mL) sliced pear, apple and cantaloupe 1 cup (250 mL) milk or milk alternative	1 cup (250 mL) sliced pear, apple and cantaloupe 1 cup (250 mL) milk or milk alternative
Lunch	Roasted Cauliflower Soup (page 223) $2\frac{1}{2}$ oz (75 g) grilled beef strips on 1 Quinoa Anzac Biscuit (page 198) $\frac{1}{2}$ cup (125 mL) carrot sticks 1 cup (250 mL) milk or milk alternative	Roasted Cauliflower Soup (page 223) $2\frac{1}{2}$ oz (75 g) grilled beef strips on 1 Quinoa Anzac Biscuit (page 198) $\frac{1}{2}$ cup (125 mL) carrot sticks 1 cup (250 mL) milk or milk alternative
Afternoon Snack	$\frac{1}{2}$ cup (125 mL) yogurt with $\frac{1}{2}$ cup (125 mL) blackberries	1 cup (250 mL) yogurt with $\frac{1}{2}$ cup (125 mL) blackberries
Dinner	Chicken and Vegetable Stew (page 280) Zucchini and Chickpea Salad (page 244) Date Cake with Coconut Topping (page 307) 1 cup (250 mL) milk or milk alternative	Chicken and Vegetable Stew (page 280) Zucchini and Chickpea Salad (page 244) Date Cake with Coconut Topping (page 307) 1 cup (250 mL) milk or milk alternative
Evening Snack	1 Millet and Flax Muffin (page 202)	2 Millet and Flax Muffins (page 202) 3 tbsp (45 mL) cream cheese
Day 15: Monday		
Breakfast	1 Sweet Potato and Quinoa Breakfast Tortilla (page 183) 1 serving of fresh fruit or $\frac{1}{2}$ cup (125 mL) 100% juice $\frac{1}{2}$ cup (125 mL) milk or milk alternative Herbal tea or decaf coffee	2 Sweet Potato and Quinoa Breakfast Tortillas (page 183) 1 serving of fresh fruit or $\frac{1}{2}$ cup (125 mL) 100% juice $\frac{1}{2}$ cup (125 mL) milk or milk alternative Herbal tea or decaf coffee
Morning Snack	Lemon Pudding (page 316)	Lemon Pudding (page 316)
Lunch	Dill Carrot Soup (page 221) $\frac{1}{2}$ cup (125 mL) salad greens tossed with 1 tbsp (15 mL) Cilantro Oil (page 249) 4 celery sticks 2 gluten-free crackers 1 cup (250 mL) milk or milk alternative	Dill Carrot Soup (page 221) 1 cup (250 mL) salad greens tossed with 2 tbsp (30 mL) Cilantro Oil (page 249) 6 celery sticks 4 gluten-free crackers 1 cup (250 mL) milk or milk alternative
Afternoon Snack	2 tbsp (30 mL) raw hazelnuts	3 tbsp (45 mL) raw hazelnuts
Dinner	Veal Braised with Onions (page 283) 1 cup (250 mL) cooked rice noodles $\frac{1}{2}$ cup (125 mL) cooked corn kernels $\frac{1}{2}$ cup (125 mL) steamed cubed zucchini 1 cup (250 mL) milk or milk alternative	Veal Braised with Onions (page 283) 1 cup (250 mL) cooked rice noodles 1 cup (250 mL) cooked corn kernels 1 cup (250 mL) steamed cubed zucchini 1 cup (250 mL) milk or milk alternative

Meal	Menu Plan for Women	Menu Plan for Men
Evening Snack	1 slice Old-Fashioned Cornbread (page 196) (optional: spread with 1 tbsp/15 mL maple syrup)	1 slice Old-Fashioned Cornbread (page 196) (optional: spread with 1 tbsp/15 mL maple syrup) 1 oz (30 g) mild cheese

Day 16: Tuesday

Meal	Menu Plan for Women	Menu Plan for Men
Breakfast	Easy Eggs (page 178) 1 slice toasted Brown Sandwich Bread (page 190) with 1 tsp (5 mL) butter 1 serving of fresh fruit or 1/2 cup (125 mL) 100% juice 1/2 cup (125 mL) milk or milk alternative Herbal tea or decaf coffee	Easy Eggs (page 178) 2 slices toasted Brown Sandwich Bread (page 190) with 2 tsp (10 mL) butter 1 serving of fresh fruit or 1/2 cup (125 mL) 100% juice 1/2 cup (125 mL) milk or milk alternative Herbal tea or decaf coffee
Morning Snack	1/2 cup (125 mL) yogurt with 1/2 cup (125 mL) blackberries	1 cup (250 mL) yogurt with 1 cup (250 mL) blackberries
Lunch	Greens and Grains Gratin (page 266) Bulgur Pilaf (page 302) 4 celery sticks 1/2 cup (125 mL) pear juice 1 cup (250 mL) milk or milk alternative	Greens and Grains Gratin (page 266) Bulgur Pilaf (page 302) 6 celery sticks 1/2 cup (125 mL) pear juice 1 cup (250 mL) milk or milk alternative
Afternoon Snack	1 Berry Cheesecake Bar (page 308)	2 Berry Cheesecake Bars (page 308)
Dinner	Halibut with Coconut Lime Sauce (page 255) Sweet Potato Chips (page 211) 1/2 cup (125 mL) steamed peas 1/2 cup (125 mL) steamed carrot coins 1 cup (250 mL) milk or milk alternative	Halibut with Coconut Lime Sauce (page 255) Sweet Potato Chips (page 211) 1 cup (250 mL) steamed peas 1 cup (250 mL) steamed carrot coins 1 cup (250 mL) milk or milk alternative
Evening Snack	6 Oven-Dried Apple Slices (page 212) 1/4 cup (60 mL) Mint Yogurt Dip (page 207)	12 Oven-Dried Apple Slices (page 212) 1/2 cup (125 mL) Mint Yogurt Dip (page 207)

Day 17: Wednesday

Meal	Menu Plan for Women	Menu Plan for Men
Breakfast	Not Your Same Old Oats (page 177) 1 Millet and Flax Muffin (page 202) 1 serving of fresh fruit or 1/2 cup (125 mL) 100% juice 1/2 cup (125 mL) milk or milk alternative Herbal tea or decaf coffee	Not Your Same Old Oats (page 177) 2 Millet and Flax Muffins (page 202) 1 serving of fresh fruit or 1/2 cup (125 mL) 100% juice 1/2 cup (125 mL) milk or milk alternative Herbal tea or decaf coffee
Morning Snack	Iron-Builder Juice (page 216)	Iron-Builder Juice (page 216)
Lunch	Zucchini Stuffed with Rice and Mushrooms (page 263) 1/2 cup (125 mL) salad greens tossed with 1 tbsp (15 mL) Cilantro Oil (page 249) 1/4 cup (60 mL) Quick Roasted Red Pepper Dip (page 206) 5 rice crackers 1 cup (250 mL) Blueberry Lemon Elixir (page 214)	Zucchini Stuffed with Rice and Mushrooms (page 263) 1 cup (250 mL) salad greens tossed with 2 tbsp (30 mL) Cilantro Oil (page 249) 1/2 cup (125 mL) Quick Roasted Red Pepper Dip (page 206) 10 rice crackers 1 cup (250 mL) Blueberry Lemon Elixir (page 214)
Afternoon Snack	1/4 cup (60 mL) Coconut Quinoa Oat Granola (page 175) 1 cup (250 mL) milk or milk alternative	1/2 cup (125 mL) Coconut Quinoa Oat Granola (page 175) 1 cup (250 mL) milk or milk alternative
Dinner	Lemon-Thyme Roast Chicken (page 272) Braised Baby Bok Choy (page 286) 1 medium baked potato 1/2 cup (125 mL) mashed baked acorn squash 1 cup (250 mL) milk or milk alternative	Lemon-Thyme Roast Chicken (page 272) Braised Baby Bok Choy (page 286) 1 medium baked potato 1 cup (250 mL) mashed baked acorn squash 1 cup (250 mL) milk or milk alternative

Meal	Menu Plan for Women	Menu Plan for Men
Evening Snack	1 Scottish Oat Cake (page 200)	2 Scottish Oat Cakes (page 200)
Day 18: Thursday		

Breakfast	1 Crispy Brown Rice Treat (page 309)
	1 slice toasted Brown Sandwich Bread
	  (page 190) with 1 tsp (5 mL) butter
	1 serving of fresh fruit or ½ cup (125 mL)
	  100% juice
	½ cup (125 mL) milk or milk alternative
	Herbal tea or decaf coffee
		2 Crispy Brown Rice Treats (page 309)
		2 slices toasted Brown Sandwich Bread
		  (page 190) with 2 tsp (10 mL) butter
		1 serving of fresh fruit or ½ cup (125 mL)
		  100% juice
		½ cup (125 mL) milk or milk alternative
		Herbal tea or decaf coffee

Morning Snack	1 Baked Granola Apple (page 312)	1 Baked Granola Apple (page 312)
Lunch	Gingered Carrot and Quinoa Salad (page 239) 1 slice Old-Fashioned Cornbread (page 196) ½ cup (125 mL) apple juice 1 cup (250 mL) milk or milk alternative	Gingered Carrot and Quinoa Salad (page 239) 2 slices Old-Fashioned Cornbread (page 196) ½ cup (125 mL) apple juice 1 cup (250 mL) milk or milk alternative
Afternoon Snack	1 pear	1 pear

Dinner	Oven-Baked Beef Stew (page 281)
	Mashed Sweet Potatoes with Rosemary
	  (page 298)
	Cool Cucumber Salad (page 240)
	1 cup (250 mL) milk or milk alternative
		Oven-Baked Beef Stew (page 281)
		Mashed Sweet Potatoes with Rosemary
		  (page 298)
		Cool Cucumber Salad (page 240)
		1 cup (250 mL) milk or milk alternative

Evening Snack	Cold Maple Mousse (page 315)	Cold Maple Mousse (page 315)
Day 19: Friday		

Breakfast	1 Easy Breakfast Cookie (page 188)
	1 boiled egg
	1 serving of fresh fruit or ½ cup (125 mL)
	  100% juice
	½ cup (125 mL) milk or milk alternative
	Herbal tea or decaf coffee
		2 Easy Breakfast Cookies (page 188)
		1 boiled egg
		1 serving of fresh fruit or ½ cup (125 mL)
		  100% juice
		½ cup (125 mL) milk or milk alternative
		Herbal tea or decaf coffee

Morning Snack	Mango Lassi (page 215)	Mango Lassi (page 215)

Lunch	Chickpea Soup (page 233)
	1 Chapati (page 194)
	½ cup (125 mL) ricotta cheese
	¼ cup (60 mL) Quick Roasted Red Pepper Dip
	  (page 206)
	6 carrot and/or celery sticks
	1 cup (250 mL) milk or milk alternative
		Chickpea Soup (page 233)
		2 Chapati (page 194)
		1 cup (250 mL) ricotta cheese
		½ cup (125 mL) Quick Roasted Red Pepper Dip
		  (page 206)
		8 carrot and/or celery sticks
		1 cup (250 mL) milk or milk alternative

Afternoon Snack	1 Millet and Flax Muffin (page 202)	1 Millet and Flax Muffin (page 202)

Dinner	Red Pepper and Goat Cheese Pizza (page 270)
	  made with Quinoa Pizza Dough (page 195)
	Grilled Vegetable Salad (page 242)
	1 cup (250 mL) milk or milk alternative
		Red Pepper and Goat Cheese Pizza (page 270)
		  made with Quinoa Pizza Dough (page 195)
		Grilled Vegetable Salad (page 242)
		1 cup (250 mL) milk or milk alternative

Evening Snack	Sweet Potato Chips (page 211) with 1 tbsp
	  (15 mL) Mint Yogurt Dip (page 207)
		Sweet Potato Chips (page 211) with 3 tbsp
		  (45 mL) Mint Yogurt Dip (page 207)

Meal	Menu Plan for Women	Menu Plan for Men
Day 20: Saturday		

Breakfast	Crustless Zucchini Quiche (page 182)
	6 Oven-Dried Apple Slices (page 212)
	1 serving of fresh fruit or ½ cup (125 mL)
	  100% juice
	½ cup (125 mL) milk or milk alternative
	Herbal tea or decaf coffee
		Crustless Zucchini Quiche (page 182)
		12 Oven-Dried Apple Slices (page 212)
		1 serving of fresh fruit or ½ cup (125 mL)
		  100% juice
		½ cup (125 mL) milk or milk alternative
		Herbal tea or decaf coffee

Morning Snack	1 Oatmeal Raisin Cookie (page 310)	2 Oatmeal Raisin Cookies (page 310)
Lunch	Kasha with Summer Vegetables (page 265) 2 oz (60 g) farmer's cheese Agua de Manzana (Apple Water) (page 213) 1 cup (250 mL) milk or milk alternative	Kasha with Summer Vegetables (page 265) 2 oz (60 g) farmer's cheese Agua de Manzana (Apple Water) (page 213) 1 cup (250 mL) milk or milk alternative
Afternoon Snack	4 pear and/or melon slices	6 pear and/or melon slices

Dinner	Pepper-Stuffed Chicken with Cantaloupe Sauce
	  (page 275)
	Quick Sautéed Kale (page 292)
	Gingered Carrot and Quinoa Salad (page 239)
	½ cup (125 mL) steamed cauliflower
	1 cup (250 mL) milk or milk alternative
		Pepper-Stuffed Chicken with Cantaloupe Sauce
		  (page 275)
		Quick Sautéed Kale (page 292)
		Gingered Carrot and Quinoa Salad (page 239)
		1 cup (250 mL) steamed cauliflower
		1 cup (250 mL) milk or milk alternative

Evening Snack	½ cup (125 mL) gluten-free ice cream	1 cup (250 mL) gluten-free ice cream
Day 21: Sunday		

Breakfast	1 Crêpe (page 184) with 1 tbsp (15 mL)
	  maple syrup
	2 tbsp (30 mL) ricotta cheese
	1 serving of fresh fruit or ½ cup (125 mL)
	  100% juice
	½ cup (125 mL) milk or milk alternative
	Herbal tea or decaf coffee
		2 Crêpes (page 184) with 2 tbsp (30 mL)
		  maple syrup
		3 tbsp (45 mL) ricotta cheese
		1 serving of fresh fruit or ½ cup (125 mL)
		  100% juice
		½ cup (125 mL) milk or milk alternative
		Herbal tea or decaf coffee

Morning Snack	½ cup (125 mL) yogurt with ½ cup (125 mL)
	  grapes
		1 cup (250 mL) yogurt with 1 cup (250 mL)
		  grapes

Lunch	Quinoa and Black Bean Salad (page 246) 1 Traditional Tea Biscuit (page 197) Cool Cucumber Salad (page 240) 1 cup (250 mL) milk or milk alternative	Quinoa and Black Bean Salad (page 246) 2 Traditional Tea Biscuits (page 197) Cool Cucumber Salad (page 240) 1 cup (250 mL) milk or milk alternative
Afternoon Snack	1 medium apple	1 medium apple

Dinner	2½ oz (75 g) roasted beef
	Baked Parsnip Fries (page 299)
	½ cup (125 mL) salad greens and sliced
	  cucumber tossed with a splash of olive oil and
	  lemon juice
	Rhubarb Bread Pudding (page 318)
	1 cup (250 mL) milk or milk alternative
		3½ oz (105 g) roasted beef
		Baked Parsnip Fries (page 299)
		1 cup (250 mL) salad greens and sliced
		  cucumber tossed with a splash of olive oil
		  and lemon juice
		Rhubarb Bread Pudding (page 318)
		1 cup (250 mL) milk or milk alternative

Evening Snack	1 Lemon Almond Biscotti (page 311) ¼ cup (60 mL) Mint Yogurt Dip (page 207)	1 Lemon Almond Biscotti (page 311) ½ cup (125 mL) Mint Yogurt Dip (page 207)

Meal	Menu Plan for Women	Menu Plan for Men
Day 22: Monday		
Breakfast	1 Honey Whole Wheat Muffin (page 201) 1 tbsp (15 mL) cream cheese 1 serving of fresh fruit or ½ cup (125 mL) 100% juice ½ cup (125 mL) milk or milk alternative Herbal tea or decaf coffee	2 Honey Whole Wheat Muffins (page 201) 3 tbsp (45 mL) cream cheese 1 serving of fresh fruit or ½ cup (125 mL) 100% juice ½ cup (125 mL) milk or milk alternative Herbal tea or decaf coffee
Morning Snack	Quick Roasted Red Pepper Dip (page 206) 1 Crispy Brown Rice Treat (page 309)	Quick Roasted Red Pepper Dip (page 206) 1 Crispy Brown Rice Treat (page 309)
Lunch	Capellini with Watercress, Carrots and Almonds (page 268) 4 zucchini spears 1 cup (250 mL) low-fat cottage cheese ½ cup (125 mL) grape juice	Capellini with Watercress, Carrots and Almonds (page 268) 6 zucchini spears 1 cup (250 mL) low-fat cottage cheese ½ cup (125 mL) grape juice
Afternoon Snack	Fresh Fruit Tart (page 305)	Fresh Fruit Tart (page 305)
Dinner	One-Hour Roast Chicken with Sage and Garlic (page 273) Mashed Sweet Potatoes with Rosemary (page 298) ½ cup (125 mL) steamed green beans ½ cup (125 mL) steamed carrot coins 1 cup (250 mL) milk or milk alternative	One-Hour Roast Chicken with Sage and Garlic (page 273) Mashed Sweet Potatoes with Rosemary (page 298) 1 cup (250 mL) steamed green beans 1 cup (250 mL) steamed carrot coins 1 cup (250 mL) milk or milk alternative
Evening Snack	Ricotta Cheese with Pear (page 305)	Ricotta Cheese with Pear (page 305)
Day 23: Tuesday		
Breakfast	Apple Berry Muesli (page 174) 1 serving of fresh fruit or ½ cup (125 mL) 100% juice ½ cup (125 mL) milk or milk alternative Herbal tea or decaf coffee	Apple Berry Muesli (page 174) 1 serving of fresh fruit or ½ cup (125 mL) 100% juice ½ cup (125 mL) milk or milk alternative Herbal tea or decaf coffee
Morning Snack	2 dates	4 dates
Lunch	Harvest Vegetable Barley Soup (page 230) 1 Blueberry Lemon Cornmeal Muffin (page 203) 2 oz (60 g) mild cheese ½ cup (125 mL) salad greens tossed with 1 tbsp (15 mL) Cilantro Oil (page 249) 1 cup (250 mL) milk or milk alternative	Harvest Vegetable Barley Soup (page 230) 1 Blueberry Lemon Cornmeal Muffin (page 203) 2 oz (60 g) mild cheese 1 cup (250 mL) salad greens tossed with 2 tbsp (30 mL) Cilantro Oil (page 249) 1 cup (250 mL) milk or milk alternative
Afternoon Snack	1 Oatmeal Raisin Cookie (page 310)	2 Oatmeal Raisin Cookies (page 310)
Dinner	Quinoa and Black Bean Salad (page 246) 1 Traditional Tea Biscuit (page 197) Braised Baby Bok Choy (page 286) 1 cup (250 mL) milk or milk alternative	Quinoa and Black Bean Salad (page 246) 2 Traditional Tea Biscuits (page 197) Braised Baby Bok Choy (page 286) 1 cup (250 mL) milk or milk alternative
Evening Snack	Black Sticky Rice Pudding (page 317)	Black Sticky Rice Pudding (page 317)
Day 24: Wednesday		
Breakfast	Cheese-Baked Eggs (page 180) 1 slice toasted Brown Sandwich Bread (page 190) with 1 tsp (5 mL) butter 1 serving of fresh fruit or ½ cup (125 mL) 100% juice ½ cup (125 mL) milk or milk alternative Herbal tea or decaf coffee	Cheese-Baked Eggs (page 180) 2 slices toasted Brown Sandwich Bread (page 190) with 2 tsp (10 mL) butter 1 serving of fresh fruit or ½ cup (125 mL) 100% juice ½ cup (125 mL) milk or milk alternative Herbal tea or decaf coffee

Meal	Menu Plan for Women	Menu Plan for Men
Morning Snack	Rhubarb Bread Pudding (page 318)	Rhubarb Bread Pudding (page 318)
Lunch	Chicken Soup with Roasted Vegetables (page 232) 2 gluten-free crackers 1/2 cup (125 mL) pear juice 1 cup (250 mL) milk or milk alternative	Chicken Soup with Roasted Vegetables (page 232) 4 gluten-free crackers 1/2 cup (125 mL) pear juice 1 cup (250 mL) milk or milk alternative
Afternoon Snack	Lemon Sherbet (page 320)	Lemon Sherbet (page 320)
Dinner	Broiled Herbed Trout Fillets (page 261) Basic Brown Rice Pilaf (page 301) 1/2 cup (125 mL) steamed peas 1/2 cup (125 mL) steamed sliced beets 1 cup (250 mL) milk or milk alternative	Broiled Herbed Trout Fillets (page 261) 2 servings Basic Brown Rice Pilaf (page 301) 1 cup (250 mL) steamed peas 1 cup (250 mL) steamed sliced beets 1 cup (250 mL) milk or milk alternative
Evening Snack	1 cup (250 mL) air-popped popcorn with 2 tbsp (30 mL) butter or preferred oil and a pinch of salt (optional: add a pinch of ground turmeric)	2 cups (500 mL) air-popped popcorn with 1/4 cup (60 mL) butter or preferred oil and a pinch of salt (optional: add a pinch of ground turmeric)

Day 25: Thursday

Meal	Menu Plan for Women	Menu Plan for Men
Breakfast	Coconut Quinoa Oat Granola (page 175) 4 apple and/or pear slices 1/2 cup (125 mL) milk or milk alternative Herbal tea or decaf coffee	Coconut Quinoa Oat Granola (page 175) 6 apple and/or pear slices 1/2 cup (125 mL) milk or milk alternative Herbal tea or decaf coffee
Morning Snack	Iron-Builder Juice (page 216)	Iron-Builder Juice (page 216)
Lunch	2 1/2 oz (75 g) roasted chicken Rosemary Quinoa Focaccia (page 192) 6 cucumber and red bell pepper spears 1/2 cup (125 mL) grape juice 1 cup (250 mL) milk or milk alternative	3 1/2 oz (105 g) roasted chicken Rosemary Quinoa Focaccia (page 192) 8 cucumber and red bell pepper spears 1/2 cup (125 mL) grape juice 1 cup (250 mL) milk or milk alternative
Afternoon Snack	1/2 cup (125 mL) applesauce	1 cup (250 mL) applesauce
Dinner	Oven-Baked Beef Stew (page 281) Herbed Parsnips (page 294) 1 medium baked potato 1/2 cup (125 mL) steamed cauliflower florets 1 cup (250 mL) milk or milk alternative	Oven-Baked Beef Stew (page 281) Herbed Parsnips (page 294) 1 medium baked potato 1 cup (250 mL) steamed cauliflower florets 1 cup (250 mL) milk or milk alternative
Evening Snack	Blueberry Honey Cake (page 306)	Blueberry Honey Cake (page 306)

Day 26: Friday

Meal	Menu Plan for Women	Menu Plan for Men
Breakfast	Best-Ever Scrambled Eggs (page 179) 1 slice toasted Multigrain Sandwich Bread (page 191) with 1 tsp (5 mL) butter 1 serving of fresh fruit or 1/2 cup (125 mL) 100% juice 1/2 cup (125 mL) milk or milk alternative Herbal tea or decaf coffee	Best-Ever Scrambled Eggs (page 179) 2 slices toasted Multigrain Sandwich Bread (page 191) with 2 tsp (10 mL) butter 1 serving of fresh fruit or 1/2 cup (125 mL) 100% juice 1/2 cup (125 mL) milk or milk alternative Herbal tea or decaf coffee
Morning Snack	1 Sweet Potato Muffin (page 204) 1 oz (30 g) farmer's cheese or fresh cheese curd	2 Sweet Potato Muffins (page 204) 2 oz (60 g) farmer's cheese or fresh cheese curd
Lunch	Harvest Vegetable Barley Soup (page 230) 1 Chapati (page 194) with 1/4 cup (60 mL) hummus 1/2 cup (125 mL) salad greens tossed with a splash of olive oil and cider vinegar 1 cup (250 mL) milk or milk alternative	Harvest Vegetable Barley Soup (page 230) 2 Chapati (page 194) with 1/4 cup (60 mL) hummus 1 cup (250 mL) salad greens tossed with a splash of olive oil and cider vinegar 1 cup (250 mL) milk or milk alternative
Afternoon Snack	2 tbsp (30 mL) raw almonds	3 tbsp (45 mL) raw almonds

Meal	Menu Plan for Women	Menu Plan for Men
Dinner	Red Pepper and Goat Cheese Pizza (page 270) 1 cup (250 mL) milk or milk alternative	2 servings Red Pepper and Goat Cheese Pizza (page 270) 1 cup (250 mL) milk or milk alternative
Evening Snack	1/2 cup (125 mL) yogurt with 1/4 cup (60 mL) blueberries (optional: add 1 tbsp/15 mL maple syrup)	1 cup (250 mL) yogurt with 1/2 cup (125 mL) blueberries (optional: add 1 tbsp/15 mL maple syrup)
Day 27: Saturday		
Breakfast	1 slice Old-Fashioned Cornbread (page 196) 1 tbsp (15 mL) cream cheese 1 serving of fresh fruit or 1/2 cup (125 mL) 100% juice 1/2 cup (125 mL) milk or milk alternative Herbal tea or decaf coffee	2 slices Old-Fashioned Cornbread (page 196) 3 tbsp (45 mL) cream cheese 1 serving of fresh fruit or 1/2 cup (125 mL) 100% juice 1/2 cup (125 mL) milk or milk alternative Herbal tea or decaf coffee
Morning Snack	1/2 Veggie Sandwich (page 207)	1 Veggie Sandwich (page 207)
Lunch	1 boiled egg, sliced 1 slice Brown Sandwich Bread (page 190) spread with 1 tbsp (15 mL) Quick Roasted Red Pepper Dip (page 206) Crispy Shallots (page 211) 1/2 cup (125 mL) grape juice 1 cup (250 mL) milk or milk alternative	1 boiled egg, sliced 2 slices Brown Sandwich Bread (page 190) spread with 2 tbsp (30 mL) Quick Roasted Red Pepper Dip (page 206) Crispy Shallots (page 211) 1/2 cup (125 mL) grape juice 1 cup (250 mL) milk or milk alternative
Afternoon Snack	1 tbsp (15 mL) Date Paste (page 319) 1 medium pear	2 tbsp (30 mL) Date Paste (page 319) 1 medium pear
Dinner	Veal Braised with Onions (page 283) Garlicky Cauliflower Purée (page 289) Cabbage and Carrot Slaw (page 238) 1 cup (250 mL) milk or milk alternative	Veal Braised with Onions (page 283) Garlicky Cauliflower Purée (page 289) Cabbage and Carrot Slaw (page 238) 1 cup (250 mL) milk or milk alternative
Evening Snack	1 cup (250 mL) air-popped popcorn with 1 tbsp (15 mL) butter or preferred oil and a pinch of salt (optional: add a pinch of ground turmeric)	2 cups (500 mL) air-popped popcorn with 2 tbsp (30 mL) butter or preferred oil and a pinch of salt (optional: add a pinch of ground turmeric)
Day 28: Sunday		
Breakfast	Finnish Apple Pancake (page 187) with 1 tbsp (15 mL) maple syrup 1 serving of fresh fruit or 1/2 cup (125 mL) 100% juice 1/2 cup (125 mL) milk or milk alternative Herbal tea or decaf coffee	Finnish Apple Pancake (page 187) with 1 tbsp (15 mL) maple syrup 1 serving of fresh fruit or 1/2 cup (125 mL) 100% juice 1/2 cup (125 mL) milk or milk alternative Herbal tea or decaf coffee
Morning Snack	1 medium apple	1 medium apple
Lunch	Grilled Vegetable Salad (page 242) 1 Quinoa Anzac Biscuit (page 198) 1/2 cup (125 mL) apple juice 1 cup (250 mL) milk or milk alternative	Grilled Vegetable Salad (page 242) 2 Quinoa Anzac Biscuits (page 198) 1/2 cup (125 mL) apple juice 1 cup (250 mL) milk or milk alternative
Afternoon Snack	Mango Lassi (page 215)	Mango Lassi (page 215)
Dinner	Lemon-Thyme Roast Chicken (page 272) Mashed Sweet Potatoes with Rosemary (page 298) Braised Green Beans and Fennel (page 291) Lemon Blueberry Panna Cotta (page 314) 1 cup (250 mL) milk or milk alternative	Lemon-Thyme Roast Chicken (page 272) Mashed Sweet Potatoes with Rosemary (page 298) Braised Green Beans and Fennel (page 291) Lemon Blueberry Panna Cotta (page 314) 1 cup (250 mL) milk or milk alternative
Evening Snack	Cold Maple Mousse (page 315)	Cold Maple Mousse (page 315)

Part 4

Recipes for Primary Headache Relief

Introduction to the Recipes

The meal plan on page 158 is built from these healthy and nutritious migraine-relief recipes. While there is no magic bullet to make migraines go away altogether, following the meal plan, keeping to a regular meal and snack schedule, and drinking lots of fluids throughout the day will help you manage your headaches.

Scattered throughout the recipes are tips that will teach you how to reduce the histamine levels in your favorite recipes. It is not possible to have a totally histamine-free diet, and a small amount of histamine is unlikely to trigger a headache. Each person has histamine responses to different foods; keeping track of the foods you eat and your headache pattern will help you learn which foods to avoid or reduce.

About the Nutrient Analyses

Computer-assisted nutrient analysis of the meal plans and recipes was prepared using Food Processor® SQL, version 10.9, ESHA Research Inc., Salem OR (this software contains over 35,000 food items based largely on the latest USDA data and the entire Canadian Nutrient File, 2007b). The database was supplemented when necessary with data from the Canadian Nutrient File (version 2010) and documented data from other reliable sources.

The analyses were based on:
- imperial weights and measures (except for foods typically packaged and used in metric quantities);
- the larger number of servings (i.e., the smaller portion) when there is a range;
- the smaller ingredient quantity when there is a range;
- the first ingredient listed when there is a choice of ingredients.

Calculations involving meat and poultry use lean portions without skin and with visible fat trimmed. A pinch of salt was calculated as $\frac{1}{8}$ tsp (0.5 mL). All recipes were analyzed prior to cooking. Optional ingredients and garnishes, and ingredients that are not quantified, were not included in the calculations.

Breakfast

Apple Berry Muesli

This hearty breakfast is a version of muesli, a traditional Swiss breakfast cereal. Adding almonds will not raise the histamine level.

Tips

If you're using frozen berries, defrost in the microwave until thawed. Check frequently to prevent cooking. Drain liquid before adding to the yogurt mixture.

Lemon juice has low levels of histamine, but small amounts are unlikely to trigger headache.

Reduce the Histamine
Wait to grate and add the apples until you're ready to serve.

2 cups	quick-cooking rolled oats	500 mL
2 cups	low-fat plain yogurt	500 mL
1 cup	milk	250 mL
3 tbsp	granulated sugar or liquid honey	45 mL
2	large apples, cored	2
	Juice of 1/2 lemon	
1 cup	chopped berries	250 mL
	Raisins and nuts (optional)	

1. In a medium bowl, combine oats, yogurt, milk and sugar. Set aside.

2. Grate apples, leaving the skin on. Sprinkle with lemon juice to prevent browning. Add apples and berries to yogurt mixture. Gently mix together. Refrigerate overnight. Serve topped with raisins and/or nuts, if desired.

This recipe courtesy of dietitian Sandra Gabriele.

Make-Your-Own Breakfast Cereal

To banish those breakfast blahs, try making your own nutritious cereal. It's a nice comfort food, a great energy source and a perfect start to any morning. It's also an excellent recipe for the young chefs in your household. You can involve your family in creating their own breakfast cereal blend from start to finish, including the bulk food shopping, where they choose a variety of grains. Your children will love being involved in selecting the ingredients for their custom breakfast.

Nutrients per 1 of 8 servings	
Calories	201
Fat	3 g
Carbohydrate	36 g
Protein	8 g

Coconut Quinoa Oat Granola

Outcast in the 1990s as an artery-clogging villain, virgin coconut oil has been newly embraced by health-conscious eaters everywhere. It's praised for its high levels of lauric acid, which is believed to help increase levels of "good" cholesterol, but it's the oil's delicate, sweet, tropical, almost vanilla-like flavor that has really won people over. Here, it enhances oats and quinoa, coaxing out their natural nuttiness in a most delicious way.

- Preheat oven to 300°F (150°C)
- Large rimmed baking sheet, lined with parchment paper

2 cups	large-flake (old-fashioned) rolled oats (certified gluten-free, if needed)	500 mL
1 cup	quinoa, rinsed	250 mL
1 cup	unsweetened flaked coconut	250 mL
¾ cup	almonds, coarsely chopped	175 mL
1½ tsp	ground cardamom or ginger	7 mL
½ cup	coconut oil, warmed	125 mL
½ cup	liquid honey or brown rice syrup	125 mL
⅔ cup	chopped dried apricots or golden raisins	150 mL

1. In a large bowl, combine oats, quinoa, coconut, almonds and cardamom.

2. In a medium bowl, whisk together oil and honey until well blended.

3. Add the honey mixture to the oats mixture and stir until well coated. Spread mixture in a single layer on prepared baking sheet.

4. Bake in preheated oven for 20 to 25 minutes or until oats are golden brown. Let cool completely on pan.

5. Transfer granola to an airtight container and stir in apricots. Store at room temperature for up to 2 weeks.

Nutrients per ½ cup (125 mL)	
Calories	385
Fat	21 g
Carbohydrate	43 g
Protein	6 g

Quinoa Crunch

Here, quinoa is transformed into a crispy-sweet topping that's heavenly sprinkled on yogurt, cereal or muffins, mixed into trail mix or simply eaten out of hand.

Tip

An equal amount of pure maple syrup, brown rice syrup or agave nectar may be used in place of the honey.

- Preheat oven to 375°F (190°C)
- Rimmed baking sheet, lined with parchment paper

1 cup	quinoa, rinsed	250 mL
1 tbsp	vegetable oil	15 mL
1 tbsp	liquid honey	15 mL
$\frac{1}{8}$ tsp	fine sea salt	0.5 mL

1. In a small bowl, combine quinoa, oil, honey and salt. Spread in a single layer on prepared baking sheet.

2. Bake in preheated oven for 11 to 13 minutes, stirring occasionally, until quinoa is crisp. Transfer to a large plate and let cool completely.

3. Transfer quinoa crunch to an airtight container and store at room temperature for up to 1 month.

Nutrients per $\frac{1}{4}$ cup (60 mL)	
Calories	248
Fat	8 g
Carbohydrate	4 g
Protein	1 g

Not Your Same Old Oats

This breakfast cereal combines the goodness of oats and oat bran with high-fiber grains like cracked wheat.

Tip
To vary this recipe, try altering the proportion and types of grains.

1 cup	large-flake rolled oats	250 mL
2/3 cup	5-grain cereal	150 mL
1/2 cup	oat bran	125 mL
1/3 cup	medium bulgur (cracked wheat)	75 mL

1. In a large bowl, combine oats, cereal, oat bran and bulgur. Store in airtight container.

This recipe courtesy of Michael G. Baylis.

For 1 serving of Not Your Same old Oats

Place 1/3 cup (75 mL) of the oat mixture in a deep bowl. Add 3/4 cup (175 mL) water and a pinch of salt. Microwave on High for 2 minutes; stir. Microwave for 1 to 2 minutes longer. Or cook in small saucepan on top of stove for about 5 minutes.

Nutrients per serving	
Calories	143
Fat	2 g
Carbohydrate	27 g
Protein	6 g

Toasted Quinoa Porridge

This power breakfast is an easy bowlful of deliciousness. Not as heavy as other grain porridges, it's one of those magical breakfast dishes that works for any season of the year.

Nutrients per serving	
Calories	187
Fat	3 g
Carbohydrate	33 g
Protein	7 g

½ cup	quinoa, rinsed	125 mL
½ tsp	ground cinnamon	2 mL
⅛ tsp	fine sea salt	0.5 mL
1¼ cups	milk or plain non-dairy milk (such as soy, almond, rice or hemp), divided	300 mL
1 cup	water	250 mL

Suggested Accompaniments

Agave nectar, liquid honey, brown rice syrup or pure maple syrup

Fresh or dried fruit

1. In a small saucepan, over medium heat, toast quinoa, stirring, for 2 to 3 minutes or until golden and fragrant. Add cinnamon, salt, 1 cup (250 mL) of the milk and water; bring to a boil. Reduce heat to low, cover and simmer, stirring occasionally, for about 25 minutes or until liquid is absorbed.

2. Serve drizzled with the remaining milk and any of the suggested accompaniments, as desired.

Easy Eggs

An egg and a microwave — what could be easier than that?

Variation
Stir 1 tbsp (15 mL) shredded light Cheddar cheese into the egg before cooking.

Nutrients per serving	
Calories	63
Fat	4 g
Carbohydrate	0 g
Protein	6 g

- **Small silicone baking cup or ¾-cup (175 mL) ramekin**

1	large egg	1
	Salt and freshly ground black pepper (optional)	

1. In baking cup, stir egg lightly with a fork until blended.

2. Microwave on High for 30 seconds. Let cool for 2 minutes. If desired, season to taste with salt and pepper.

Best-Ever Scrambled Eggs

This recipe is proof that the simplest recipes are often the best.

Tips

For a little bit of spice, add a pinch of cayenne pepper with the salt and pepper.

Double or triple this recipe as required.

4	large eggs	4
1/4 cup	cream or milk	60 mL
1/4 tsp	salt	1 mL
	Freshly ground black pepper	
1 tbsp	butter	15 mL

1. In a bowl, whisk together eggs, cream, salt, and black pepper to taste. Set aside.

2. In a saucepan, melt butter over low heat. Add egg mixture and cook just until eggs begin to set, about 2 minutes. Begin to stir, scraping up set bits from the bottom, and stir constantly until the mixture is setting but still moist, about 3 minutes. Remove from heat and serve immediately.

Variations

Scrambled Eggs with Smoked Salmon: Accompany eggs with 2 slices smoked salmon per serving and garnish with 1 tbsp (15 mL) finely chopped green onion or chives.

Mexican-Style Scrambled Eggs: Add 1 tsp (5 mL) finely chopped jalapeño pepper (alternatively, add hot pepper sauce to beaten eggs, to taste), 1/4 cup (60 mL) cooked or thawed corn kernels and 1/4 cup (60 mL) diced cured chorizo sausage to saucepan along with the butter. Stir in 2 tbsp (30 mL) salsa after the eggs are cooked. Be sure to use cured cooked chorizo sausage (which is hard) as the uncooked variety will not cook in this recipe. Serve with sliced tomatoes in season.

Scrambled Eggs with Pesto: Just before serving, stir 1 to 2 tbsp (15 to 30 mL) basil pesto into the eggs.

Scrambled Eggs with Fine Herbs: Sprinkle cooked eggs with any combination of the following mixture of fresh herbs, to taste: finely chopped parsley, chives, basil, tarragon, marjoram and thyme.

Nutrients per serving	
Calories	304
Fat	27 g
Carbohydrate	2 g
Protein	13 g

Cheese-Baked Eggs

This is the easiest and the very best way to cook eggs without watching them!

Tip

Any of the hard cheeses that shred well may replace Swiss. Use Cheddar or Monterey Jack for Mexican-style, Asiago or provolone when you want to go Italian or small dollops of chèvre for a French influence. Use mild cheese for lower histamine levels.

- Preheat oven to 350°F (180°C)
- 8-inch (20 cm) baking pan, greased

¾ cup	shredded Swiss cheese	175 mL
6	large eggs	6
⅔ cup	milk or light (5%) cream	150 mL
	Salt and freshly ground black pepper	
	Finely chopped fresh parsley or basil (optional)	

1. Sprinkle cheese over bottom of prepared pan. Break eggs over cheese.

2. Whisk together milk and salt and pepper to taste. Pour over eggs.

3. Bake in a preheated oven for 15 minutes or until eggs are just set. Sprinkle with chopped parsley, if desired.

Nutrients per 1 of 6 servings	
Calories	172
Fat	12 g
Carbohydrate	3 g
Protein	13 g

Sweet Potato Omelet

This delicious and unusual omelet is reminiscent of potato pancakes. Your tummy will be smiling!

Tips

To flip the omelet, put a plate over the skillet and turn it out. Flip over into the skillet to cook the other side.

Onion has low levels of histamine. Eating it occasionally is unlikely to trigger headaches. You could replace it with an equal amount of chopped shallots, if desired.

Variation

Substitute sliced green beans, chopped bean sprouts, diced bell pepper, diced mushrooms or any combination of your favorite vegetables for the sweet potatoes.

2	large eggs	2
1 cup	shredded peeled sweet potatoes	250 mL
1/2 cup	chopped onion	125 mL
1	clove garlic, chopped	1
1 tsp	salt or soy sauce	5 mL
1 tbsp	vegetable oil	15 mL

1. In a small bowl, beat eggs with a fork. Stir in sweet potatoes, onion, garlic and salt until well combined.

2. Heat a medium skillet over medium-high heat. Add oil and swirl to coat the pan. Pour in egg mixture; cook, turning once, until lightly browned on both sides, about 2 minutes per side.

This recipe courtesy of dietitian Nena Wirth.

Nutrients per serving	
Calories	193
Fat	12 g
Carbohydrate	15 g
Protein	7 g

Crustless Zucchini Quiche

Makes 6 servings

Even without a pastry crust, this quiche is so delicious!

Tip

Onion has low levels of histamine. Eating it occasionally is unlikely to trigger headaches. You could replace it with an equal amount of chopped shallots, if desired.

Variation

Blanched broccoli could be substituted for the zucchini, and ham could be added.

Reduce the Histamine

Replace the all-purpose flour with an all-purpose gluten-free flour mix.

- Preheat oven to 350°F (180°C)
- 9-inch (23 cm) deep-dish pie plate, greased

	Vegetable cooking spray	
1 cup	chopped onion	250 mL
5	large eggs	5
1½ cups	skim milk	375 mL
2½ cups	grated zucchini, drained	625 mL
2 cups	chopped red bell peppers	500 mL
3 tbsp	all-purpose flour	45 mL
2 tsp	baking powder	10 mL
1 tsp	salt	5 mL
½ tsp	freshly ground black pepper	2 mL
Pinch	cayenne pepper	Pinch
2 cups	shredded light Cheddar cheese	500 mL
¼ cup	dry bread crumbs	60 mL

1. Heat a small frying over medium-high heat. Spray with vegetable cooking spray. Sauté onion until just softened, about 5 minutes.

2. In a large bowl, beat eggs and milk. Stir in onion, zucchini and red peppers.

3. In a small bowl, combine flour, baking powder, salt, black pepper and cayenne. Stir in cheese until thoroughly coated. Add to egg mixture along with bread crumbs. Pour mixture into prepared pie plate and smooth top.

4. Bake in preheated oven for 40 to 50 minutes or until top is lightly browned and puffed and a knife inserted in the center comes out clean.

This recipe courtesy of Erna Braun.

Nutrients per serving	
Calories	214
Fat	8 g
Carbohydrate	18 g
Protein	18 g

Sweet Potato and Quinoa Breakfast Tortilla

Sweet potatoes and quinoa are swapped in for the traditional white potatoes in this Spanish skillet dish. It's one of Spain's favorite vegetarian meals, and with these newfangled twists, it will become one of yours too. Serve with roasted pepper sauce.

- Preheat broiler, with rack set 4 to 6 inches (10 to 15 cm) from heat source
- Large ovenproof skillet

6	large eggs	6
1 tsp	fine sea salt	5 mL
1 tbsp	extra virgin olive oil	15 mL
2 cups	coarsely shredded peeled sweet potato (about 1 medium)	500 mL
1 cup	chopped green onions	250 mL
1¼ cups	cooked quinoa, cooled	300 mL

1. In a medium bowl, whisk together eggs and salt.

2. In ovenproof skillet, heat oil over medium-high heat. Add sweet potato and cook, stirring, for 8 to 10 minutes or until softened. Add egg mixture, green onions and quinoa, gently shaking pan to distribute eggs. Reduce heat to medium and cook for about 8 minutes, gently shaking pan every minute, until eggs are almost set.

3. Place skillet under preheated broiler and broil for 1 to 2 minutes or until lightly browned. Slide out of the pan onto a cutting board and cut into wedges.

Nutrients per serving	
Calories	163
Fat	7 g
Carbohydrate	17 g
Protein	8 g

Crêpes

These crêpes are so good, it's worth getting up a half-hour early to prepare them. They can be used to make enchiladas or as wraps filled with cream cheese and hot pepper slices, cream cheese and cucumber slices, cashew butter and banana slices, peanut butter and jam — the possibilities are endless.

Tip

Choose your favorite GF non-dairy milk, such as soy, rice, almond or potato-based milk, or, if you tolerate lactose, use regular 1% milk.

Make Ahead

Crêpes can be prepared ahead of time, cooled, layered between sheets of parchment paper and stored in an airtight container in the refrigerator for up to 3 days. Just before serving, reheat each crêpe on a plate in the microwave on High for about 20 seconds to soften it.

- 9-inch (23 cm) skillet

1/2 cup	sorghum flour	125 mL
1/2 cup	potato starch	125 mL
1/2 tsp	granulated raw cane sugar	2 mL
2	large eggs	2
1/2 cup	lactose-free 1% milk or fortified GF non-dairy milk	125 mL
2 tbsp	butter or vegan hard margarine, melted	30 mL
	Butter or vegan hard margarine	

1. In a large bowl, using a whisk, combine sorghum flour, potato starch and sugar.

2. In another bowl, beat eggs, milk, melted butter and 1/2 cup (125 mL) water. Stir into flour mixture until well blended.

3. In skillet, melt 1/2 tsp (2 mL) butter over medium heat, making sure to cover the bottom of the skillet. For each crêpe, pour in a scant 1/4 cup (60 mL) batter and swirl so that the batter covers the whole surface. Cook for about 1 minute or until edges start to curl up. Flip over and cook for 1 minute or until bottom is golden. Transfer to a plate and keep warm. Repeat with the remaining batter, adjusting heat and melting another 1/2 tsp (2 mL) butter between each batch as needed.

Nutrients per crêpe	
Calories	100
Carbohydrate	14 g
Protein	3 g
Fat	4 g

Quinoa Crêpes

Quinoa flour produces a light crêpe with lots of nutty flavor. You can forget what you've heard about crêpes being fussy or challenging — they're very easy to make. Moreover, a regular nonstick skillet works just as well as any crêpe pan or specialty crêpe griddle.

Tip
Refrigerating the batter before use allows the bubbles that form during blending to subside, making the crêpes less likely to tear during cooking. The batter will keep for up to 48 hours.

Make Ahead
Refrigerate crêpes between sheets of waxed paper, tightly covered in plastic wrap, for up to 2 days or freeze, enclosed in a sealable plastic bag, for up to 1 month.

- Blender

2	large eggs	2
¾ cup	milk	175 mL
½ cup	water	125 mL
3 tbsp	unsalted butter, melted and cooled	45 mL
¼ tsp	fine sea salt	1 mL
1 cup	quinoa flour	250 mL
	Nonstick cooking spray	

1. In blender, combine eggs, milk, water, butter and salt. Add quinoa flour and blend until smooth. Transfer to a bowl, cover and refrigerate for 1 hour.

2. Heat a large nonstick skillet over medium-high heat. Remove from heat and lightly coat pan with cooking spray. Whisk the batter slightly. For each crêpe, pour about ¼ cup (60 mL) batter into pan, quickly tilting in all directions to cover bottom of pan. Cook for about 45 seconds or until just golden at the edges. With a spatula, carefully lift edge of crêpe to test for doneness. The crêpe is ready to turn when it is golden brown on the bottom and can be shaken loose from the pan. Turn crêpe over and cook for about 15 to 30 seconds or until golden brown.

3. Transfer crêpe to an unfolded kitchen towel to cool completely. Repeat with the remaining batter, spraying skillet and adjusting heat as necessary between crêpes, stacking cooled crêpes between sheets of waxed paper to prevent sticking.

Crêpe Filling Ideas
Lemon juice and a drizzle of honey; a thin spread of nut or seed butter and all-fruit jam; Greek yogurt and fresh fruit or jam; ricotta or cottage cheese and a drizzle of honey or agave nectar; grated bittersweet chocolate (GF, if needed) and toasted nuts; thinly sliced ham and shredded Gruyère or Swiss cheese; thinly sliced pears and a drizzle of pure maple syrup; scrambled eggs or egg whites.

Nutrients per crêpe	
Calories	64
Fat	4 g
Carbohydrate	5 g
Protein	2 g

Oatmeal Pancakes

These tasty pancakes are so easy to make. Maple syrup or mixed berries on the side will make this a kid favorite.

Tips

These pancakes taste great topped with fresh berries and a dollop of your favorite yogurt.

Be aware that adding the optional cinnamon could raise the histamine level of this recipe.

Reduce the Histamine

Use almond extract instead of vanilla extract.

6	large egg whites	6
1 cup	large-flake (old-fashioned) rolled oats	250 mL
1 cup	fat-free cottage cheese	250 mL
2 tsp	granulated sugar	10 mL
1 tsp	ground cinnamon (optional)	5 mL
1 tsp	vanilla extract	5 mL
	Vegetable cooking spray	

1. In blender, on medium speed, blend egg whites, oats, cottage cheese, sugar, cinnamon (if using) and vanilla until smooth.

2. Heat a griddle or large nonstick skillet over medium-low heat. Spray lightly with vegetable cooking spray. For each pancake, pour ¼ cup (60 mL) batter onto griddle and cook until bubbly around the edges, about 2 minutes. Flip and cook until golden brown, about 2 minutes. Transfer to a plate and keep warm in a low oven. Repeat with remaining batter, spraying griddle with vegetable cooking spray and adjusting heat between batches as needed.

This recipe courtesy of Jorie Janzen.

Nutrients per pancake	
Calories	58
Fat	1 g
Carbohydrate	7 g
Protein	6 g

Finnish Apple Pancake

This is an easy recipe for a special breakfast. And it's a real hit as part of a brunch menu. Serve immediately with maple syrup or your favorite fruit preserves.

Variation

For variety, use peaches or pears to bake this delicious breakfast dish, keeping in mind that peaches may raise histamine levels.

Reduce the Histamine

Replace the all-purpose flour with an all-purpose gluten-free flour mix.

Omit the cinnamon from the topping.

- Preheat oven to 425°F (220°C)
- 8-inch (20 cm) square baking pan, greased

2 cups	thinly sliced cored peeled apples	500 mL
1 tbsp	butter, melted	15 mL
3	large eggs	3
½ cup	milk	125 mL
⅓ cup	all-purpose flour	75 mL
¼ tsp	baking powder	1 mL
⅛ tsp	salt	0.5 mL
Topping		
½ tsp	ground cinnamon	2 mL
1 tbsp	granulated sugar	15 mL

1. Place apples and butter in baking pan; toss to coat. Bake in preheated oven for 5 minutes.

2. Meanwhile, in a small bowl, whisk together eggs, milk, flour, baking powder and salt until smooth. Set aside.

3. *Topping:* In another small bowl, combine cinnamon and sugar. Set aside.

4. Pour egg mixture over cooked apples; sprinkle evenly with topping. Bake for 15 to 20 minutes or until pancake is puffed and golden brown. Serve immediately.

This recipe courtesy of dietitian Kimberly Green.

Nutrients per serving	
Calories	357
Fat	15 g
Carbohydrate	43 g
Protein	14 g

Easy Breakfast Cookies

Cookies for breakfast —
what a unique way to
ensure the whole family
gets a healthy start to
the day!

Tip
Look for 9-grain cereal in
the bulk food store or the
bulk food section of your
grocery store.

Variations
Substitute your favorite dried
fruits for the raisins.

Experiment by adding nuts
and seeds, making the
cookies a little bit different
every time.

For added fiber and less fat,
replace the vegetable oil with
1/4 cup (60 mL) of puréed
fruit or cooked puréed white
beans or red lentils.

Reduce the Histamine
Use almond extract
instead of vanilla extract.

- Preheat oven to 325°F (160°C)
- Baking sheet, lined with parchment paper

1 1/2 cups	whole wheat flour	375 mL
1 tsp	baking soda	5 mL
1 tsp	baking powder	5 mL
1/4 tsp	salt	1 mL
3/4 cup	lightly packed brown sugar	175 mL
1/2 cup	butter	125 mL
1/4 cup	vegetable oil	60 mL
1/4 cup	olive oil	60 mL
2	large eggs	2
1/4 cup	flax seeds (ground or whole)	60 mL
1 tsp	vanilla extract	5 mL
2 1/2 cups	9-grain cereal (see tip, at left)	625 mL
3/4 cup	unsweetened flaked coconut	175 mL
1/2 cup	raisins or dried cranberries	125 mL

1. In a small bowl, combine flour, baking soda, baking powder and salt.

2. In a large bowl, using an electric mixer, cream sugar, butter, vegetable oil and olive oil until smooth. Beat in eggs, flax seeds and vanilla. Stir in flour mixture until combined. Stir in 9-grain cereal, coconut and raisins.

3. Drop dough by tablespoonfuls (15 mL), about 2 inches (5 cm) apart, onto prepared baking sheet. Flatten with a fork.

4. Bake in preheated oven for 15 to 20 minutes or until browned. Let cool on baking sheet on a wire rack for 10 minutes, then transfer to rack to cool completely.

This recipe courtesy of dietitian Lisa Haber.

Nutrients per cookie	
Calories	138
Fat	8 g
Carbohydrate	16 g
Protein	3 g

Breads and Muffins

Brown Sandwich Bread

This moist bread, which slices with ease, is perfect for sandwiches. Or enjoy it with butter and jam.

Tips

Warm the milk in a glass measuring cup in the microwave on High for about 1 minute, or the traditional way, in a small saucepan over low heat.

If you don't have a glass loaf dish, use a metal loaf pan and increase the baking time by 5 to 10 minutes.

Let bread cool completely before slicing. Use a serrated bread knife for the best results. Wrap cooled bread and store at room temperature for up to 4 days or freeze for up to 1 month.

- Stand mixer
- 9- by 5-inch (23 by 12.5 cm) glass loaf dish, greased, bottom lined with parchment paper

1 cup	sorghum flour	250 mL
1/3 cup	psyllium husks	75 mL
1/4 cup	white rice flour	60 mL
1/4 cup	brown rice flour	60 mL
1/4 cup	tapioca starch	60 mL
2 tbsp	granulated raw cane sugar	30 mL
1 tsp	salt	5 mL
1/4 cup	cold butter, cut into cubes	60 mL
2 tsp	instant yeast	10 mL
1 cup	lactose-free 1% milk, heated to 120°F to 130°F (50°C to 55°C)	250 mL
2	large eggs, lightly beaten	2

1. In large bowl of stand mixer, combine sorghum flour, psyllium, white rice flour, brown rice flour, tapioca starch, sugar, salt and butter. Beat on low speed until butter is incorporated. Add yeast and beat for 1 minute.

2. With motor running on low, gradually pour in heated milk, beating until incorporated. Beat for 1 minute. Beat in eggs until incorporated. Beat for 5 minutes, stopping mixer and scraping down sides of bowl and beater halfway through.

3. Spread batter in prepared loaf dish. Cover with a lint-free towel and let rise in a warm, draft-free place for 1 hour or until doubled in bulk. Meanwhile, preheat oven to 350°F (180°C).

4. Bake for 35 to 40 minutes or until browned and a tester inserted in the center comes out clean. Let cool in dish on a wire rack for 5 minutes. Run a knife around edge of bread and remove from dish. Peel off paper, transfer bread to rack and let cool completely.

Nutrients per slice	
Calories	110
Fat	4 g
Carbohydrate	15 g
Protein	3 g

Multigrain Sandwich Bread

This no-nonsense, yeast-free, gluten-free sandwich loaf is guaranteed to please. Its subtle sweetness works beautifully with any number of sandwich fillings, from turkey to cream cheese to roasted vegetables.

Make Ahead

Store the cooled bread, wrapped in foil or plastic wrap, in the refrigerator for up to 5 days. Alternatively, wrap it in plastic wrap, then foil, completely enclosing bread, and freeze for up to 3 months. Defrost in the microwave until thawed. Check frequently to prevent cooking.

- 8- by 4-inch (20 by 10 cm) metal loaf pan, sprayed with nonstick cooking spray

1½ cups	multigrain hot cereal (GF, if needed)	375 mL
2 cups	buttermilk	500 mL
1⅓ cups	quinoa flour	325 mL
1 tbsp	cornstarch or arrowroot	15 mL
2 tsp	baking powder (GF, if needed)	10 mL
1¼ tsp	baking soda	6 mL
1¼ tsp	fine sea salt	6 mL
2	large eggs	2
½ cup	olive or vegetable oil	125 mL
¼ cup	dark (cooking) molasses or liquid honey	60 mL

1. In a large bowl, combine cereal and buttermilk. Let stand for 20 minutes.

2. Preheat oven to 375°F (190°C).

3. In another large bowl, whisk together quinoa flour, cornstarch, baking powder, baking soda and salt.

4. Whisk eggs, oil and molasses into cereal mixture until well blended.

5. Add the egg mixture to the flour mixture and stir until just blended.

6. Spread batter evenly in prepared pan.

7. Bake for 55 to 60 minutes or until a toothpick inserted in the center comes out clean. Let cool in pan on a wire rack for 5 minutes, then transfer to the rack. Serve warm or let cool completely.

Nutrients per slice	
Calories	140
Fat	8 g
Carbohydrate	14 g
Protein	3 g

Rosemary Quinoa Focaccia

With quinoa flour and baking powder in place of wheat flour and yeast, this focaccia is anything but traditional. Nevertheless, it is irresistible. Like the original, the dough is finished with the delicate crunch of coarse sea salt and is puckered to allow small pockets of flavorful olive oil to remain once the loaf is baked.

Make Ahead

Store the cooled focaccia, wrapped in foil or plastic wrap, in the refrigerator for up to 1 day.

- Preheat oven to 425°F (220°C)
- 13- by 9-inch (33 by 23 cm) glass or metal baking pan, oiled (preferably olive oil)

2 cups	quinoa flour	500 mL
1 tbsp	baking powder (GF, if needed)	15 mL
½ tsp	fine sea salt	2 mL
1 cup	water	250 mL
3 tbsp	olive oil, divided	45 mL
1 tbsp	chopped fresh rosemary	15 mL
1½ tsp	coarse sea salt	7 mL

1. In a large bowl, whisk together quinoa flour, baking powder and fine sea salt. Using a wooden spoon, stir in water and 1 tbsp (15 mL) of the oil until blended.

2. Turn dough out onto a work surface lightly floured with quinoa flour. Knead for 1 minute.

3. Transfer dough to prepared pan and pat into a ½-inch (1 cm) thick rectangle (it will not cover entire bottom of pan). Poke indentations all over top of bread with your fingertips. Brush or drizzle dough with the remaining oil and sprinkle with rosemary and coarse sea salt.

4. Bake in preheated oven for 20 to 25 minutes or until golden brown. Let cool in pan on a wire rack for 5 minutes, then transfer to the rack to cool. Serve warm or let cool completely.

Nutrients per slice	
Calories	55
Fat	3 g
Carbohydrate	6 g
Protein	11 g

Quinoa Tortillas

Makes 9 tortillas

An ancient Andean ingredient shines in this fantastic take on tortillas. Don't be intimated about making them from scratch: they are really quite easy to prepare and come together in minutes.

Tip

If you do not have a tortilla press, you can use a rolling pin. Place a 6-inch (15 cm) wide bowl upside down on the sealable plastic bag and trace a circle around it. Cut out the circle into two rounds. Place a round on either side of the dough ball before rolling it out. The plastic rounds help ensure that the tortillas do not stick and are all the same size.

Make Ahead

Store the cooled tortillas, wrapped in foil or plastic wrap, in the refrigerator for up to 5 days. Alternatively, wrap them in plastic wrap, then foil, completely enclosing bread, and freeze for up to 3 months. Defrost in the microwave until thawed. Check frequently to prevent cooking.

Nutrients per tortilla	
Calories	77
Fat	1 g
Carbohydrate	15 g
Protein	2 g

- Tortilla press (see tip, at left)
- Cast-iron or other heavy skillet

2 cups	quinoa flour	500 mL
1/3 cup	brown rice flour	75 mL
1/2 tsp	fine sea salt	2 mL
2/3 cup	hot (not boiling) water	150 mL
2 tsp	vegetable oil	10 mL

1. Cut two rounds from a heavy-duty sealable plastic bag to fit the shape of the tortilla press. Set aside.

2. In a large bowl, whisk together quinoa flour, brown rice flour and salt. Stir in hot water and oil until mixture comes together into a smooth dough.

3. Turn dough out onto a work surface lightly floured with quinoa flour or brown rice flour. Knead for about 1 minute. Cut dough into 9 equal pieces and shape each into a ball. Cover loosely with plastic wrap.

4. Place a plastic round on the bottom half of the tortilla press. Place a dough ball in the center. Top with the second plastic round. Close press, flattening dough to about 1/8 inch (3 mm) thick and forming a 6-inch (15 cm) round. If thickness of tortilla is uneven, lift dough round, in plastic, and rotate 180 degrees. Press tortilla lightly to even out. Peel off plastic.

5. Heat cast-iron skillet over medium-high heat. Cook tortilla, turning once, for about 45 seconds per side, until it looks slightly dry at the edges, starts to release from the surface of the skillet and is lightly browned in spots. Transfer to a plate.

6. Repeat steps 4 and 5 with the remaining dough balls.

Chapati

Chapati is a traditional Indian bread made from whole wheat flour that has been very finely milled. Here, barley flour is added for lightness. They make an excellent accompaniment to curries and stews, as they are great for soaking up the sauce.

Tip

If you have access to chapati flour, a very finely milled whole wheat flour that is available in Indian grocery stores, substitute it for the whole wheat pastry flour called for in this recipe.

1 cup	whole wheat pastry flour (approx.)	250 mL
1/2 cup	whole barley flour	125 mL
1/2 tsp	salt	2 mL
3 tbsp	melted butter or olive oil, divided (approx.)	45 mL
1/3 to 1/2 cup	lukewarm water	75 to 125 mL

1. In a bowl, combine whole wheat and barley flours and salt. Add 1 tbsp (15 mL) melted butter and mix well. Make a well in the center and gradually, in a stream, add water, stirring gently to incorporate the flour, until the mixture is crumbly. Knead until the dough is smooth and leaves the sides of the bowl, adding a bit more water if necessary. (Kneading makes the dough lighter, so the more the better.) Cover with a damp cloth and let rest for 1 hour to ensure moisture is evenly distributed.

2. Divide dough into 8 equal portions and form each into a ball. Return balls to the bowl and keep covered with the damp cloth. One at a time, on a floured surface, roll each ball out to about 6 inches (15 cm) in diameter.

3. Heat a nonstick skillet over medium-high heat until almost smoking. Add approximately 1/4 tsp (1 mL) of the butter to the pan and disperse over the surface. Add one chapati and cook until bubbles rise and brown spots appear on the underside, about 40 seconds. Turn over and cook until brown spots appear on the underside, about 30 seconds. Transfer to a plate and brush lightly with melted butter. Keep warm. Repeat until all dough is used up, adding fresh butter to pan with each chapati and adjusting heat as necessary to prevent burning.

Nutrients per chapati	
Calories	121
Fat	5 g
Carbohydrate	18 g
Protein	3 g

Quinoa Pizza Dough

Don't wait around for yeast: this baking powder version of pizza dough yields a crisp crust in a fraction of the time. Quinoa flour, with its naturally nutty, faintly sweet flavor, makes the dough a standout.

Tip

One of the secrets to great pizza is restraint with the toppings. A smear of sauce, a sprinkle of cheese and a light hand with any additional toppings is all you need.

Reduce the Histamine

Use a bit of pesto as a base rather than marinara sauce.

Choose mozzarella or brick cheese.

- Preheat oven to 400°F (200°C)
- Large pizza pan or rimmed baking sheet, oiled (preferably with olive oil)

1½ cups	quinoa flour	375 mL
1 tbsp	baking powder (GF, if needed)	15 mL
½ tsp	fine sea salt	2 mL
⅔ cup	water	150 mL
2 tbsp	olive oil	30 mL

Suggested toppings

Marinara sauce

Basil pesto

Shredded or grated cheese (such as mozzarella, Parmesan, Gouda or fontina)

Leftover grilled or roasted vegetables, coarsely chopped

Diced cooked lean meat or sausage (such as roasted chicken, Canadian bacon or chicken sausage)

Pitted ripe or brine-cured black olives, sliced or quartered (lengthwise)

1. In a large bowl, whisk together quinoa flour, baking powder and salt. Using a wooden spoon, stir in water and oil until a shaggy dough forms.

2. Turn dough out onto a work surface lightly floured with quinoa flour. Knead for 1 to 2 minutes or until smooth and cohesive. Shape into a ball. Use immediately.

To Make Pizza

3. Place ball on prepared pan and pat into a large round (if using a pizza pan) or rectangle (if using a baking sheet). Add any of the suggested toppings, as desired.

4. Bake for 19 to 24 minutes or until crust is golden and cheese is bubbly. Let cool on pan on a wire rack for 5 minutes, then transfer to a cutting board. Cut into 10 wedges or squares.

Nutrients per slice (without toppings)	
Calories	59
Fat	3 g
Carbohydrate	7 g
Protein	1 g

Old-Fashioned Cornbread

This traditional favorite is the perfect accompaniment to soups, stews and chilis that have a down-home feel. Use leftovers to make cornbread stuffing, or for a great snack, enjoy with a bit of salsa.

Tip

As with other quick breads, when making cornbread, one key to success is not to overmix the batter.

- Preheat oven to 400°F (200°C)
- 8-inch (20 cm) square baking pan, lightly greased

1 cup	stone-ground yellow cornmeal	250 mL
1 cup	whole barley flour	250 mL
2 tbsp	granulated sugar	30 mL
4 tsp	baking powder	20 mL
½ tsp	salt	2 mL
2	large eggs	2
1¼ cups	milk	300 mL
2 tbsp	melted butter	30 mL

1. In a bowl, combine cornmeal, barley flour, sugar, baking powder and salt. Whisk to blend and make a well in the center.

2. In a separate bowl, beat eggs. Add milk and butter and beat well. Pour into well and mix with dry ingredients just until blended. Spread in prepared pan and bake in preheated oven until top is golden and springs back, about 30 minutes. Let cool in pan on wire rack for 5 minutes. Serve warm.

Nutrients per serving	
Calories	197
Fat	6 g
Carbohydrate	31 g
Protein	6 g

Traditional Tea Biscuits

Makes 12 biscuits

Serve these up with butter and jam.

Tip

Choose your favorite GF non-dairy milk, such as soy, rice, almond or potato-based milk, or, if you tolerate lactose, use regular 1% milk.

Variation

Traditional Tea Biscuits with Raisins: Add ½ tsp (2 mL) ground cinnamon with the baking powder and add ½ cup (125 mL) raisins to the dough at the end of step 2. Bake as directed.

- Preheat oven to 350°F (180°C)
- Baking sheet, lined with parchment paper

½ cup	potato starch	125 mL
¼ cup	sorghum flour	60 mL
¼ cup	brown rice flour	60 mL
1 tbsp	granulated raw cane sugar	15 mL
2 tsp	GF baking powder	10 mL
2 tbsp	cold butter or vegan hard margarine, cut into pieces	30 mL
1	large egg white, lightly beaten	1
¼ cup	lactose-free 1% milk or fortified GF non-dairy milk	60 mL

1. In a large bowl, combine potato starch, sorghum flour, brown rice flour, sugar and baking powder. Using a pastry blender or two knives, cut in butter until mixture resembles coarse crumbs about the size of small peas.

2. In another bowl, whisk together egg white and milk. Pour into dry ingredients and stir until just combined.

3. Using a spoon, scoop out 12 spoonfuls of dough and place about 2 inches (5 cm) apart on prepared baking sheet. Bake in preheated oven for 10 to 12 minutes or until firm to the touch. Let cool on pan on a wire rack for 5 minutes. Transfer biscuits to rack to cool slightly. Serve warm.

Nutrients per biscuit	
Calories	70
Fat	2 g
Carbohydrate	13 g
Protein	1 g

Quinoa Anzac Biscuits

Anzac biscuits were
popularized by World War
I care packages to soldiers
of the Australian and
New Zealand Army Corps
(ANZAC), because they
kept well on the overseas
voyage to Europe. These
cookies are refashioned
with quinoa flakes and
quinoa flour, as they, too,
are excellent travelers!

Make Ahead
Store the cooled biscuits in
an airtight container in the
refrigerator for up to 1 week.

Variation
Tropical Anzac Biscuits: Add
⅓ cup (75 mL) golden raisins,
¼ cup (60 mL) chopped
macadamia nuts and ¾ tsp
(3 mL) ground allspice with
the coconut.

- **Preheat oven to 325°F (160°C)**
- **Large baking sheet, lined with parchment paper**

1 cup	quinoa flakes or quick-cooking rolled oats (certified GF, if needed)	250 mL
1 cup	quinoa flour	250 mL
1 cup	natural cane sugar or packed light brown sugar	250 mL
½ cup	unsweetened flaked coconut	125 mL
½ tsp	baking soda	2 mL
¼ tsp	fine sea salt	1 mL
¼ cup	unrefined virgin coconut oil, warmed, or unsalted butter, melted and cooled slightly	60 mL
3 tbsp	water	45 mL
2 tbsp	brown rice syrup, pure maple syrup or liquid honey	30 mL

1. In a large bowl, whisk together quinoa flakes, quinoa flour, sugar, coconut, baking soda and salt. Stir in oil, water and brown rice syrup until well blended.

2. Drop dough by tablespoonfuls (15 mL) onto prepared baking sheet, spacing them 2 inches (5 cm) apart.

3. Bake in preheated oven for 11 to 13 minutes or until golden brown. Let cool on pan on a wire rack for 2 minutes, then transfer to the rack to cool.

4. Repeat steps 2 and 3 with the remaining dough.

Nutrients per biscuit	
Calories	82
Fat	3 g
Carbohydrate	14 g
Protein	1 g

Quinoa Popovers

Makes 6 popovers

Offering tremendous home-style appeal, these light, airy popovers make a wonderful complement to almost any meal. No matter how tempting the aroma coming from your oven as they bake, resist opening the oven to check them until about 5 minutes before they're finished baking; check too soon, and they will deflate.

Tips

These popovers may also be made in a 12-cup muffin pan with 6 cups buttered. Reduce the second baking time by about 5 minutes.

If using a 12-cup popover pan or muffin pan, butter every other cup for even baking.

- Preheat oven to 450°F (230°C)
- Blender or food processor
- 6-cup nonstick popover pan, generously buttered

1 cup	quinoa flour	250 mL
¼ tsp	fine sea salt	1 mL
3	large eggs, at room temperature	3
1 cup	milk	250 mL
1 tbsp	unsalted butter, melted, or olive oil	15 mL

1. In blender, combine flour, salt, eggs, milk and butter; process until smooth.

2. Divide batter equally among prepared popover cups.

3. Bake in preheated oven for 10 minutes. Without opening oven door, reduce heat to 375°F (190°C). Bake for 15 to 20 minutes or until puffed and golden brown. Run a thin knife between the edge of each popover and the cup to loosen. Lift popovers from cups and serve immediately.

> **Variation**
> *Parmesan Sage Quinoa Popovers:* Add ¼ cup (60 mL) freshly grated Parmesan cheese and 1 tsp (5 mL) rubbed dried sage in step 1. Sprinkle popovers with an additional ¼ cup (60 mL) Parmesan before the final 5 minutes of baking.

Nutrients per popover	
Calories	109
Fat	5 g
Carbohydrate	10 g
Protein	6 g

Scottish Oat Cakes

Combining the crunch of a cracker with the tenderness of an oat scone, these little numbers are especially delectable. Spread them with jam or marmalade in the morning, top them with cheese at lunch, or serve them alongside soup at supper. And for heaven's sake, make sure they are present at teatime.

Make Ahead

Store the cooled oat cakes in an airtight container at room temperature for up to 5 days or in the freezer for up to 3 months. Defrost in the microwave until thawed. Check frequently to prevent cooking.

Variations

For an extra touch of sweetness, sprinkle the rounds with turbinado (raw) sugar before baking.

For a more savory finish, sprinkle the unbaked rounds with sea salt flakes.

- Preheat oven to 325°F (160°C)
- Food processor
- $2\frac{1}{2}$-inch (6 cm) round cookie cutter
- Large rimmed baking sheet, lined with parchment paper

2 cups	large-flake (old-fashioned) rolled oats	500 mL
$\frac{1}{2}$ cup	whole wheat flour	125 mL
$\frac{1}{2}$ tsp	baking powder	2 mL
$\frac{1}{2}$ tsp	fine sea salt	2 mL
1	large egg, lightly beaten	1
2 tbsp	unsalted butter, melted	30 mL
2 tbsp	liquid honey	30 mL

1. In food processor, process oats until coarsely ground.

2. In a large bowl, whisk together ground oats, flour, baking powder and salt. Using a wooden spoon, stir in egg, butter and honey until just blended.

3. Turn dough out onto a floured surface and roll out to a $\frac{1}{4}$-inch (0.5 cm) thick rectangle. Using the cookie cutter, cut dough into circles, rerolling scraps. Place 1 inch (2.5 cm) apart on prepared baking sheet.

4. Bake in preheated oven for 20 to 25 minutes or until golden and set at the edges. Let cool on pan on a wire rack for 5 minutes, then transfer to the rack. Serve warm or let cool completely.

Nutrients per oat cake	
Calories	51
Fat	2 g
Carbohydrate	8 g
Protein	1 g

Honey Whole Wheat Muffins

Makes 12 muffins

These easy muffins are simply delicious.

- Preheat oven to 400°F (200°C)
- 12-cup muffin tin, sprayed with low-fat cooking spray or paper-lined

1 cup	whole wheat flour	250 mL
1 cup	all-purpose flour	250 mL
3 tsp	baking powder	15 mL
1 tsp	salt	5 mL
1	large egg	1
1 cup	milk	250 mL
¼ cup	vegetable oil	60 mL
¼ cup	liquid honey	60 mL

1. In a large bowl, combine whole wheat flour, all-purpose flour, baking powder and salt. Make a well in the center.

2. In another bowl, whisk together egg, milk and oil. Add the honey. Stir into flour mixture until moist and lumpy.

3. Spoon batter into prepared muffin tin, dividing evenly. Bake in preheated oven for 20 to 25 minutes or until lightly browned.

Nutrients per muffin	
Calories	152
Fat	5 g
Carbohydrate	23 g
Protein	4 g

Millet and Flax Muffins

When muffins have great flavor, as these do, it's easy to forget they're a healthier alternative. Serve these to accompany any chicken dish when you want to wow your friends.

Tip

Choose your favorite GF non-dairy milk, such as soy, rice, almond or potato-based milk, or, if you tolerate lactose, use regular 1% milk.

- Preheat oven to 350°F (180°C)
- 12-cup muffin pan, 9 cups lined with paper liners

½ cup	millet grits	125 mL
¼ cup	brown rice flour	60 mL
¼ cup	ground flax seeds (flaxseed meal)	60 mL
2 tsp	GF baking powder	10 mL
1	large egg	1
2 tbsp	granulated raw cane sugar	30 mL
½ cup	lactose-free 1% milk or fortified GF non-dairy milk	125 mL
2 tbsp	unsweetened applesauce	30 mL

1. In a large bowl, whisk together millet grits, brown rice flour, flax seeds and baking powder.

2. In a medium bowl, whisk together egg, sugar, milk and applesauce until well combined. Pour over dry ingredients and stir until combined.

3. Spoon batter into prepared muffin cups, dividing equally. Bake in preheated oven for 15 to 20 minutes or until a tester inserted in the center comes out clean. Let cool in pan on a wire rack for 5 minutes. Transfer muffins to rack to cool.

Nutrients per muffin	
Calories	100
Fat	3 g
Carbohydrate	18 g
Protein	4 g

Blueberry Lemon Cornmeal Muffins

This blueberry-lemon combo is a winner!

Tips

Fresh blueberries are always best tasting, especially the small ones available in the summer. If using frozen berries, do not thaw. The flour will help to absorb the excess liquid.

When using margarine, choose a soft (non-hydrogenated) version.

Lemon has low histamine levels. Occasional or small amounts are unlikely to trigger headaches.

Make Ahead

Bake up to 2 days in advance; store in an airtight container. Freeze for up to 6 weeks.

- Preheat oven to 350°F (180°C)
- 12 muffin cups sprayed with vegetable spray

¾ cup	granulated sugar	175 mL
¼ cup	margarine or butter	60 mL
1	large egg	1
1½ tsp	grated lemon zest	7 mL
3 tbsp	freshly squeezed lemon juice	45 mL
3 tbsp	2% milk	45 mL
1 cup	all-purpose flour	250 mL
¼ cup	cornmeal	60 mL
1½ tsp	baking powder	7 mL
1 tsp	baking soda	5 mL
½ cup	2% plain yogurt	125 mL
1¼ cups	fresh or frozen blueberries	300 mL
2 tsp	all-purpose flour	10 mL

1. In a large bowl with an electric mixer, beat sugar, margarine, egg, lemon zest, lemon juice and milk until well blended. (Mixture may appear curdled.)

2. In another bowl, stir together flour, cornmeal, baking powder and baking soda. Add flour mixture and yogurt alternately to creamed mixture. In a small bowl, toss blueberries with flour; fold into batter. Divide batter among muffin cups.

3. Bake for 20 to 25 minutes or until tops are firm to the touch and tester inserted in center comes out clean.

Nutrients per muffin	
Calories	149
Fat	4 g
Carbohydrate	26 g
Protein	3 g

Sweet Potato Muffins

Start your day off well with one of these moist and delicious muffins.

Tip

For the mixed dried fruit, try raisins, blueberries, cherries and cranberries.

Reduce the Histamine

Replace the orange zest with lemon zest.

- **Preheat oven to 400°F (200°C)**
- **12-cup muffin tin, lightly greased or lined with paper cups**

1 cup	quick-cooking rolled oats	250 mL
1 cup	buttermilk (approx.)	250 mL
1/2 cup	all-purpose flour	125 mL
1/2 cup	whole wheat flour	125 mL
1/4 cup	granulated sugar	60 mL
1 tbsp	wheat germ	15 mL
1 tbsp	baking powder	15 mL
1 tsp	salt	5 mL
1/2 tsp	baking soda	2 mL
1 cup	mixed dried fruit (see tip, at left)	250 mL
1	large egg, beaten	1
1/2 cup	grated sweet potato	125 mL
1/4 cup	lightly packed brown sugar	60 mL
1/4 cup	vegetable oil	60 mL
1 tsp	grated orange zest	5 mL

1. Place oatmeal in a large bowl and pour in buttermilk; stir to combine. Cover and let stand for 10 minutes.

2. Meanwhile, in a small bowl, combine all-purpose flour, whole wheat flour, granulated sugar, wheat germ, baking powder, salt and baking soda. Stir in dried fruit.

3. In another small bowl, combine egg, sweet potato, brown sugar, oil and orange zest. Stir into oatmeal mixture. Gradually fold in flour mixture until just moistened. If too stiff, add a little more buttermilk.

4. Divide batter evenly among prepared muffin cups, filling almost to the top (these muffins do not rise much).

5. Bake for 20 minutes or until a tester inserted in the center of a muffin comes out clean. Let cool in tin for 10 minutes, then remove to a wire rack to cool completely.

This recipe courtesy of Eileen Campbell.

Nutrients per muffin	
Calories	194
Fat	6 g
Carbohydrate	33 g
Protein	4 g

Appetizers, Snacks and Beverages

Quick Roasted Red Pepper Dip

Roasted red peppers are flavorful and offer key nutrients. No wonder they often appear as an ingredient in recipes. You can roast them yourself and freeze them for later use or purchase them already prepared in a jar.

Tip

Red peppers are high in vitamin C, vitamin A and antioxidants. To increase fiber, serve this delicious dip with raw vegetables, whole wheat pita bread triangles or whole wheat crackers.

Reduce the Histamine

Omit the hot pepper flakes.

3	roasted red bell peppers (see box, page 241), skins and seeds removed	3
¾ cup	feta cheese, drained and crumbled (about 6 oz/175 g)	175 mL
½ tsp	minced garlic	2 mL
¼ tsp	hot pepper flakes	1 mL

1. In a food processor or blender, purée peppers, feta cheese, garlic and hot pepper flakes. Chill before serving.

This recipe courtesy of dietitian Helen Haresign.

Nutrients per ¼ cup (60 mL)	
Calories	58
Fat	3 g
Carbohydrate	5 g
Protein	3 g

Mint Yogurt Dip

Enjoy as a vegetable dip or a dipping sauce for grilled vegetables and meats.

Nutrients per 2 tbsp (30 mL)	
Calories	40
Fat	1 g
Carbohydrate	5 g
Protein	3 g

½	clove garlic, minced	½
2 cups	plain yogurt	500 mL
2 tbsp	chopped fresh mint (or 1 tbsp/ 15 mL dried mint or dill)	30 mL

1. In a medium bowl, combine garlic, yogurt and mint.

This recipe courtesy of dietitian Marketa Graham.

Veggie Sandwich

Makes 1 serving

This snack is quick and fun to make and is good any time of the day.

Tip
Keep washed lettuce in the fridge, along with a few carrot slivers, so kids can make this sandwich on their own when they are hungry.

Nutrients per serving	
Calories	22
Fat	2 g
Carbohydrate	1 g
Protein	1 g

1	piece red leaf lettuce (or lettuce of your choice)	1
1 tsp	cream cheese	5 mL
1	baby carrot, cut into 4 slivers	1

1. Wash lettuce and pat dry. Spread cream cheese on lettuce. Place carrot slivers up the middle of the lettuce on top of the cream cheese. Roll up lettuce.

This recipe courtesy of dietitian Patricia Wright.

Frittata di Menta

Swiss chard or peppery greens like rapini are often used as frittata fillings, as are artichoke hearts and zucchini flowers.

Tips

Adding leafy herbs to recipes reduces histamine levels.

Onion has low levels of histamine. Eating it occasionally is unlikely to trigger headaches. You could replace it with an equal amount of chopped shallots, if desired.

- **Large ovenproof skillet**

3 tbsp	olive oil, divided	45 mL
1	onion, finely chopped	1
1 cup	whole fresh mint leaves, washed and dried thoroughly	250 mL
1/4 cup	chopped flat-leaf (Italian) parsley	60 mL
8	large eggs	8
3 tbsp	fresh bread crumbs	45 mL
3 tbsp	grated pecorino Romano	45 mL
2 tsp	light (10%) cream	10 mL
2 tsp	all-purpose flour	10 mL
1/2 tsp	salt	2 mL
1/4 tsp	freshly ground black pepper	1 mL

1. In a large ovenproof skillet, heat 4 tsp (20 mL) of the olive oil over medium heat. Add onion and cook for 6 minutes or until softened. Remove from heat. Stir in mint and parsley. Transfer to a bowl and let cool. Wipe skillet clean with paper towel.

2. In another bowl, whisk together eggs, bread crumbs, pecorino Romano, cream, flour, salt and pepper. Stir in cooled onion-herb mixture.

3. Preheat broiler. Return skillet to medium heat. Add remaining olive oil, swirling to coat surface of skillet. Pour egg mixture into skillet; cook, gently running a narrow metal spatula around the edges to lift cooked egg up and allow uncooked egg to run beneath for 5 minutes or until frittata is set and cooked on the bottom.

4. Place skillet 6 inches (15 cm) beneath broiler. Cook for 2 minutes or until top is set and golden brown. Serve immediately or cooled to room temperature, cut into squares or strips.

Nutrients per 1 of 6 servings	
Calories	213
Fat	17 g
Carbohydrate	11 g
Protein	4 g

Summer Corn and Quinoa Griddle Cakes

A bite-size celebration of New World crops, these griddle cakes capture the golden sweetness of corn cut from the cob and elevate the flavor with the fragrant foundation of quinoa.

Tip
Adding leafy herbs to recipes reduces histamine levels.

⅔ cup	quinoa flour	150 mL
1 tsp	fine sea salt	5 mL
¼ tsp	freshly cracked black pepper	1 mL
3	large eggs, lightly beaten	3
1	small red bell pepper, chopped	1
1½ cups	fresh or thawed frozen corn kernels	375 mL
1 cup	cooked quinoa, cooled	250 mL
½ cup	packed fresh basil leaves, chopped	125 mL
	Olive oil	

1. In a medium bowl, whisk together quinoa flour, salt, black pepper and eggs. Gently stir in red pepper, corn, quinoa and basil.

2. In a large nonstick skillet, heat 2 tsp (10 mL) oil over medium heat. For each griddle cake, drop about ¼ cup (60 mL) batter into skillet and flatten slightly. Cook for 2 to 3 minutes per side or until browned. Transfer to a plate lined with paper towels. Repeat with the remaining batter, adding more oil and adjusting heat as necessary between batches. Serve warm or at room temperature.

Nutrients per cake	
Calories	50
Fat	2 g
Carbohydrate	6 g
Protein	2 g

Chewy Coconut Quinoa Bars

How could something that tastes so good also be good for you? Eating is believing.

Tips

Any other variety of natural nut or seed butter, such as peanut, sunflower seed or cashew butter, may be used in place of the almond butter.

If the bars crumble while you're cutting them, refrigerate for 15 to 30 minutes, until they are more firm.

Make Ahead

Store cooled bars in an airtight container at room temperature for up to 5 days. Or wrap them in plastic wrap, then foil, completely enclosing them, and freeze for up to 6 months. Defrost in the microwave until thawed. Check frequently to prevent cooking.

- Preheat oven to 350°F (180°C)
- 8-inch (20 cm) square metal baking pan, lined with foil and sprayed with nonstick cooking spray

2 cups	quinoa flakes	500 mL
2 cups	unsweetened flaked coconut	500 mL
1 tsp	ground ginger	5 mL
1/2 tsp	fine sea salt	2 mL
3/4 cup	liquid honey or brown rice syrup	175 mL
6 tbsp	coconut oil, warmed, or vegetable oil	90 mL
1/3 cup	unsweetened natural almond butter	75 mL

1. In a large bowl, combine quinoa flakes, coconut, ginger and salt.

2. In a medium bowl, whisk together honey, oil and almond butter until blended.

3. Add the honey mixture to the quinoa mixture and stir until evenly coated. Using your hands, a spatula or a large piece of waxed paper, press mixture firmly into prepared pan.

4. Bake in preheated oven for 30 to 40 minutes or until browned at the edges but still slightly soft at the center. Let cool completely in pan on a wire rack. Using foil liner, lift mixture from pan and invert onto a cutting board. Peel off foil and cut into 15 bars.

Nutrients per bar	
Calories	200
Fat	12 g
Carbohydrate	21 g
Protein	2 g

Sweet Potato Chips

Cut super-thin slices for crispy, delicious sweet potato chips!

Make Ahead
Store chips in an airtight container at room temperature for up to 1 week.

Nutrients per serving	
Calories	25
Fat	0 g
Carbohydrate	6 g
Protein	1 g

- Preheat oven to 375°F (190°C)
- 2 rimmed baking sheets, lined with parchment paper

2	medium-large sweet potatoes	2
	Nonstick cooking spray (preferably olive oil)	
¼ tsp	fine sea salt	1 mL

1. Using a very sharp knife or a mandoline, cut sweet potatoes into $1/16$-inch (2 mm) thick slices. Arrange in a single layer on prepared baking sheets. Spray with cooking spray and sprinkle with salt.

2. Bake in preheated oven for 11 to 16 minutes or until edges are golden brown. Transfer chips to a wire rack and let cool completely (they will crisp more as they cool).

Crispy Shallots

These crisp treats make a great garnish for soup or grilled meat.

- Candy/deep-fry thermometer

1½ cups	vegetable oil	375 mL
6	shallots, thinly sliced	6
	Salt	

1. In a saucepan, heat oil over medium heat until it registers 350°F (180°C) on thermometer. Add shallots, in two batches, and fry, stirring frequently, until golden brown, 3 to 4 minutes. Using a slotted spoon, remove shallots to a plate lined with paper towels. Season to taste with salt. Serve hot or let cool and use within 3 hours.

Nutrients per serving	
Calories	93
Fat	9 g
Carbohydrate	3 g
Protein	0 g

Fried Sage Leaves

These are great as a snack or as a garnish for soup.

| ¼ cup | unsalted butter | 60 mL |
| 18 | fresh sage leaves | 18 |

1. In a skillet, melt butter over medium heat. Add sage leaves and cook, turning once, until lightly browned and crispy on both sides, about 2 minutes per side. Using a slotted spoon, remove leaves to a plate lined with paper towels. The butter can be drizzled over soup or reserved for another use.

Nutrients per leaf	
Calories	27
Fat	3 g
Carbohydrate	0 g
Protein	0 g

Oven-Dried Apple Slices

Makes 12 slices

These dried apple slices make a super snack-on-the-go. Try adding them to trail mix.

Make Ahead
Store in an airtight container for up to 4 days.

- Preheat oven to 300°F (150°C)
- Baking sheet, lined with parchment paper or Silpat

| 1 | Granny Smith apple | 1 |

1. Thinly slice apple into round slices, so that you have a cross-section of the apple, leaving the core and seeds intact. (You should have at least 12 slices. Don't worry if some of the slices are not whole. They can be patched together.)

2. Arrange slices on prepared baking sheet and patch together any incomplete rounds. Bake in preheated oven until dried, 30 to 45 minutes. Check frequently and, if slices are coloring too much, reduce heat by 25°F (5°C). Let cool on sheet on a wire rack.

Nutrients per slice	
Calories	8
Fat	0 g
Carbohydrate	2 g
Protein	0 g

Agua de Manzana (Apple Water)

This fruit water has a subtle and refreshing flavor. The preparation couldn't be simpler. Make a pitcher every morning, refrigerate and watch it disappear.

Tips

For the best flavor, choose tart apples, such as Jonathan or Granny Smith.

In Peru, people leave the cores, seeds and apple pieces in the water and let them settle on the bottom of the pitcher, decanting just the water as they pour. If this troubles you, strain out the solids after the flavor has infused for 2 or 3 hours, then refrigerate the strained water.

Choose organic apples whenever possible. Pesticides, herbicides and other chemicals used on non-organic produce burden the liver and can add to hormonal and metabolic imbalances.

2	apples	2
8 cups	spring water	2 L
	Prickly pear juice	

1. Cut apples into small chunks and place in a pitcher (you can include the core, seeds and/or skin, if desired). Add spring water. Cover and refrigerate for about 2 hours, until chilled and flavor is infused, or for up to 2 days.

2. To serve, pour water into a glass and add 1 to 3 tsp (5 to 15 mL) prickly pear juice, to taste.

Nutrients per serving	
Calories	84
Fat	0 g
Carbohydrate	21 g
Protein	0 g

Blueberry Lemon Elixir

This juice is sweet and slightly spicy — a perfect thirst-quencher!

Nutrients per serving	
Calories	120
Fat	0 g
Carbohydrate	32 g
Protein	0 g

- **Blender**

1/2 cup	filtered water	125 mL
1/2 cup	blueberries	125 mL
1/4 cup	freshly squeezed lemon juice	60 mL
3 tbsp	agave nectar	45 mL
2 tsp	chopped gingerroot	10 mL

1. In blender, combine water, blueberries, lemon juice, agave nectar and ginger. Blend on high speed until smooth.

Mango Mint Mojo

The sweetness of mango and the freshness of lime juice and mint make a dynamite combination. This sauce tastes so good that you might want to eat it right out of the bowl!

Tip

If possible, prepare early in the day to allow the flavors to develop. It keeps well in the refrigerator for up to 2 days.

Nutrients per serving	
Calories	21
Fat	0 g
Carbohydrate	6 g
Protein	0 g

12	fresh mint leaves	12
1	ripe mango, peeled, pitted and chopped	1
1/2 cup	freshly squeezed lime juice	125 mL

1. In blender, on high speed, purée mint, mango and lime juice until smooth.

This recipe courtesy of Eileen Campbell.

Mango Lassi

Makes 2 servings

This refreshing drink is a favorite at Indian restaurants. Now you can make it at home to serve with the spicy recipes in this book.

Tips

If fresh mangos are not available, you may be able to find frozen mangos in the freezer section of your grocery store. Substitute 1 cup (250 mL) frozen mango chunks.

This drink keeps well in the refrigerator overnight.

1	ripe mango, peeled, pitted and chopped	1
½ cup	low-fat plain or vanilla yogurt	125 mL
½ cup	milk	125 mL
	Liquid honey	
½ cup	ice cubes	125 mL

1. In blender, on high speed, blend mango, yogurt, milk, honey to taste and ice for 2 minutes or until smooth.

This recipe courtesy of Eileen Campbell.

Mangos

If you'll be using the mango right away, be sure to buy a ripe one. Mangos are ripe when they can be easily indented with your thumb. Avoid mangos that are so ripe they feel mushy.

Mangos have large, flat stones in the middle. It is a little tricky to remove the fruit, but if you follow these simple instructions, the task should be easier: Make an initial cut about ½ inch (1 cm) from the center and cut off a long slice of mango. Do the same on the other side. For each of these pieces, use a sharp knife to score the flesh in long lines, first lengthwise, then crossways, cutting almost through to the skin to create small cubes. Using a spoon, scoop cubes from skin. Peel the stone section, remove any flesh from the outside edges and cut into cubes.

Nutrients per serving	
Calories	190
Fat	3 g
Carbohydrate	39 g
Protein	6 g

Iron-Builder Juice

Juicers make it so easy to get a ton of nutrients in a tasty drink!

Variation

Substitute 1 head of romaine lettuce or 1 bunch spinach or arugula for the Swiss chard.

Nutrients per serving	
Calories	50
Fat	0 g
Carbohydrate	11 g
Protein	1 g

- Juicer

3	large red beets, sliced, divided	3
4	carrots, sliced, divided	4
1/2	bunch Swiss chard or beet greens, divided	1/2
1	small apple, sliced, divided	1

1. In juicer, process one-quarter of the beets, 1 carrot, one-quarter of the chard and one-quarter of the apple. Repeat until all the vegetables have been juiced. Whisk well and serve immediately.

Eat Your Greens Smoothie

Makes 3 servings

This smoothie is an excellent source of bone-building nutrients.

Variations

Substitute chopped papaya or pear for the mango.

Replace the lettuce with arugula, spinach or mustard greens.

Nutrients per serving	
Calories	110
Fat	2 g
Carbohydrate	23 g
Protein	3 g

- Blender

1 cup	enriched hemp milk	250 mL
1/2 cup	chopped peeled mango	125 mL
1/2 cup	chopped trimmed kale	125 mL
1/4 cup	chopped romaine lettuce	60 mL
1/4 cup	chopped fresh parsley or cilantro	60 mL
1	banana	1
1	chopped pitted date	1

1. In blender, combine hemp milk, mango, kale, lettuce, parsley, banana and date. Blend on high speed until smooth.

Soups

Vegetable Stock

Here's the perfect stock for vegetarians. It keeps for up to 6 months if frozen in airtight containers.

Tip

Onion has low levels of histamine. Eating it occasionally is unlikely to trigger headaches. You could replace it with an equal amount of chopped shallots, if desired.

6 cups	water	1.5 L
1	large sweet potato, diced	1
2	large celery stalks, chopped	2
2	large leeks, cleaned and sliced	2
1	large onion, chopped	1
½ cup	chopped parsley	125 mL
2	large cloves garlic	2
2	bay leaves	2
¼ tsp	freshly ground black pepper	1 mL
⅛ tsp	salt	0.5 mL

1. In a saucepan over medium-high heat, combine water, potato, celery, leeks, onion, parsley, garlic, bay leaves, pepper and salt; bring to a boil. Reduce heat to low; simmer, covered, for $1\frac{1}{2}$ hours.

2. Pour mixture through a strainer; discard solids. Refrigerate stock until cold. Stock can be kept, refrigerated, for up to 3 days or frozen in an airtight container.

Nutrients per 1 cup (250 mL)	
Calories	8
Fat	0 g
Carbohydrate	2 g
Protein	0 g

Chilled Melon Soup with Ginger and Lime

This delicious soup is perfect for a hot summer day. It can be the main dish in an elegant lunch or poured into a tall glass for a nutrient-packed cocktail. For an impressive presentation, garnish with edible flower petals.

Tip

Purée melon in a food processor or blender to make about 4 cups (1 L) when making this recipe.

2 cups	white wine	500 mL
¼ cup	grated lime zest	60 mL
2 tbsp	lime juice	30 mL
2 tbsp	liquid honey	30 mL
3 tbsp	grated gingerroot	45 mL
1	large honeydew melon, peeled, seeded, cut into chunks and puréed	1

1. In a saucepan, combine wine, lime zest and juice, honey and ginger; bring to a boil. Reduce heat and simmer, uncovered, until reduced by half. Cool to room temperature. Strain through a fine sieve.

2. Add melon purée to wine mixture. Chill thoroughly.

This recipe courtesy of chef Kenneth Peace and dietitian Maye Musk.

Nutrients per serving	
Calories	97
Fat	0 g
Carbohydrate	22 g
Protein	1 g

Cold Mango Soup

This refreshing soup showcases sweet mangos.

Tips

Try to ensure that the mango is ripe. If not, add some sugar to taste.

This soup can be frozen for up to 3 weeks.

Onion has low levels of histamine. Eating it occasionally is unlikely to trigger headaches. You could replace it with an equal amount of chopped shallots, if desired.

Make Ahead

Prepare and refrigerate up to 2 days before.

- **Food processor**

2 tsp	vegetable oil	10 mL
½ cup	chopped onions	125 mL
2 tsp	minced garlic	10 mL
2 cups	Vegetable Stock (page 218) or ready-to-use vegetable broth	500 mL
2½ cups	chopped ripe mango (about 2 large), divided	625 mL

Garnish (Optional)

2% plain yogurt
Fresh cilantro leaves

1. In a nonstick saucepan, heat oil over medium heat. Add onions and garlic; cook, stirring, for 4 minutes or until browned.

2. Add stock. Bring to a boil; reduce heat to medium-low and cook for 5 minutes or until onions are soft.

3. Transfer mixture to a food processor. Add 2 cups (500 mL) of the mango. Purée until smooth. Stir in remaining chopped mango.

4. Chill 2 hours or until cold. If desired, serve with a dollop of yogurt and garnish with cilantro.

Nutrients per serving	
Calories	99
Fat	3 g
Carbohydrate	20 g
Protein	1 g

Dill Carrot Soup

This delicious soup is great for keeping colds away.

Tips

This soup can be served hot or cold.

A dollop of yogurt on each bowlful enhances both the appearance and flavor.

Make Ahead

Make and refrigerate up to a day before. If serving warm, reheat gently.

- Food processor

1 lb	carrots, sliced (6 to 8 medium)	500 g
2 tsp	vegetable oil	10 mL
2 tsp	crushed garlic	10 mL
1 cup	chopped onion	250 mL
3½ cups	ready-to-use chicken broth	875 mL
¾ cup	2% milk	175 mL
2 tbsp	chopped fresh dill (or 1 tsp/5 mL dried dillweed)	30 mL
2 tbsp	chopped fresh chives or green onions	30 mL

1. In large saucepan of boiling water, cook carrots just until tender. Drain and return to saucepan; set aside.

2. In nonstick skillet, heat oil; sauté garlic and onion until softened, approximately 5 minutes. Add to carrots along with broth; cover and simmer for 25 minutes.

3. Purée in food processor until smooth, in batches if necessary. Return to saucepan; stir in milk, dill and chives.

Nutrients per 1 of 6 servings	
Calories	96
Fat	3 g
Carbohydrate	12 g
Protein	5 g

Carrot, Sweet Potato and Parsnip Soup

Here's a smooth-textured soup with beautiful color. It is full of vitamins and will stick to your ribs!

Tips

You can substitute all carrots for the parsnips or vice versa.

Onion has low levels of histamine. Eating it occasionally is unlikely to trigger headaches. You could replace it with an equal amount of chopped shallots, if desired.

Adding leafy herbs to recipes reduces histamine levels.

Make Ahead

Make and refrigerate up to a day before and reheat before serving, adding more broth if too thick.

- Food processor

2 tsp	vegetable oil	10 mL
1 tsp	crushed garlic	5 mL
1 cup	chopped onion	250 mL
3½ cups	ready-to-use chicken broth	825 mL
1	small potato, peeled and chopped	1
¾ cup	chopped carrots	175 mL
¾ cup	chopped peeled sweet potato	175 mL
½ cup	chopped peeled parsnip	125 mL
2 tbsp	chopped fresh dill (or 1 tsp/5 mL dried dillweed)	30 mL

1. In medium nonstick saucepan, heat oil; sauté garlic and onion for approximately 5 minutes or until softened.

2. Add broth, potato, carrots, sweet potato and parsnip; reduce heat, cover and simmer for 30 to 40 minutes or until vegetables are tender.

3. Purée in food processor until creamy and smooth. Stir in dill.

Nutrients per serving	
Calories	149
Fat	4 g
Carbohydrate	23 g
Protein	6 g

Roasted Cauliflower Soup

Get ready: with its sublime balance of spices, subtle sweetness and buttery, velvety texture, this seemingly simple soup has a serious wow factor.

Tips

When puréeing the soup in a food processor or blender, fill the bowl no more than halfway full at a time.

Store the cooled soup in an airtight container in the refrigerator for up to 2 days or in the freezer for up to 6 months. Thaw in the microwave using the Defrost function. Warm soup in a medium saucepan over medium-low heat.

Lemon has low histamine levels. Occasional or small amounts are unlikely to trigger headaches.

- Preheat oven to 450°F (230°C)
- Large rimmed baking sheet, lined with foil and sprayed with nonstick cooking spray (preferably olive oil)
- Food processor, blender or immersion blender

6 cups	cauliflower florets (about 1 large head)	1.5 L
4 tsp	extra virgin olive oil, divided	20 mL
½ tsp	fine sea salt, divided	2 mL
2 cups	chopped onions	500 mL
2 tsp	ground cumin	10 mL
2 cups	ready-to-use reduced-sodium chicken or vegetable broth	500 mL
4 cups	water	1 L
1 tbsp	freshly squeezed lemon juice	15 mL
¼ cup	packed fresh parsley leaves, roughly chopped	60 mL

1. On prepared baking sheet, toss cauliflower with half the oil and half the salt. Spread in a single layer. Roast in preheated oven for 35 to 40 minutes, stirring occasionally, until golden-brown and tender.

2. Meanwhile, in a large saucepan, heat the remaining oil over medium-high heat. Add onions and cook, stirring, for 6 to 8 minutes or until softened.

3. Stir in roasted cauliflower, cumin, the remaining salt, broth and water. Bring to a boil. Reduce heat and simmer, stirring occasionally, for 20 minutes or until cauliflower is very soft.

4. Working in batches, transfer soup to food processor (or use immersion blender in pot) and purée until smooth. Return soup to pan (if necessary) and whisk in lemon juice. Warm over medium heat, stirring, for 1 minute. Serve sprinkled with parsley.

Nutrients per serving	
Calories	63
Fat	3 g
Carbohydrate	9 g
Protein	2 g

Red Onion and Grilled Red Pepper Soup

This naturally sweet soup is high in fiber.

Tips

Sweet bell peppers and red onions make this a naturally sweet-tasting soup. Sugar may not be necessary.

Start with the lesser amount of stock, adding more to reach the consistency you prefer.

Adding leafy herbs to recipes reduces histamine levels.

Make Ahead

Prepare up to 2 days in advance. Add more stock if too thick. Freeze up to 4 weeks.

• **Preheat oven to broil**

3	large red bell peppers	3
2 tsp	vegetable oil	10 mL
2 tsp	minced garlic	10 mL
1 tbsp	packed brown sugar	15 mL
5 cups	thinly sliced red onions	1.25 L
3 to 3½ cups	Vegetable Stock (page 218) or ready-to-use vegetable broth	750 to 875 mL

Garnish

⅓ cup	chopped fresh basil or parsley	75 mL
	Light sour cream (optional)	

1. Arrange oven rack 6 inches (15 cm) under element. Cook peppers on baking sheet, turning occasionally, 20 minutes or until charred. Cool. Discard stem, skin and seeds; cut peppers into thin strips. Set aside.

2. In a large nonstick saucepan, heat oil over medium-low heat. Add garlic, brown sugar and red onions; cook, stirring occasionally, for 15 minutes or until onions are browned. Stir in stock and red pepper strips; cook for 15 minutes longer.

3. In a blender or food processor, purée soup until smooth. Serve hot, garnished with chopped basil or parsley and a dollop of sour cream, if desired.

Nutrients per serving	
Calories	129
Fat	3 g
Carbohydrate	25 g
Protein	3 g

Red and Yellow Bell Pepper Soup

Two soups in one bowl!

Tips

If desired, cilantro can be added before puréeing for a more intense flavor.

Orange peppers can be used instead of red or yellow.

Roasted peppers in a jar (packed in water) can replace fresh peppers. Use about 4 oz (125 g) peppers in a jar for each fresh pepper required.

Make Ahead

Roast peppers earlier in the day and set aside.

Prepare both soups earlier in the day, and keep them separate until serving.

Reduce the Histamine
Substitute sweet potatoes for the potatoes.

- Preheat broiler
- Food processor

2	red bell peppers	2
2	yellow bell peppers	2
2 tsp	vegetable oil	10 mL
2 tsp	minced garlic	10 mL
1½ cups	chopped onions	375 mL
1¼ cups	chopped carrots	300 mL
½ cup	chopped celery	125 mL
4 cups	ready-to-use chicken or vegetable broth	1 L
1½ cups	diced peeled potatoes	375 mL
	Freshly ground black pepper	
¼ cup	chopped fresh cilantro, dill or basil	60 mL

1. Roast the peppers under the broiler for 15 to 20 minutes, turning several times until charred on all sides. Place in a bowl covered tightly with plastic wrap; let stand until cool enough to handle. Remove skin, stem and seeds.

2. In a nonstick saucepan sprayed with vegetable spray, heat oil over medium heat. Add garlic, onion, carrots and celery; cook for 8 minutes or until vegetables are softened, stirring occasionally. Add broth and potatoes; bring to a boil. Reduce heat to low; cover and let cook for 20 to 25 minutes or until carrots and potatoes are tender.

3. Put the red peppers in food processor and process until smooth. Add half of the soup mixture to the red pepper purée and process until smooth. Season with pepper and pour into serving bowl. Rinse out food processor. Put yellow peppers in food processor and process until smooth; add remaining soup to yellow pepper purée and process until smooth. Season to taste with pepper and pour into another serving bowl. To serve, ladle some of the red pepper soup into one side of individual bowl while at the same time ladling some of the yellow pepper soup into the other side of the bowl. Add cilantro to soup and serve.

Nutrients per serving	
Calories	99
Fat	2 g
Carbohydrate	19 g
Protein	3 g

Thai-Style Squash Soup

Garlic, ginger, lemongrass, lime and coconut milk bring the flavors of Thailand to your dinner table.

Tips

For convenience, buy a jar of minced ginger.

If you can't find wild lime leaves locally, substitute grated lime zest (3 leaves = the zest of 1 lime).

Variation

If you are lucky enough to have any leftovers, this soup is great as a sauce over grilled fish, chicken or pork.

● **Preheat oven to 350°F (180°C)**

1	head garlic	1
1 tbsp	olive oil	15 mL
2 tbsp	vegetable oil	30 mL
1	onion, diced	1
2 tbsp	finely minced gingerroot	30 mL
2 tbsp	finely minced lemongrass	30 mL
1	large butternut squash, peeled, seeded and diced	1
3¼ cups	ready-to-use reduced-sodium chicken broth	800 mL
1	can (14 oz/398 mL) light coconut milk	1
	Salt and freshly ground black pepper	
4	wild lime leaves (optional)	4

1. Cut top off head of garlic to expose the cloves. Place on a small piece of foil. Drizzle with olive oil. Cover with foil and bake in preheated oven for 30 minutes or until cloves are soft.

2. Meanwhile, in a large saucepan, heat vegetable oil over medium heat. Sauté onion, ginger and lemongrass until tender, about 5 minutes. Add squash and broth; bring to a boil. Reduce heat, cover and simmer for 30 minutes. Remove from heat. Squeeze roasted garlic into soup, making sure not to get any skin in soup.

3. Working in batches, transfer soup to blender and purée on high speed until smooth.

4. Return soup to saucepan and stir in coconut milk. Season to taste with salt and pepper. Add wild lime leaves, if using. Heat over low heat for 10 minutes or until heated through and lime flavor infuses soup.

This recipe courtesy of Eileen Campbell.

Nutrients per serving	
Calories	118
Fat	6 g
Carbohydrate	16 g
Protein	2 g

Squash and Carrot Soup

You're sure to enjoy this warm and creamy root-based soup.

Tips

Start with the smaller amount of broth, adding more if soup is too thick.

Choose yogurt over light sour cream for the garnish, as sour cream can increase histamine levels.

Make Ahead

Prepare up to 2 days in advance. Reheat, adding extra broth if necessary. Freeze up to 4 weeks.

2 tsp	vegetable oil	10 mL
1½ tsp	minced garlic	7 mL
1½ cups	sliced leeks	375 mL
6 cups	chopped butternut squash (about 1¾ lb/875 g)	1.5 L
3½ to 4½ cups	Vegetable Stock (page 218) or ready-to-use vegetable broth	875 mL to 1.125 L
1 cup	diced carrots	250 mL
½ tsp	dried thyme	2 mL

Garnish (Optional)

2% plain yogurt or light sour cream

1. In a nonstick saucepan sprayed with vegetable spray, heat oil over medium-low heat. Stir in garlic and leeks; cook, covered, for 5 minutes or until softened.

2. Stir in squash, broth (see tip, at left), carrots and thyme. Bring to a boil; reduce heat to medium-low, cover and cook for 12 to 15 minutes or until vegetables are tender.

3. Transfer soup to a food processor or blender. Purée until smooth. If desired, serve with a dollop of yogurt or sour cream.

Nutrients per 1 of 6 servings	
Calories	106
Fat	2 g
Carbohydrate	23 g
Protein	2 g

Winter Squash Quinoa Bisque

This easy-to-prepare squash soup is a delicious way to warm up on a cold day.

Tip

Onion has low levels of histamine. Eating it occasionally is unlikely to trigger headaches. You could replace it with an equal amount of chopped shallots, if desired.

Make Ahead

Store the cooled soup in an airtight container in the refrigerator for up to 2 days or in the freezer for up to 6 months. Thaw in the microwave using the Defrost function. Warm soup in a medium saucepan over medium-low heat.

Variation

Use 3 cups (750 mL) canned pumpkin purée (not pie filling) in place of the frozen winter squash purée.

1 tbsp	unsalted butter	15 mL
1¼ cups	minced onions	300 mL
½ cup	quinoa flakes or quinoa flour	125 mL
1½ tsp	dried thyme	7 mL
2	packages (each 12 oz/375 g) frozen winter squash purée, thawed	2
4 cups	ready-to-use reduced-sodium chicken or vegetable broth	1 L
	Fine sea salt and freshly ground black pepper	
3 tbsp	minced fresh chives (optional)	45 mL

1. In a large pot, melt butter over medium-high heat. Add onions and cook, stirring, for 5 to 6 minutes or until softened.

2. Stir in quinoa flakes, thyme, squash and broth; bring to a boil. Reduce heat to low, cover and simmer, stirring occasionally, for 25 to 30 minutes or until thickened. Season to taste with salt and pepper. Serve sprinkled with chives, if desired.

Nutrients per serving	
Calories	187
Fat	3 g
Carbohydrate	34 g
Protein	6 g

Santa Fe Sweet Potato Soup

This yummy soup has a gorgeous color and is sure to satisfy the heat-lovers in your family.

Make Ahead

This soup can be assembled the night before it is cooked. Follow preparation directions in steps 1 and 2. Cover and refrigerate overnight. The next day, continue cooking as directed in steps 3 and 4.

Reduce the Histamine

Slow cooking increases histamine levels in food, so if you have a response to a slow-cooked recipe, try cooking it on the stovetop or in the oven instead.

Omit the chile peppers. Place the hot pepper sauce, hot pepper flakes or pepper grinder on the table so diners can spice up their soup to taste.

- **Slow cooker**

2	dried New Mexico chile peppers	2
2 cups	boiling water	500 mL
1 tbsp	vegetable oil	15 mL
2	onions, finely chopped	2
4	cloves garlic, minced	4
1	finely chopped jalapeño pepper (optional)	1
1 tsp	salt (optional)	5 mL
1 tsp	dried oregano	5 mL
4 cups	cubed peeled sweet potatoes (½-inch/1 cm cubes)	1 L
6 cups	ready-to-use vegetable or chicken broth	1.5 L
2 cups	corn kernels (thawed if frozen)	500 mL
1 tsp	grated lime zest	5 mL
2 tbsp	freshly squeezed lime juice	30 mL
2	roasted red bell peppers (see box, page 241), cut into thin strips	2
	Finely chopped cilantro	

1. In a heatproof bowl, soak chiles in boiling water for 30 minutes. Drain, discarding soaking liquid and stems. Pat dry, chop finely and set aside.

2. In a skillet, heat oil over medium heat. Add onions and cook, stirring, until softened. Add garlic, jalapeño (if using), salt (if using), oregano and reserved chiles and cook, stirring, for 1 minute. Transfer mixture to slow cooker stoneware. Add sweet potatoes and broth and stir to combine.

3. Cover and cook on Low for 8 to 10 hours or on High for 4 to 6 hours, until sweet potatoes are tender. Strain vegetables, reserving broth. In a blender or food processor, purée vegetables with 1 cup (250 mL) reserved broth until smooth. Return mixture, along with reserved broth, to slow cooker stoneware. Or, using a hand-held blender, purée the soup in stoneware. Add corn, lime zest and juice. Cover and cook on High for 20 minutes, until corn is tender.

4. When ready to serve, ladle soup into individual bowls and garnish with red pepper strips and cilantro.

Nutrients per serving	
Calories	175
Fat	3 g
Carbohydrate	31 g
Protein	7 g

Harvest Vegetable Barley Soup

Here's a hearty soup that will both fill you up and warm you up.

Tips

Using a commercially prepared low-sodium chicken or vegetable broth reduces the sodium content of this recipe from 1051 mg to 727 mg.

If you have time to make the Vegetable Stock on page 218, you can reduce the sodium to 127 mg/serving — a savings of 600 mg!

2 tbsp	margarine or butter	30 mL
1	large onion, chopped	1
3	cloves garlic, finely chopped	3
1½ cups	diced peeled rutabaga	375 mL
½ tsp	dried thyme or marjoram	2 mL
8 cups	ready-to-use reduced-sodium chicken or vegetable broth (approx.)	2 L
½ cup	pearl barley, rinsed	125 mL
1½ cups	diced peeled sweet potatoes	375 mL
1½ cups	diced zucchini	375 mL
	Salt and freshly ground black pepper	

1. In a large Dutch oven or stockpot, melt butter over medium heat. Add onion, garlic, rutabaga and thyme; cook, stirring often, for 5 minutes or until vegetables are lightly colored.

2. Stir in broth and barley; bring to a boil. Reduce heat, cover and simmer for 20 minutes. Add sweet potatoes and zucchini; simmer, covered, for 15 minutes or until barley is tender. Season to taste with salt and pepper.

Nutrients per serving	
Calories	231
Fat	6 g
Carbohydrate	34 g
Protein	11 g

Black Bean Soup

No recipe collection is complete without a black bean soup recipe!

Tip

Canned black beans can sometimes be difficult to find. Use 12 oz (375 g) cooked beans. One cup (250 mL) of dry beans yields approximately 3 cups (750 mL) cooked. Plan to soak the beans overnight before cooking them, as this will help reduce the histamine.

Make Ahead

Prepare and refrigerate up to a day ahead and reheat gently before serving, adding more broth if too thick.

- Food processor

2 tsp	vegetable oil	10 mL
2 tsp	minced garlic	10 mL
1 cup	chopped onions	250 mL
1 cup	chopped carrots	250 mL
1	can (19 oz/540 mL) black beans, drained (or 12 oz/375 g cooked beans)	1
3 cups	ready-to-use chicken broth	750 mL
¾ tsp	ground cumin	3 mL
¼ cup	chopped fresh cilantro or parsley	60 mL

1. In a nonstick saucepan sprayed with vegetable spray, heat oil over medium heat; add garlic, onions and carrots and cook, stirring occasionally, for 4 minutes or until the onion is softened.

2. Add beans, broth and cumin; bring to a boil. Cover, reduce heat to medium-low and simmer for 20 minutes or until carrots are softened. Transfer to food processor and purée until smooth.

3. Ladle into bowls; sprinkle with cilantro.

Nutrients per 1 of 5 servings	
Calories	147
Fat	3 g
Carbohydrate	25 g
Protein	8 g

Chicken Soup
with Roasted Vegetables

Roasted root vegetables are sweet and hearty and make this soup the perfect ending to a cold fall or winter day.

Tips

Size really does matter in this recipe. With disciplined dice, the vegetables cook more evenly, and the uniformly chopped vegetables make for a nice texture and a more attractive soup.

Soup will stay hot much longer in a heated bowl.

Onion has low levels of histamine. Eating it occasionally is unlikely to trigger headaches. You could replace it with an equal amount of chopped shallots, if desired.

- Preheat oven to 450°F (230°C)
- 2 large rimmed baking sheets

1	whole chicken (about 3 lbs/1.5 kg) or 3 lbs (1.5 kg) skinless chicken thighs	1
2	stalks celery, including leafy tops, cut into large chunks	2
1	large onion (unpeeled), halved	1
1	large carrot, quartered	1
8 cups	ready-to-use chicken broth	2 L
4	sprigs fresh thyme	4
1	bay leaf	1
1/3 cup	olive oil	75 mL
2	parsnips, cut into 1/2-inch (1 cm) dice	2
2	carrots, cut into 1/2-inch (1 cm) dice	2
2	onions, cut into 1/2-inch (1 cm) thick wedges	2
1	large sweet potato, cut into 1/2-inch (1 cm) dice	1
1	large bulb fennel, cut into 1/2-inch (1 cm) thick wedges	1
1 tsp	salt	5 mL
1/2 tsp	freshly ground black pepper	2 mL
1/2 cup	chopped fresh parsley	125 mL
	Garlic Croutons (see variation, page 250)	

1. In a large pot, combine chicken, celery, halved onion, quartered carrot, broth, thyme and bay leaf. If chicken isn't immersed, add water or broth to cover. Bring to a boil over medium-high heat. Partially cover, reduce heat to low and simmer gently until a thermometer inserted into the thickest part of a breast registers 170°F (77°C), about 45 minutes. Skim the soup if any scum develops on the surface.

Nutrients per serving	
Calories	417
Fat	17 g
Carbohydrate	51 g
Protein	15 g

2. Meanwhile, drizzle baking sheets evenly with oil. Divide parsnips, carrots, onion wedges, sweet potato and fennel between the two sheets. Season with salt and pepper; toss to coat and spread in a single layer. Roast in preheated oven, turning occasionally, until just tender and brown in spots, about 40 minutes.

3. Using tongs, transfer chicken to a large plate and let cool slightly. Remove skin and bones and discard. Shred the meat into bite-size pieces. Set aside.

4. Strain the stock and discard all solids. Skim the surface of the stock and remove fat, if desired. Return stock to pot and bring to a simmer over medium heat. Add roasted vegetables and simmer until tender, about 10 minutes. Add reserved chicken and parsley; heat until steaming, about 5 minutes.

5. Ladle into heated bowls and garnish with croutons.

Chickpea Soup

Makes 6 to 8 servings

This simple recipe is a great accompaniment to any meal.

Tip
A 19-oz (540 mL) can of chickpeas will yield about 2 cups (500 mL) once the beans are drained and rinsed.

Nutrients per 1 of 8 servings	
Calories	190
Fat	1 g
Carbohydrate	40 g
Protein	6 g

8	small potatoes, cut into bite-size pieces	8
4 cups	ready-to-use reduced-sodium vegetable or chicken broth	1 L
2 cups	rinsed drained canned chickpeas	500 mL
1/2 tsp	dried rosemary	2 mL

1. In a large pot, combine potatoes, broth, chickpeas, rosemary and 4 cups (1 L) water. Bring to a boil over medium-high heat. Cover, leaving lid ajar, reduce heat to low and simmer, stirring occasionally, for 30 minutes or until potatoes are tender (or for up to 1 hour if you prefer a very soft texture).

Gingery Chicken and Wild Rice Soup

The addition of a flavorful whole grain, leeks and a hint of ginger is a particularly delicious spin on classic chicken and rice soup. Make the stock a day ahead so it can be refrigerated, which makes easy work of skimming off the fat (see tip, below). This makes a great light dinner accompanied by whole-grain rolls and a tossed salad.

Tip

For best results, make the stock and cook the chicken the day before you plan to serve the soup. Cover and refrigerate stock and chicken separately. The fat will rise to the surface of the stock and can be easily removed. It will be easy to remove the skin and chop the cold chicken. Save the excess chicken to make sandwiches or a salad.

1	whole chicken (about 3 lbs/1.5 kg), cut into pieces	1
1	onion, coarsely chopped	1
2	carrots, peeled and diced	2
2	stalks celery, diced	2
4	sprigs parsley	4
1	clove garlic	1
1	bay leaf	1
1/2 tsp	salt	2 mL
1/2 tsp	cracked black peppercorns	2 mL
12 cups	water	3 L
1 tbsp	olive oil	15 mL
2	large leeks, white parts only, cleaned and sliced	2
2	cloves garlic, minced	2
2 tbsp	minced gingerroot	30 mL
1 cup	brown and wild rice mixture, rinsed and drained	250 mL

1. In a stockpot, combine chicken, onion, carrots, celery, parsley, whole garlic, bay leaf, salt, peppercorns and water. Bring to a boil over high heat. Using a slotted spoon, skim off foam. Reduce heat to medium-low and simmer, uncovered, until chicken is falling off the bone, about 1 1/2 hours. Drain, reserving chicken and liquid separately. Let cool. Cut the chicken into bite-size pieces, discarding skin and bones. Skim off fat from the stock (see tip, at left).

Nutrients per serving	
Calories	269
Fat	8 g
Carbohydrate	27 g
Protein	22 g

Onion has low levels of histamine. Eating it occasionally is unlikely to trigger headaches. You could replace it with an equal amount of chopped shallots, if desired.

Variation

Substitute an equal quantity of rinsed wild rice for the mixture. You may need to increase the cooking time, depending upon the size of the grains.

2. Measure 2 cups (500 mL) of chicken and set aside in the refrigerator. (Refrigerate remainder for other uses; see tip, at left.) In a large saucepan or stockpot, heat oil over medium heat for 30 seconds. Add leeks and cook, stirring, until softened, about 5 minutes. Add minced garlic and ginger and cook, stirring, for 1 minute. Add rice and toss to coat. Add reserved stock and bring to a boil. Reduce heat and simmer, uncovered, until rice is quite tender, about 1 hour. Add reserved chicken. Cover and simmer until chicken is heated through, about 15 minutes.

Chicken and Corn Chowder

The evaporated milk gives this creamy soup a richness that suggests it is higher in fat than it actually is. The addition of sweet potato and red pepper helps increase your intake of beta carotene and vitamin C.

Tips

When using margarine, choose a non-hydrogenated version to limit consumption of trans fats.

Onion has low levels of histamine. Eating it occasionally is unlikely to trigger headaches. You could replace it with an equal amount of chopped shallots, if desired.

1 tbsp	margarine	15 mL
1 cup	diced onion	250 mL
1 cup	diced celery	250 mL
½ cup	diced red bell pepper	125 mL
1	boneless skinless chicken breast (about 4 oz/125 g), cubed	1
4 cups	ready-to-use reduced-sodium chicken broth	1 L
1 cup	diced peeled sweet potato	250 mL
1 cup	frozen corn kernels, thawed	250 mL
1	can (14 oz/385 mL) evaporated milk	1
1 tbsp	chopped fresh parsley	15 mL

1. In a large saucepan, melt margarine over medium heat. Sauté onion, celery and red pepper until softened, about 5 minutes. Add chicken, broth, sweet potato and corn; bring to a boil. Reduce heat, cover and simmer for 25 minutes or until chicken and potatoes are cooked through. Add evaporated milk and parsley; heat over low heat (do not boil or milk will curdle).

This recipe courtesy of Eileen Campbell.

Reduce the Histamine

Replace the evaporated milk with 1½ cups (375 mL) half-and-half (10%) or light (5%) cream.

Cut the kernels off cooked fresh corn instead of using frozen corn.

Nutrients per serving	
Calories	118
Fat	3 g
Carbohydrate	14 g
Protein	10 g

Salads and Dressings

Cabbage and Carrot Slaw

This traditional coleslaw is an especially great salad to make for a potluck — it travels well because it does not contain any mayonnaise.

2 cups	thinly sliced cabbage	500 mL
1 cup	small carrot strips	250 mL
2 tbsp	cider vinegar	30 mL
1 tbsp	extra virgin olive oil	15 mL
	Salt and freshly ground black pepper	

1. In a salad bowl, combine cabbage and carrots.

2. Add vinegar and oil and toss to combine. Season lightly with salt and pepper. Cover and refrigerate for at least 1 hour before serving.

Nutrients per serving

Calories	60
Fat	4 g
Carbohydrate	5 g
Protein	1 g

Shaved Beet Salad with Pistachios and Goat Cheese

Here's a fantastic salad for any beet-lover!

Reduce the Histamine

Replace the pistachios with almonds.

Use farmer's cheese or mozzarella instead of goat cheese.

2 tbsp	freshly squeezed lemon juice	30 mL
2 tbsp	extra virgin olive oil	30 mL
2 tsp	agave nectar or liquid honey	10 mL
1/4 tsp	fine sea salt	1 mL
4	orange, yellow or red beets	4
4 cups	packed arugula	1 L
1/4 cup	crumbled soft goat cheese	60 mL
2 tbsp	chopped toasted pistachios	30 mL

1. In a small bowl, whisk together lemon juice, oil, agave nectar and salt.

2. Using a vegetable peeler, peel beets, then shave them into ribbons.

3. Arrange arugula on a large platter. top with beets, goat cheese and pistachios. Drizzle with dressing.

Nutrients per serving

Calories	161
Fat	11 g
Carbohydrate	13 g
Protein	4 g

Gingered Carrot and Quinoa Salad

Carrots and quinoa take on an exotic twist with the flavors of ginger and chile pepper in this easy-to-prepare salad. Quinoa has a subtle sesame flavor already; adding toasted sesame seeds to the salad enhances it.

Tip

For a spicier salad, leave in some or all of the serrano seeds.

Reduce the Histamine

Omit the serrano or jalapeño pepper.

Replace the rice vinegar with cider vinegar.

2 cups	cooked quinoa, cooled	500 mL
2 cups	coarsely shredded carrots	500 mL
1 cup	thinly sliced green onions	250 mL
1 tbsp	grated gingerroot	15 mL
1 tsp	minced seeded serrano or jalapeño pepper	5 mL
3 tbsp	unseasoned rice vinegar	45 mL
1½ tbsp	vegetable oil	22 mL
2 tsp	liquid honey	10 mL
	Fine sea salt and freshly cracked black pepper	
2 tbsp	toasted sesame seeds (optional)	30 mL

1. In a large bowl, combine quinoa, carrots and green onions.

2. In a small bowl, whisk together ginger, serrano pepper, vinegar, oil and honey. Add to quinoa mixture and gently toss to coat. Season to taste with salt and pepper. Cover and refrigerate for at least 30 minutes, until chilled, or for up to 2 hours.

3. Just before serving, sprinkle with sesame seeds, if desired.

Nutrients per serving	
Calories	205
Fat	1 g
Carbohydrate	46 g
Protein	3 g

Cool Cucumber Salad

This creamy salad is a perfect palate cooler to serve with any spicy meat or poultry dish.

Tips

Yogurt cheese, which is lower in fat than traditional cream cheese, has many uses. Use it instead of cream cheese in dips and salad dressings or as a spread for bagels.

Use this salad as an accompaniment to spicy dishes.

3 cups	thinly sliced English cucumber (unpeeled), about 1 large	750 mL
½ tsp	salt	2 mL
½ cup	yogurt cheese (see box, below)	125 mL
½ tsp	lemon juice	2 mL
¼ tsp	minced garlic	1 mL
¼ tsp	ground ginger	1 mL

1. Place cucumber slices in a large colander; sprinkle with salt. Let stand for 10 to 15 minutes over a large bowl (or in the sink) to drain. Rinse well under cold water. Pat dry and transfer to a bowl. Set aside.

2. In a separate bowl, blend together yogurt cheese, lemon juice, garlic and ginger. Add mixture to cucumber; toss gently. Chill before serving.

This recipe courtesy of Erna Braun.

To Make 1 cup (250 mL) Yogurt Cheese

Use 2 cups (500 mL) lower-fat plain yogurt (Balkan-style, not stirred, made without gelatin). Line a sieve with a double thickness of paper towel or cheesecloth. Pour yogurt into the sieve and place over a bowl. Cover well with plastic wrap and refrigerate for at least 2 hours. Discard liquid and keep solids in an airtight container in the refrigerator for up to 1 week.

If you want to drain the yogurt overnight, use 3 cups (750 mL) yogurt to get 1 cup (250 mL) yogurt cheese. The longer you drain the yogurt, the more tart it becomes.

Nutrients per serving	
Calories	27
Fat	1 g
Carbohydrate	3 g
Protein	2 g

Roasted Red Pepper Salad

This attractive salad makes a great accompaniment to any grilled meat. Red peppers are rich in phytochemicals and antioxidants such as beta-carotene and vitamin C.

Tips

Keep roasted red peppers in your freezer and you can make this salad anytime.

Adding leafy herbs to recipes reduces histamine levels.

6	roasted red bell peppers (see box, below), each cut into 6 strips	6
1 tbsp	balsamic or red wine vinegar	15 mL
2 tsp	olive oil	10 mL
2 tbsp	chopped fresh basil (optional)	30 mL
	Freshly ground black pepper	

1. Arrange peppers in the bottom of a serving dish.

2. In a bowl, whisk together vinegar and olive oil; drizzle over peppers. Sprinkle with basil (if using). Season with pepper to taste. Chill for 1 hour.

This recipe courtesy of Nikola Ajdacic.

To Roast Peppers

Heat barbecue or broiler; place peppers on grill or broiling pan and cook. Keep turning peppers until skins are blistered and black. Place roasted peppers in large pot with lid. Steam will make them sweat, and skin will be easier to peel off. Let peppers cool. Remove stems, seeds and skin.

Nutrients per serving	
Calories	48
Fat	2 g
Carbohydrate	8 g
Protein	1 g

Grilled Vegetable Salad

1	medium zucchini	1
1	red bell pepper	1
½	large red onion	½
12	small mushrooms	12
3 cups	mixed lettuce leaves (Boston, romaine, radicchio)	750 mL

Dressing

2 tbsp	lemon juice	30 mL
2 tbsp	water	30 mL
1 tbsp	brown sugar	15 mL
4 tsp	balsamic vinegar	20 mL
1 tsp	crushed garlic	5 mL
2 tbsp	olive oil	30 mL
	Salt and freshly ground black pepper	

Makes 4 servings

Super-easy grilled veggies make a tasty addition to any meal. Make sure to use button mushrooms, which are low in histamine.

Tips

If using wooden skewers, soak them in water for at least 30 minutes before using to prevent scorching.

Lemon has low histamine levels. Occasional or small amounts are unlikely to trigger headaches.

Reduce the Histamine
Replace the balsamic vinegar with cider vinegar.

1. Cut zucchini, red pepper and onion into 2-inch (5 cm) chunks. Alternately thread along with mushrooms onto barbecue skewers.

2. *Dressing:* In a small bowl, combine lemon juice, water, sugar, vinegar and garlic; gradually whisk in oil. Season to taste with salt and pepper. Pour into dish large enough to hold skewers.

3. Add skewers to dressing; marinate for 20 minutes, turning often. Meanwhile, preheat barbecue.

4. Grill vegetables until tender, basting with dressing and rotating often, approximately 15 minutes.

5. Remove vegetables from skewers and place on lettuce-lined serving platter. Pour any remaining dressing over vegetables.

Nutrients per serving	
Calories	107
Fat	7 g
Carbohydrate	10 g
Protein	2 g

Southwestern Sweet Potato Salad

Here's a healthy alternative to traditional potato salad.

Tip
Adding leafy herbs to recipes reduces histamine levels.

Reduce the Histamine
Omit the hot pepper sauce from the recipe. Place it on the table so diners can add it to taste.

2 lbs	sweet potatoes, peeled and cut into 1-inch (2.5 cm) pieces	1 kg
2 tsp	ground cumin	10 mL
1/4 tsp	fine sea salt	1 mL
2 tbsp	extra virgin olive oil	30 mL
2 tbsp	freshly squeezed lime juice	30 mL
1/4 tsp	hot pepper sauce	1 mL
1	red bell pepper, finely chopped	1
3/4 cup	packed fresh cilantro leaves, chopped	175 mL
1/2 cup	thinly sliced green onions	125 mL

1. Place potatoes in a large pot and cover with cold water. Bring to a boil over medium-high heat. Boil for 9 to 11 minutes or until tender. Drain and let cool completely.

2. In a small bowl, whisk together cumin, salt, oil, lime juice and hot pepper sauce.

3. In a large bowl, combine cooled sweet potatoes, red pepper, cilantro and green onions. Add dressing and gently toss to coat.

Nutrients per serving	
Calories	128
Fat	4 g
Carbohydrate	22 g
Protein	2 g

Zucchini and Chickpea Salad

This tasty salad is a good source of vitamin C, vitamin B₅, riboflavin and manganese.

Tip

Adding leafy herbs to recipes reduces histamine levels.

½ tsp	fine sea salt	2 mL
½ tsp	freshly ground black pepper	2 mL
1 tbsp	finely grated lemon zest	15 mL
3 tbsp	freshly squeezed lemon juice	45 mL
2 tbsp	extra virgin olive oil	30 mL
3	small zucchini, trimmed, quartered lengthwise and diced	3
2	cans (14 to 19 oz/398 to 540 mL) chickpeas, drained and rinsed	2
½ cup	fresh basil leaves, chopped	125 mL
½ cup	crumbled feta cheese	125 mL

1. In a small bowl, whisk together salt, pepper, lemon zest, lemon juice and oil.

2. In a medium bowl, combine zucchini, chickpeas, basil and feta. Add dressing and gently toss to coat.

Nutrients per serving	
Calories	107
Fat	6 g
Carbohydrate	10 g
Protein	4 g

Rice, Black Bean and Red Pepper Salad

With a good amount of high-quality protein, this salad is a great addition to a vegetarian meal.

Tips

Warning: Snow peas may be a trigger for migraines for some people.

Lemon has low histamine levels. Occasional or small amounts are unlikely to trigger headaches.

Reduce the Histamine

Replace the red wine vinegar with cider vinegar.

Cut the kernels off cooked fresh corn instead of using canned or frozen.

2 cups	ready-to-use chicken broth or water	500 mL
½ cup	wild rice	125 mL
½ cup	white rice	125 mL
1 cup	chopped red bell peppers	250 mL
1 cup	chopped snow peas	250 mL
1 cup	canned black beans, drained and rinsed	250 mL
½ cup	corn kernels	125 mL
⅓ cup	chopped red onions	75 mL
⅓ cup	chopped fresh cilantro or parsley	75 mL
1	medium green onion, chopped	1

Dressing

3 tbsp	olive oil	45 mL
2 tbsp	lemon juice	30 mL
1 tbsp	red wine vinegar	15 mL
1 tsp	minced garlic	5 mL

1. Bring broth to boil in a saucepan; add wild rice and white rice. Cover, reduce heat to medium-low and simmer for 20 minutes or until rice is tender. Remove from heat and let stand for 5 minutes, or until all liquid is absorbed. Rinse with cold water and put in large serving bowl.

2. Add red peppers, snow peas, black beans, corn, red onions, cilantro and green onion to rice and toss to combine.

3. *Dressing:* In a small bowl, whisk together olive oil, lemon juice, red wine vinegar and garlic; pour over salad and toss well.

Nutrients per serving	
Calories	251
Fat	8 g
Carbohydrate	40 g
Protein	8 g

Quinoa and Black Bean Salad

With black beans, tomatoes, cumin and cilantro, this quick quinoa salad takes a delectable Tex-Mex detour.

Reduce the Histamine
Replace the tomatoes with slightly under-ripe mangos.

1 cup	quinoa, rinsed	250 mL
2 cups	water	500 mL
1½ tsp	ground cumin	7 mL
½ tsp	fine sea salt	2 mL
3 tbsp	extra virgin olive oil	45 mL
2 tsp	finely grated lime zest	10 mL
2 tbsp	freshly squeezed lime juice	30 mL
1 tsp	agave nectar or liquid honey	5 mL
1	can (14 to 19 oz/398 to 540 mL) black beans, drained and rinsed	1
2 cups	chopped tomatoes	500 mL
½ cup	thinly sliced green onions	125 mL
½ cup	packed fresh cilantro leaves, chopped	125 mL

1. In a medium saucepan, combine quinoa and water. Bring to a boil over medium-high heat. Reduce heat to low, cover and simmer for 15 to 18 minutes or until water is absorbed. Remove from heat and let cool completely.

2. In a small bowl, whisk together cumin, salt, oil, lime zest, lime juice and agave nectar.

3. In a large bowl, combine cooled quinoa, beans, tomatoes, green onions and cilantro. Add dressing and gently toss to coat. Cover and refrigerate for at least 30 minutes, until chilled, or for up to 4 hours.

Nutrients per serving	
Calories	357
Fat	14 g
Carbohydrate	47 g
Protein	12 g

Quinoa Salad

This simple, delicious salad packs a nutritional punch. Thanks to the quinoa, it even provides a complete protein, so it's a great choice for vegetarians. Whether it serves two people or four depends on how much you're willing to share!

Tip

Lemon has low histamine levels. Occasional or small amounts are unlikely to trigger headaches.

Variation

If you're making this salad for non-vegetarians, you can substitute reduced-sodium GF chicken or turkey broth for the vegetable broth.

1 1/4 cups	Vegetable Stock (page 218) or ready-to-use reduced-sodium vegetable broth	300 mL
3/4 cup	quinoa, rinsed	175 mL
1/2 cup	thawed frozen peas	125 mL
1/4 cup	finely chopped orange bell pepper	60 mL
1/4 cup	finely chopped yellow bell pepper	60 mL
1 tbsp	finely chopped red onion	15 mL
2 tbsp	extra virgin olive oil	30 mL
1 tbsp	chopped fresh parsley	15 mL
1 tsp	dried thyme	5 mL
1 tsp	freshly squeezed lemon juice	5 mL
	Salt and freshly ground black pepper	

1. In a saucepan, bring broth to a boil over high heat. Add quinoa, reduce heat to low, cover and simmer for 20 minutes or until quinoa is tender and liquid is almost absorbed. Remove from heat and let stand, covered, for 5 minutes or until liquid is absorbed.

2. In a large bowl, combine quinoa, peas, orange pepper, yellow pepper and red onion.

3. In a small bowl, whisk together oil, parsley, thyme and lemon juice. Drizzle over salad and toss to coat. Season to taste with salt and pepper. Serve warm or cover and refrigerate for 1 hour, until chilled, and serve cold.

Nutrients per 1 of 4 servings	
Calories	210
Fat	9 g
Carbohydrate	26 g
Protein	6 g

Tabbouleh

This intriguing, healthy, delicious salad is packed with parsley, which is, in turn, packed with antioxidant nutrients, including vitamin C. However, parsley also contains a significant amount of vitamin K, so if you are taking blood thinners, check with your dietitian before eating this salad.

Tips

This recipe uses a minimum quantity of oil. If you prefer a sweeter taste, add 2 tbsp (30 mL) more oil.

Leftover tabbouleh can be kept in the refrigerator, covered, for up to 3 days. Be sure to bring it back up to room temperature before serving.

Reduce the Histamine
Replace the tomato with finely chopped zucchini, yellow summer squash or cucumber.

2 cups	packed chopped fresh parsley	500 mL
1	onion, finely chopped	1
1	tomato, finely chopped	1
½ cup	bulgur wheat	125 mL
6 tbsp	freshly squeezed lemon juice	90 mL
¼ cup	olive oil	60 mL
	Salt and freshly ground black pepper	

1. In a bowl, combine parsley, onion and tomato. Mix well. Set aside.

2. In a saucepan, boil bulgur wheat in plenty of water for 6 to 8 minutes, until tender. Drain and refresh with cold water. Drain again completely and add cooked bulgur to the vegetables in the bowl. Mix well.

3. Sprinkle lemon juice and olive oil over the salad. Season to taste with salt and pepper. Toss to mix thoroughly. Transfer to a serving plate. The salad can be served immediately, although it'll be better if it waits up to 2 hours, covered and unrefrigerated.

Nutrients per serving	
Calories	118
Fat	10 g
Carbohydrate	9 g
Protein	2 g

Lemon Vinaigrette

Makes about
½ cup (125 mL)

This very useful vinaigrette is one to keep on hand in the refrigerator. Enjoy it with cooked vegetables such as green beans or broccoli or drizzled over fish fillets before baking or grilling.

⅓ cup	extra virgin olive oil	75 mL
3 tbsp	freshly squeezed lemon juice	45 mL
2 tbsp	chopped fresh dill	30 mL
	Salt and freshly ground black pepper	

1. In a container with a tight-fitting lid, combine oil, lemon juice and dill. Season to taste with salt and pepper. Cover and shake well to blend.

> **Make Ahead**
> Store in the refrigerator for up to 2 weeks.

Nutrients per 1 tbsp (15 mL)	
Calories	78
Fat	9 g
Carbohydrate	1 g
Protein	0 g

Cilantro Oil

Makes about
1 cup (250 mL)

This healthy and delicious oil is a great choice for salad dressings and marinades.

2 cups	packed fresh cilantro leaves	500 mL
½ cup	olive oil	125 mL
½ cup	vegetable oil	125 mL

1. Bring a large saucepan of water to a boil. Add cilantro and blanch for 5 seconds. Drain and immediately plunge into a bowl of ice water. Drain well and squeeze out all liquid.

2. In a blender, purée cilantro, olive oil and vegetable oil until smooth. Strain through several layers of cheesecloth or a paper coffee filter into a squeeze bottle, discarding solids.

> **Make Ahead**
> Store in an airtight container in the refrigerator for up to 3 days.

Nutrients per 1 tbsp (15 mL)	
Calories	126
Fat	14 g
Carbohydrate	0 g
Protein	0 g

Buttery Croutons

Makes about 3 cups (750 mL)

Add some crunch to your salad. Try making buttery croutons, pumpernickel croutons and garlic croutons (see variations, below) and mixing them all together.

Variations

Pumpernickel Croutons: Substitute pumpernickel bread for the white bread and olive oil for the melted butter.

Garlic Croutons: In a small skillet, melt ¼ cup (60 mL) butter over medium heat. Add 3 cloves garlic, minced, and sauté until sizzling, about 2 minutes. Remove from heat. Use garlic butter in place of the melted butter.

Reduce the Histamine
Use gluten-free bread.

- **Preheat oven to 400°F (200°C)**
- **Large rimmed baking sheet**

3 cups	cubed rustic white bread (½-inch/1 cm cubes)	750 mL
¼ cup	unsalted butter, melted	60 mL
½ tsp	salt	2 mL

1. On baking sheet, combine bread, butter and salt; toss to coat evenly and spread in a single layer. Bake, stirring once, until crisp, about 10 minutes. Let cool on sheet on a wire rack and use within 3 hours.

Nutrients per ½ cup (125 mL)	
Calories	375
Fat	11 g
Carbohydrate	59 g
Protein	10 g

Fish and Vegetarian Mains

Simple Grilled Fish

Makes 4 servings

Sometimes the best-tasting food comes from simple ingredients with the right accompaniments. Serve this dish with steamed broccoli and whole wheat rolls — you'll have a complete meal ready within minutes so you can get on with your busy schedule.

Variation

Substitute tilapia, sole, haddock or halibut for the orange roughy.

- Preheat broiler
- Rimmed baking sheet, lightly greased

1 tbsp	chopped fresh parsley	15 mL
1 tbsp	butter, melted	15 mL
	Juice of 1 lemon	
4	orange roughy fillets (about 1¾ lbs/875 g total)	4

1. In a small bowl, combine parsley, butter and lemon juice.

2. Place fish fillets on prepared baking sheet and baste both sides with butter mixture.

3. Broil for 5 to 10 minutes or until fish is opaque and flakes easily with a fork.

This recipe courtesy of Eileen Campbell.

Nutrients per serving	
Calories	170
Fat	4 g
Carbohydrate	1 g
Protein	30 g

Fish Fillets with Corn and Red Pepper Salsa

Makes 4 servings

A savory salsa adds zest and tang to perfectly cooked fish.

Tips

After broiling bell pepper, put in small bowl and cover tightly with plastic wrap; this allows the skin to be removed easily.

Roasted corn gives an exceptional flavor in this recipe. Either barbecue or broil until just cooked and charred, along with pepper. Remove kernels with a sharp knife.

Lemon has low histamine levels. Occasional or small amounts are unlikely to trigger headaches.

Make Ahead

Prepare salsa earlier in the day and refrigerate.

- Preheat broiler
- Baking dish, sprayed with vegetable spray

Salsa

1	large red bell pepper	1
1½ cups	corn kernels	375 mL
⅓ cup	chopped red onions	75 mL
¼ cup	chopped fresh cilantro	60 mL
2 tbsp	fresh lime or lemon juice	30 mL
3 tsp	olive oil, divided	15 mL
2 tsp	minced garlic, divided	10 mL
1 lb	fish fillets	500 g

1. *Salsa*: Broil red pepper for 15 to 20 minutes, turning occasionally, until charred on all sides. Remove pepper and set oven at 425°F (220°C). When pepper is cool, remove skin, seeds and stem. Chop and put in small bowl along with corn, onions, cilantro, lime juice, 2 tsp (10 mL) of olive oil and 1 tsp (5 mL) of the garlic; mix well.

2. Put fish in single layer in prepared baking dish and brush with remaining 1 tsp (5 mL) garlic and 1 tsp (5 mL) oil. Bake uncovered for 10 minutes per inch (2.5 cm) thickness of fish or until fish flakes easily when pierced with a fork. Serve with salsa.

Nutrients per serving	
Calories	81
Fat	5 g
Carbohydrate	6 g
Protein	3 g

Baked Fish and Vegetables en Papillote

Cooking "en papillote" preserves the flavor of the fish and leaves the vegetables crisp but tender

Tip

Warning: Snow peas may be a trigger for migraines for some people.

Reduce the Histamine

Use 8 button mushrooms instead of 4 large white mushrooms.

● **Preheat oven to 450°F (230°C)**

	Nonstick cooking spray	
4	fish fillets (each about 4 oz/125 g)	4
4	large white mushrooms, sliced	4
2	green onions, sliced	2
20	snow peas, trimmed	20
	Salt and freshly ground black pepper	

1. Cut four pieces of parchment paper or foil 4 inches (10 cm) larger than fish fillets. Lightly spray with cooking spray. Place each fillet in center of paper. Top each with 1 sliced mushroom, a quarter of the onions and 5 snow peas. Season lightly with salt and pepper.

2. Fold long ends of paper or foil twice so mixture is tightly enclosed. Lift short ends, bring together on top and fold twice. Place seam side up on baking pan.

3. Bake for 20 minutes or until fish is opaque and flakes easily when tested with a fork and vegetables are tender. Open each package and serve contents on dinner plates.

Nutrients per serving	
Calories	135
Fat	2 g
Carbohydrate	4 g
Protein	25 g

Halibut with Coconut Lime Sauce

Highly prized for its firm, mild flesh, halibut is well worth the occasional splurge at the fish counter. Here, it heads to the islands in a splendid ginger- and lime-infused coconut sauce.

Tips

Sea bass, cod or any other firm white fish fillets may be used in place of the halibut.

Warning: If serving peas with this dish, as in the menu plan on page 165, be aware that peas have low histamine levels. Include peas in small amounts on days when your other headache triggers are low. Otherwise, serve green beans instead.

Reduce the Histamine

Omitting the cayenne will reduce the histamine.

- Preheat oven to 350°F (180°C)
- 9-inch (23 cm) glass baking dish, sprayed with nonstick cooking spray (preferably olive oil)

1 tsp	vegetable oil	5 mL
2	cloves garlic, minced	2
1 tbsp	minced gingerroot	15 mL
½ tsp	fine sea salt	2 mL
⅛ tsp	cayenne pepper	0.5 mL
½ cup	light coconut milk	125 mL
1 tsp	grated lime zest	5 mL
2 tbsp	freshly squeezed lime juice	30 mL
4	skinless Pacific halibut fillets (each about 5 oz/150 g)	4
½ cup	packed fresh cilantro leaves, chopped	125 mL

1. In a medium skillet, heat oil over medium heat. Add garlic and ginger; cook, stirring, for 2 minutes. Add salt, cayenne, coconut milk, lime zest and lime juice; reduce heat and simmer, stirring occasionally, for 5 minutes.

2. Place fish in prepared baking dish and spoon coconut sauce over top. Bake in preheated oven for 13 to 16 minutes or until fish is opaque and flakes easily when tested with a fork.

3. Place a fillet on each plate and spoon sauce over top. Sprinkle with cilantro.

Nutrients per serving	
Calories	149
Fat	5 g
Carbohydrate	2 g
Protein	24 g

Herb-Roasted Salmon

Makes 6 servings

Salmon has such a marvelous flavor that little else is needed in the way of seasoning. This simple herb-oil mixture makes it easy.

- Preheat oven to 450°F (230°C)
- Shallow oblong pan, greased

1	large salmon fillet (about 2 lbs/1 kg)	1
1 tbsp	olive oil	15 mL
2 tbsp	chopped fresh chives	30 mL
1 tbsp	chopped fresh tarragon (or 1 tsp/5 mL dried)	15 mL
	Salt and freshly ground black pepper	

1. Place fish, skin side down, in prepared pan.

2. In a small bowl, combine oil, chives and tarragon. Rub half into flesh of salmon.

3. Bake for 10 minutes per inch (2.5 cm) of thickness or until fish is opaque and flakes easily when tested with a fork.

4. To serve, cut salmon in half crosswise. Lift flesh from skin with a spatula. Transfer to a platter. Discard skin, and then drizzle fish with remaining herbs and oil. Season lightly with salt and pepper.

Nutrients per serving	
Calories	178
Fat	6 g
Carbohydrate	0 g
Protein	31 g

Salmon with Roasted Vegetables

Here's a great dish for parents who want to savor a quiet meal together after the children have been fed and put to bed. With or without the kids, it's a perfect meal for two.

Tips

The tail end of the salmon, which contains the fewest bones, is used in this recipe. However, you can substitute two 4-oz (125 g) salmon fillets, if desired.

This recipe provides a serving of fish and 3 servings of vegetables. To complete the meal, serve with rice and finish with yogurt.

Lemon has low histamine levels. Occasional or small amounts are unlikely to trigger headaches.

- Preheat oven to 425°F (220°C)
- 11- by 7-inch (28 by 18 cm) baking dish

1 tbsp	olive oil	15 mL
2 tsp	minced garlic	10 mL
2 tsp	dried thyme, divided	10 mL
1 cup	diced peeled sweet potatoes	250 mL
1 cup	diced zucchini or red bell peppers	250 mL
1 cup	diced peeled parsnips or potatoes	250 mL
2 tbsp	lemon juice	30 mL
1/4 tsp	freshly ground black pepper	1 mL
1	salmon tail (8 to 12 oz/250 to 375 g), patted dry	1

1. In a small bowl, stir together olive oil, garlic and 1 tsp (5 mL) of the thyme. Place sweet potatoes, zucchini and parsnips in baking dish and sprinkle with oil mixture; toss to coat. Spread out vegetables in a single layer and roast in preheated oven for 15 minutes.

2. In the bowl used for oil mixture, combine remaining thyme, lemon juice and pepper. Brush mixture over salmon tail.

3. Remove vegetables from oven and stir. Place salmon skin side down on top of vegetables. Bake for 10 to 15 minutes or until fish is opaque and flakes easily with a fork. Remove skin from salmon before serving.

This recipe courtesy of dietitian Lynn Roblin.

Nutrients per serving	
Calories	415
Fat	20 g
Carbohydrate	34 g
Protein	25 g

Barbecued Stuffed Salmon

Makes 6 servings

This quick and easy-to-make dish is perfect for entertaining. Your guests will be impressed, and you'll be relaxed at serving time.

Tips

To cook fish on the barbecue, put it in a fish cooker or wrap it loosely in foil left open at the top. This way the fish will remain moist yet have that great barbecue flavor.

Make this recipe the centerpiece of a summer dinner on the deck. Roast an assortment of vegetables on the grill with the salmon.

Reduce the Histamine
Replace the crabmeat with cooked white fish, such as pollock.

- **Preheat barbecue or oven to 450°F (230°C)**

1	small onion, finely chopped	1
2	cloves garlic, minced	2
1	stalk celery, finely chopped	1
1 tbsp	butter or margarine	15 mL
1	can (4½ oz/128 g) crabmeat, drained	1
1 cup	cooked rice	250 mL
1 tsp	grated lemon zest	5 mL
2 tbsp	lemon juice	30 mL
1 tbsp	finely chopped parsley	15 mL
½ tsp	salt	2 mL
¼ tsp	freshly ground black pepper	1 mL
2	salmon fillets (1½ lbs/750 g total)	2
½	lemon, sliced	½

1. In a medium skillet over high heat, cook onion, garlic and celery in butter until softened. Stir in crabmeat, rice, lemon zest, lemon juice, parsley, salt and pepper.

2. Place stuffing over 1 fish fillet; top with second fillet. Secure with string or toothpicks. Arrange lemon slices on top. Wrap loosely in several thicknesses of aluminum foil.

3. Place on barbecue grill. Cook for about 45 minutes or until fish flakes easily with fork. Or bake in preheated oven for 10 minutes per inch (2.5 cm) of thickness.

This recipe courtesy of Maureen Prairie.

Nutrients per serving	
Calories	238
Fat	9 g
Carbohydrate	9 g
Protein	28 g

Salmon in a Parcel

Do you avoid cooking fish because you are worried about the smell it sometimes leaves in the kitchen? In this recipe, the fish is enclosed in foil, and no smell escapes at all.

Tip

The rule of thumb for cooking fish is 10 minutes per inch (2.5 cm) of thickness. The thicker the fish, the longer you need to cook it.

- Preheat oven to 450°F (230°C)
- Rimmed baking sheet

4	salmon fillets (about 1 lb/500 g total)	4
1	lemon, thinly sliced	1
½ cup	chopped fresh dill	125 mL
1 tbsp	olive oil	15 mL

1. Cut 4 pieces of foil big enough to completely wrap each piece of fish. Place 1 salmon fillet in the center of each piece of foil. Top each with lemon slices, sprinkle with dill and drizzle with olive oil. Fold foil over fish and crimp in the center. Tuck excess foil under, pinching to seal edges. Place foil packets on baking sheet.

2. Bake in preheated oven for about 20 minutes or until salmon is opaque and flakes easily with a fork.

This recipe courtesy of Eileen Campbell.

Nutrients per serving	
Calories	218
Fat	14 g
Carbohydrate	3 g
Protein	20 g

Fish for the Sole

You'll forgive the pun, but this cracker-crusted fish really is comfort food for the soul — and it does your body good too!

Tips

To crush the crackers, place them in a sealable plastic bag. Seal and use a rolling pin to crush them to the consistency of dry bread crumbs. Alternatively, you can crush them in a blender.

Lemon has low histamine levels. Occasional or small amounts are unlikely to trigger headaches.

- **Preheat oven to 350°F (180°C)**
- **13- by 9-inch (33 by 23 cm) glass baking dish, greased**

2	cloves garlic, minced	2
1/4 cup	GF cracker crumbs	60 mL
2 tbsp	chopped fresh parsley	30 mL
2 tbsp	olive oil (approx.)	30 mL
	Juice of 1/2 lemon	
3	pieces skinless sole fillet (each about 3 1/2 oz/100 g)	3

1. In a small bowl, combine garlic, cracker crumbs, parsley, oil and lemon juice; stir until a paste forms, adding more oil if mixture is too dry.

2. Arrange sole in prepared baking dish. Spread paste over fish.

3. Cover dish with foil and bake in preheated oven for 20 to 30 minutes or until fish flakes easily when tested with a fork. Uncover and bake for 5 minutes or until crust is crispy.

Nutrients per serving	
Calories	220
Fat	10 g
Carbohydrate	8 g
Protein	23 g

Broiled Herbed Trout Fillets

Butterflied trout fillets enhanced by a fresh herb dressing cook quickly under the broiler, delivering a light, satisfying entrée.

Tips

Other mild, lean white fish, such as orange roughy, snapper, cod, tilefish or striped bass, may be used in place of the trout.

Warning: If serving peas with this dish, as in the menu plan on page 169, be aware that peas have low histamine levels. Include peas in small amounts on days when your other headache triggers are low. Otherwise, serve green beans instead.

Reduce the Histamine
Remove the skin before cooking the fish.

- Preheat broiler, with rack set 4 to 6 inches (10 to 15 cm) from the heat source
- Broiler pan, sprayed with nonstick cooking spray (preferably olive oil)

1	clove garlic, minced	1
1 tbsp	minced fresh flat-leaf (Italian) parsley	15 mL
1 tbsp	minced fresh chives	15 mL
2 tsp	minced fresh oregano	10 mL
1/2 tsp	fine sea salt	2 mL
1/4 tsp	freshly cracked black pepper	1 mL
1 tbsp	extra virgin olive oil	15 mL
1 tbsp	freshly squeezed lemon juice	15 mL
4	skin-on trout fillets (each about 6 oz/175 g)	4

1. In a medium bowl, whisk together garlic, parsley, chives, oregano, salt, pepper, oil and lemon juice.

2. Place fish, skin side down, on prepared pan. Generously brush with dressing. Broil for 4 to 6 minutes or until fish is opaque and flakes easily when tested with a fork.

Nutrients per serving	
Calories	216
Fat	10 g
Carbohydrate	1 g
Protein	30 g

Zucchini Frittata

Makes 6 servings

Zucchini is a sweet summer squash, North American in origin, that has been warmly embraced in Italian cooking. Make this Italian-style omelet when zucchini is in season or vary the recipe using other vegetables — mushrooms, red or green bell peppers and broccoli would also work well.

Tips

If the handle of your skillet is not ovenproof, wrap it in foil for protection.

If you don't have ground fennel in your cupboard, use a generous teaspoon (5 mL) of fennel seeds in this recipe. Toast them over medium heat in a dry pan until they release their aroma, then crush finely before adding to the eggs. The flavor will be even better than if you had used the ground spice.

This meatless light meal is best served with lower-fat accompaniments. A side salad, crusty bread and a fruit dessert will complete the meal.

- Preheat broiler
- Ovenproof skillet

2 cups	sliced zucchini	500 mL
1	small onion, minced	1
1 tbsp	butter or margarine	15 mL
1½ tsp	olive oil	7 mL
6	large eggs, beaten	6
1 tbsp	chopped fresh parsley	15 mL
1 tsp	ground fennel (see tip, at left)	5 mL
½ tsp	ground dried rosemary	2 mL
½ tsp	salt	2 mL
¼ tsp	freshly ground black pepper	1 mL
2 tbsp	shredded Cheddar cheese	30 mL

1. In a large ovenproof skillet over medium-high heat, cook zucchini and onion in butter and olive oil for about 5 minutes or until tender.

2. In another bowl, combine eggs, parsley, fennel, rosemary, salt and pepper; pour over vegetables. Cook over medium heat, without stirring, until bottom of mixture has set but top is still soft. Sprinkle cheese on top. Place under preheated broiler for about 3 minutes or until cheese is melted and top is brown.

This recipe courtesy of Ruth Borthwick.

Reduce the Histamine
Use farmer's cheese or mozzarella instead of Cheddar cheese.

Nutrients per serving	
Calories	126
Fat	9 g
Carbohydrate	3 g
Protein	7 g

Zucchini Stuffed with Rice and Mushrooms

Makes 4 servings

Try this dish on days when your headache triggers are low, since it includes tomato sauce — a higher-histamine food. Make sure to choose button mushrooms, which have a low histamine level.

Tips

Wild rice can be replaced with brown or white rice or a combination. Cook white rice for only 15 to 20 minutes; allow 35 minutes for brown rice.

Wild rice is expensive, so you may want to use it only for special meals — or use less by combining it with white rice, brown rice or mixed greens.

Make Ahead

Prepare up to 1 day in advance and bake just before serving.

Reduce the Histamine

Do not add the optional Parmesan cheese.

Nutrients per serving	
Calories	135
Fat	2 g
Carbohydrate	27 g
Protein	6 g

- 13- by 9-inch (33 by 23 cm) glass baking dish, sprayed with vegetable spray

3 cups	Vegetable Stock (page 218) or ready-to-use vegetable broth	750 mL
½ cup	wild rice	125 mL
2	large zucchini (each about 8 oz/250 g)	2
1 tsp	vegetable oil	5 mL
2 tsp	minced garlic	10 mL
¾ cup	chopped onions	175 mL
2 cups	sliced mushrooms	500 mL
1½ tsp	drained capers	7 mL
1 tsp	dried basil	5 mL
½ tsp	dried oregano	2 mL
¾ cup	prepared tomato pasta sauce	175 mL
3 tbsp	grated Parmesan cheese, divided (optional)	45 mL

1. In a small saucepan, bring stock to a boil; stir in rice, cover, reduce heat to low and cook for 35 to 40 minutes or until rice is tender. Drain excess liquid.

2. Meanwhile, cut each zucchini in half lengthwise. In a large pot of boiling water, cook zucchini for 4 minutes; drain. When cool enough to handle, carefully scoop out pulp, leaving shells intact. Chop pulp and set aside. Put zucchini shells into prepared baking dish.

3. Preheat oven to 350°F (180°C). In a large nonstick frying pan sprayed with vegetable spray, heat oil over medium-high heat. Add garlic and onions; cook for 3 minutes or until softened. Stir in mushrooms, capers, basil and oregano; cook for 5 minutes or until mushrooms are browned. Stir in zucchini pulp; cook for 2 minutes. Remove from heat.

4. Stir cooked rice, tomato sauce and 1 tbsp (15 mL) of the Parmesan cheese (if using) into vegetable mixture. Stuff mixture evenly into zucchini boats, mounding filling high. Sprinkle with remaining Parmesan (if using). Cover dish tightly with foil.

5. Bake for 15 minutes or until heated through.

Spanish Vegetable Paella

Traditional paella is made in a wide shallow pan, but today's nonstick skillet makes a very good substitute and reduces the amount of oil needed for this dish.

Tip
Try a variety of different vegetables, including bite-size pieces of broccoli, cauliflower, green beans, bell peppers and zucchini.

Reduce the Histamine
Omit the hot pepper flakes from the recipe. Place hot pepper sauce or hot pepper flakes on the table so diners can add heat to taste.

- **Preheat oven to 375°F (190°C)**

4 cups	assorted prepared vegetables (see tip, at left)	1 L
3½ cups	ready-to-use reduced-sodium chicken or vegetable broth	875 mL
¼ tsp	saffron threads, crushed	1 mL
Pinch	hot pepper flakes	Pinch
2 tbsp	olive oil	30 mL
4	green onions, chopped	4
3	large cloves garlic, finely chopped	3
1½ cups	short-grain white rice, such as Arborio	375 mL

1. Cook vegetables (except peppers and zucchini) in a saucepan of boiling, lightly salted water for 1 minute. Rinse under cold water to chill; drain well.

2. In the same saucepan, bring broth to a boil. Add saffron and hot pepper flakes. Keep warm.

3. In a large nonstick skillet, heat oil over medium-high heat. Add green onions and garlic; cook, stirring, for 1 minute. Add vegetables to skillet; cook, stirring often, for 4 minutes or until lightly colored. Stir in rice and hot broth mixture. Reduce heat so rice cooks at a gentle boil; cook, uncovered, without stirring, for 10 minutes or until most of the liquid is absorbed.

4. Cover skillet with lid or foil. (If skillet handle is not ovenproof, wrap in double layer of foil.) Bake in preheated oven for 15 minutes or until all liquid is absorbed and rice is tender. Remove; let stand, covered, for 5 minutes before serving.

Nutrients per serving	
Calories	226
Fat	6 g
Carbohydrate	35 g
Protein	8 g

Kasha with Summer Vegetables

With its assortment of tender spring vegetables, this quick-to-the-table side dish also makes a great meat-free lunch.

Tip

Onion has low levels of histamine. Eating it occasionally is unlikely to trigger headaches. You could replace it with an equal amount of chopped shallots, if desired.

2 cups	ready-to-use reduced-sodium vegetable or chicken broth	500 mL
1	large egg, beaten lightly	1
1 cup	whole kasha (toasted buckwheat groats)	250 mL
3 tsp	extra virgin olive oil, divided	15 mL
2	cloves garlic, minced	2
1	red bell pepper, chopped	1
1 cup	chopped onion	250 mL
1	zucchini, cut into ¼-inch (0.5 cm) dice	1
1 cup	fresh or thawed frozen corn kernels	250 mL
¼ tsp	fine sea salt	1 mL
	Nonfat plain yogurt (optional)	

1. In a medium saucepan, bring broth to a boil over medium-high heat.

2. Meanwhile, in a small bowl, combine egg and kasha.

3. In a large, deep skillet, heat 1 tsp (5 mL) of the oil over medium heat. Add kasha mixture and cook, stirring to separate the grains, for 2 to 4 minutes or until golden. Remove from heat and gradually stir in broth. Reduce heat, cover tightly and simmer for 12 to 15 minutes or until liquid is absorbed.

4. Meanwhile, in a large skillet, heat the remaining oil over medium-high heat. Add garlic, red pepper and onion; cook, stirring, for 6 to 8 minutes or until softened. Add zucchini, corn and salt; cook, stirring, for 3 minutes or until zucchini is slightly softened.

5. Stir vegetable mixture into kasha mixture. Serve warm, with yogurt on the side, if desired.

Nutrients per serving	
Calories	153
Fat	3 g
Carbohydrate	31 g
Protein	5 g

Greens and Grains Gratin

Get glowing reviews for greens! This hearty dish makes a delicious meal when served with a baked potato, or stands out as a superb side dish.

Make Ahead

The gratin can be made ahead through step 4; cover and refrigerate for up to 8 hours. You may need to increase the baking time by 10 minutes, but check it after 30 minutes.

Reduce the Histamine

Use farmer's cheese or mozzarella instead of Cheddar cheese.

Replace the dry bread crumbs with gluten-free bread crumbs.

- Preheat oven to 350°F (180°C)
- Ovenproof skillet

⅓ cup	bulgur	75 mL
⅓ cup	millet (or more bulgur)	75 mL
1⅓ cup	boiling water	325 mL
1	bunch greens (such as spinach, collard greens, Swiss chard)	1
4 tsp	olive oil, divided	20 mL
6	cloves garlic, minced	6
	Salt and freshly ground black pepper	
2 cups	shredded sharp (old) Cheddar cheese, divided	500 mL
¼ cup	dry bread crumbs	60 mL
¼ cup	finely chopped nuts (such as almonds)	60 mL
2 tbsp	minced fresh flat-leaf (Italian) parsley	30 mL

1. In a heatproof bowl, combine bulgur and millet. Pour in boiling water, cover and let stand for 15 minutes. Drain off any excess water.

2. Meanwhile, clean greens and tear into small pieces.

3. In ovenproof skillet, heat 1 tbsp (15 mL) of the olive oil over medium-low heat. Sauté garlic until golden, about 2 minutes. Add grains and greens; sauté until grains are slightly browned and greens are wilted, about 5 minutes. Season to taste with salt and pepper. Remove from heat. Transfer half of the mixture to a bowl and set aside.

4. Spread the remaining mixture in the bottom of the skillet. Top with 1 cup (250 mL) of the cheese. Spread reserved half of mixture over cheese.

5. In a small bowl, combine the remaining 1 tsp (5 mL) oil, the remaining 1 cup (250 mL) cheese, bread crumbs, nuts and parsley. Spread evenly over grains mixture.

6. Bake in preheated oven for 30 minutes or until cheese is bubbly and top is golden brown.

This recipe courtesy of Nicole Fetterly.

Nutrients per serving	
Calories	308
Fat	15 g
Carbohydrate	22 g
Protein	15 g

Pasta with Roasted Vegetables and Goat Cheese

This dish is a great way to increase your vegetable intake. Leftovers are delicious served cold or reheated for lunch the next day.

Tip

When choosing vegetables for roasting, select those with darker colors of red, orange and green; they are richest in nutrients and phytochemicals.

Reduce the Histamine

Use gluten-free pasta.

Replace the eggplant with more zucchini, celeriac or a not-too-sweet winter squash.

Replace the dried Italian seasoning with 1½ tbsp (22 mL) chopped fresh herbs, such as marjoram, thyme, rosemary, sage, oregano and/or basil. Add the fresh herbs in step 3, when tossing the pasta with the vegetables.

Omit the optional Parmesan cheese.

Nutrients per serving

Calories	395
Fat	13 g
Carbohydrate	56 g
Protein	14 g

- Preheat oven to 425°F (220°C)
- Large rimmed baking sheet, greased

4 cups	cubed zucchini	1 L
2 cups	cubed eggplant	500 mL
2 cups	coarsely chopped red bell peppers	500 mL
1 cup	coarsely chopped sweet white or red onions	250 mL
2 tbsp	olive oil	30 mL
1½ tsp	dried Italian seasoning or French herbs	7 mL
8 oz	rotini, penne or other pasta	250 g
3½ to 4 oz	soft crumbled goat cheese	100 to 125 g
	Grated Parmesan cheese (optional)	

1. Combine zucchini, eggplant, peppers and onions in a large bowl. Add oil and Italian seasoning; toss to coat. Place vegetables in a single layer on prepared baking sheet; roast in preheated oven, stirring occasionally, for 30 to 40 minutes or until vegetables are golden and slightly softened.

2. Meanwhile, in a pot of boiling water, cook pasta according to package directions or until tender but firm; drain.

3. Toss vegetables with pasta. Sprinkle goat cheese over top; toss to combine or leave as is. Sprinkle with Parmesan cheese, if desired.

This recipe courtesy of dietitian Renée Crompton.

Whole Wheat Pizza with Roasted Vegetables

The vegetable mixture in this recipe is equally spectacular on a pizza crust covered with a thin layer of pesto or pizza sauce. Spread whole wheat pizza dough with sauce and roasted vegetables. Add crumbled goat cheese and grated Parmesan, if desired. (To reduce the histamine, use a gluten-free pizza crust and omit the Parmesan or replace it with farmer's cheese or mozzarella.)

Capellini with Watercress, Carrots and Almonds

"Refreshing" may not be a word that comes up much when discussing pasta, but that's exactly how these noodles will strike you. A handful of almonds — rich in protein, minerals and vitamins E and B — in combination with toothsome multigrain pasta makes this dish main course–worthy, while watercress adds piquant emerald verve, vitamins and antioxidants.

Tips

An equal amount of arugula, roughly torn or chopped, may be used in place of the watercress.

To toast sliced almonds, place up to ½ cup (125 mL) almonds in a medium skillet set over medium heat. Cook, shaking the skillet, for 2 to 3 minutes or until almonds are golden brown and fragrant. Let cool completely before use.

Reduce the Histamine
Use gluten-free pasta.

Nutrients per serving	
Calories	334
Fat	11 g
Carbohydrate	57 g
Protein	11 g

8 oz	multigrain or whole wheat capellini (angel hair) pasta	250 g
1½ tbsp	extra virgin olive oil	22 mL
2	cloves garlic, thinly sliced	2
2 cups	shredded carrots	500 mL
6 cups	packed tender watercress sprigs	1.5 L
¼ tsp	fine sea salt	1 mL
¼ tsp	freshly cracked black pepper	1 mL
¼ cup	freshly squeezed lemon juice	60 mL
¼ cup	sliced almonds, toasted (see tip, at left)	60 mL

1. In a large pot of boiling salted water, cook pasta according to package directions until al dente. Drain, reserving 2 tbsp (30 mL) pasta water. Return pasta to pot.

2. Meanwhile, in a large skillet, heat oil over medium-high heat. Add garlic and carrots; cook, stirring, for 1 to 2 minutes or until carrots are slightly softened. Remove from heat and stir in watercress.

3. To the pasta, add watercress mixture, salt, pepper, lemon juice and the reserved pasta water, tossing to combine. Serve sprinkled with almonds.

Quinoa Spaghetti with Kale

This dish could easily pass muster as the definitively healthy pasta recipe. But it's the synchronicity of flavors that makes it worth making (often). A good-quality extra virgin olive oil makes all the difference, adding a mellow, grassy flavor that ties the other ingredients together.

Tip

Quinoa pastas are available in health food stores and in the health food section of well-stocked supermarkets. If you can't find quinoa spaghetti, use multigrain or whole wheat spaghetti.

Reduce the Histamine

Omit the hot pepper flakes from the recipe. Place hot pepper sauce or hot pepper flakes on the table so diners can add heat to taste.

Use cider vinegar instead of sherry or white wine vinegar.

Omit the Parmesan cheese.

1 lb	kale, stems and ribs removed, leaves very thinly sliced crosswise (about 8 cups/2 L)	500 g
8 oz	quinoa spaghetti pasta	250 g
1 1/2 tbsp	extra virgin olive oil	22 mL
2 cups	thinly sliced red onions	500 mL
2	cloves garlic, minced	2
1/8 tsp	hot pepper flakes	0.5 mL
1/2 tsp	fine sea salt	2 mL
2 tsp	sherry vinegar or white wine vinegar	10 mL
1/4 cup	freshly grated Parmesan cheese	60 mL

1. In a large pot of boiling salted water, cook kale for about 10 minutes or until just tender. Using a slotted spoon, transfer kale to a medium bowl.

2. In the same pot, return water to a boil. Cook pasta according to package directions until al dente. Drain, reserving 1/4 cup (60 mL) pasta water. Return pasta to pot.

3. Meanwhile, in a large skillet, heat oil over medium-high heat. Add red onions and cook, stirring, for 6 to 8 minutes or until softened. Add garlic and hot pepper flakes; cook, stirring, for 1 minute. Add kale, reduce heat to medium and cook, stirring, for 2 minutes or until heated through. Remove from heat and stir in salt and vinegar.

4. To the pasta, add kale mixture and the reserved pasta water, tossing to combine. Cook, tossing, over medium-low heat for 1 minute. Serve sprinkled with cheese.

Nutrients per serving	
Calories	385
Fat	9 g
Carbohydrate	66 g
Protein	15 g

Red Pepper and Goat Cheese Pizza

Here's a fast and tasty treat that makes a great change from the standard pepperoni pizza. Served warm or cold, it's terrific for lunch or a light supper — or even breakfast!

Tip

Onion has low levels of histamine. Eating it occasionally is unlikely to trigger headaches. You could replace it with an equal amount of chopped shallots, if desired.

Reduce the Histamine

Use gluten-free pizza dough.

Replace the tomato with thinly sliced zucchini, button mushrooms, broccoli or fennel.

Omit the black olives.

- Preheat oven to 400°F (200°C) if using flatbread or 450°F (230°C) if using pizza dough
- Pizza pan or baking sheet

1	12-inch (30 cm) round flatbread or enough pizza dough for a 12-inch (30 cm) pizza	1
1 tbsp	olive oil	15 mL
1 cup	shredded mozzarella cheese	250 mL
¼ cup	soft crumbled goat cheese	60 mL
1	large red bell pepper, thinly sliced	1
1	large tomato, sliced	1
¼ cup	sliced black olives	60 mL
¼ cup	sweet Vidalia onion, sliced (optional)	60 mL
1 tsp	dried basil (or 2 tbsp/30 mL chopped fresh basil)	5 mL

1. Place flatbread on baking sheet. Alternatively, if using pizza dough, spread out dough on lightly greased pizza pan to make a 12-inch (30 cm) circle.

2. Brush olive oil on top of flatbread or pizza dough. Sprinkle with mozzarella cheese. Top with goat cheese, red pepper, tomato, black olives, onion (if using) and basil.

3. Bake pizza in bottom half of preheated oven for 10 to 15 minutes or until crust is golden and filling is bubbly.

This recipe courtesy of dietitian Lynn Roblin.

Nutrients per serving	
Calories	373
Fat	18 g
Carbohydrate	40 g
Protein	14 g

Chicken, Beef and Veal

Lemon-Thyme Roast Chicken

Makes 8 servings

A roast chicken that is crispy on the outside and juicy on the inside is hard to beat.

Tip

Using a V-shaped rack is an excellent and healthy way to roast chicken. The open cavity of the chicken is placed over the rack, allowing the chicken to roast upright. If you don't have a V-shaped rack, you can just place the chicken in the roasting pan. However, the overall result is better with the rack — the chicken skin crisps all around, and any excess fat drips off into the pan.

Variations

Try other seasoning combinations for this roast chicken. Make it international by using tandoori paste or a mixture of hoisin and chili sauces, keeping in mind that these may increase the histamine levels.

For a one-dish meal, add cubed root vegetables, such as sweet potatoes, carrots, potatoes and turnips, around the chicken for the last hour of cooking. For the last 10 minutes of cooking, add apple or pear slices.

Nutrients per serving	
Calories	231
Fat	15 g
Carbohydrate	1 g
Protein	24 g

- **Roasting pan with V-shaped rack**

1	whole roasting chicken (5 to 6 lbs/ 2.5 to 3 kg)	1
4	cloves garlic, minced	4
¼ cup	olive oil	60 mL
2 tbsp	chopped fresh thyme	30 mL
1 tsp	freshly ground black pepper	5 mL
	Grated zest and juice of 1 lemon	
	Salt	

1. Prepare chicken by trimming excess fat from body or cavity.

2. In a bowl large enough to hold the chicken, whisk together garlic, olive oil, thyme, pepper, lemon zest, lemon juice and salt to taste. Place chicken in bowl and turn to coat completely, inside and out. Cover and refrigerate for at least 1 hour or overnight. Preheat oven to 450°F (230°C) and remove top rack.

3. Place chicken on rack in roasting pan and baste with marinade. Roast for 15 to 20 minutes. Reduce heat to 375°F (190°C) and roast for $1\frac{1}{2}$ to 2 hours (depending on the size of the chicken) or until skin is dark golden and crispy, drumsticks wiggle when touched, and a meat thermometer inserted into the thickest part of a thigh registers 185°F (85°C). Remove from oven and let rest, tented with foil, for 10 to 15 minutes before carving. (This allows the juices to redistribute and provides a much moister chicken.)

This recipe courtesy of Eileen Campbell.

One-Hour Roast Chicken with Sage and Garlic

Who has time to wait around for a chicken to roast when you're in a hurry? Take an hour off the roasting time by cutting the bird open along the backbone, placing it flat on the broiler pan and then boosting the oven temperature. The result? A golden, succulent bird in about half the time.

Tip

In this recipe, the chicken is "butterflied," or "spatchcocked." Cooking time is reduced when the bird is cut along the backbone and flattened.

Reduce the Histamine

Brush the seasoned oil on only half the chicken, or omit the paprika altogether.

- **Preheat oven to 400°F (200°C)**
- **Broiler pan, sprayed with vegetable cooking spray**

1	chicken (about 3½ lbs/1.75 kg)	1
1 tbsp	butter, softened	15 mL
2	cloves garlic, minced	2
1 tbsp	minced fresh sage (or 1 tsp/5 mL dried)	15 mL
1½ tsp	grated lemon zest	7 mL
½ tsp	salt	2 mL
½ tsp	freshly ground black pepper	2 mL
2 tsp	olive oil	10 mL
¼ tsp	paprika	1 mL

1. Remove giblets and neck from chicken. Using heavy-duty kitchen scissors, cut chicken open along backbone; press down on breast bone to flatten slightly and arrange skin-side up on rack of a broiler pan.

2. In a bowl, blend butter with garlic, sage, lemon zest, salt and pepper. Gently lift breast skin; using a knife or spatula, spread butter mixture under skin to coat breasts and part of legs. Press down on outside skin to smooth and spread butter mixture.

3. In a small bowl, combine olive oil and paprika; brush over chicken.

4. Roast chicken for 1 hour or until juices run clear and a meat thermometer inserted in the thickest part of the thigh registers 185°F (85°C). Transfer chicken to a platter. Tent with foil; let rest 5 minutes before carving.

Nutrients per serving	
Calories	242
Fat	10 g
Carbohydrate	1 g
Protein	37 g

Just-for-Kids Honey Lemon Chicken

Kids love simple dishes like this one, with its straightforward flavors. And this chicken dish is simple enough that even young cooks can make it.

Tips

This recipe also works well with a whole cut-up chicken or bone-in chicken breasts. With its tang of lemon and sweetness of honey, this dish is sure to become a family favorite.

Lemon has low histamine levels. Occasional or small amounts are unlikely to trigger headaches.

- Preheat oven to 350°F (180°C)
- 13- by 9-inch (33 by 23 cm) glass baking dish

8	chicken thighs, skin removed	8
2 tbsp	liquid honey	30 mL
2 tsp	grated lemon zest	10 mL
1 tsp	freshly squeezed lemon juice	5 mL
1	large clove garlic, minced	1
1/4 tsp	salt	1 mL
1/4 tsp	freshly ground black pepper	1 mL

1. Arrange chicken in baking dish. In a bowl, combine honey, lemon zest, lemon juice, garlic, salt and pepper; spoon over chicken.

2. Bake in oven, basting once, for 45 to 55 minutes or until juices run clear when chicken is pierced.

Nutrients per serving	
Calories	201
Fat	5 g
Carbohydrate	12 g
Protein	27 g

Pepper-Stuffed Chicken with Cantaloupe Sauce

Makes 4 servings

Roasted peppers add flavor and color to this unusual dish.

Tips

Remove the bay leaf before serving as it might cause someone to choke if eaten.

The red pepper and cantaloupe boost the vitamin A and C content of this dish. Team it up with a salad for a meal with eye appeal.

Onion has low levels of histamine. Eating it occasionally is unlikely to trigger headaches. You could replace it with an equal amount of chopped shallots, if desired.

● **Preheat broiler**

½	large red bell pepper	½
½	large green bell pepper	½
4	boneless skinless chicken breasts (4 oz/125 g each)	4
	Salt and freshly ground black pepper	
2 cups	water	500 mL
1	stalk celery, cut into ½-inch (1 cm) pieces	1
1	small onion, sliced	1
1	bay leaf	1
¼	large cantaloupe, peeled	¼
2 tsp	lemon juice	10 mL
	Chopped fresh parsley	

1. Roast red and green peppers (see box, page 241). Cut each into 4 long strips.

2. Place chicken between plastic wrap; flatten with mallet. Sprinkle with salt and pepper to taste. Place 1 green and 1 red pepper strip on each chicken breast; roll up tightly and secure with toothpick.

3. In a skillet, bring water, celery, onion, bay leaf and ¼ tsp (1 mL) each salt and pepper to a boil; add chicken rolls. Cover and simmer for 10 to 15 minutes or until chicken is no longer pink inside. Remove from liquid; drain.

4. In a food processor or blender, purée cantaloupe with lemon juice. Heat gently in small saucepan. Divide among 4 plates. Slice each chicken breast into 3 diagonal pieces. Place on cantaloupe purée. Sprinkle with parsley.

This recipe courtesy of chef Vern Dean and dietitian Jane Thornthwaite.

Nutrients per serving	
Calories	169
Fat	2 g
Carbohydrate	10 g
Protein	28 g

Chicken Breasts with Sweet Potatoes and Onions

A breeze to prepare, this easy-to-assemble dish is elegant enough to serve to company. The herb and lemon butter tucked under the skins keeps the chicken moist and imparts a wonderful flavor to the vegetables layered on the bottom.

Tips

Make extra batches of rosemary butter, shape into small logs, wrap in plastic wrap and store in the freezer. Cut into slices and use to tuck under the breast skins of whole roasting chickens or Cornish hens, or to top grilled meats.

If you purchased whole breasts with backs on, cut away backbone using poultry shears.

This recipe can easily be halved to serve 2.

- Preheat oven to 375°F (190°C)
- 13- by 9-inch (33 by 23 cm) glass baking dish, greased

2	sweet potatoes (about 1½ lbs/750 g)	2
1	onion	1
1½ tsp	chopped fresh rosemary (or ½ tsp/2 mL dried rosemary, crumbled)	7 mL
	Salt and freshly ground black pepper	
4	skinless bone-in chicken breasts	4

Rosemary Butter

2 tbsp	butter	30 mL
1	large clove garlic, minced	1
1 tsp	grated lemon zest	5 mL
2 tsp	chopped fresh rosemary (or ¾ tsp/3 mL dried rosemary, crumbled)	10 mL
¼ tsp	salt	1 mL
¼ tsp	freshly ground black pepper	1 mL

1. Peel sweet potatoes and onion; cut into thin slices. Layer in prepared baking dish. Season with rosemary and salt and pepper to taste.

2. *Rosemary Butter:* In a small bowl, mash together butter, garlic, lemon zest, rosemary, salt and pepper. Divide into four portions.

3. Place chicken breasts, skin side up, on work surface. Remove any fat deposits under skins. Press down on breast bone to flatten slightly. Carefully loosen the breast skins and tuck rosemary butter under skins, patting to distribute evenly.

4. Arrange chicken on top of vegetables in baking dish. Roast for 45 to 55 minutes or until vegetables are tender and chicken is cooked through and nicely colored.

Nutrients per serving	
Calories	220
Fat	8 g
Carbohydrate	19 g
Protein	18 g

Grilled Garlic-Ginger Chicken Breasts

This simple grilled chicken can be enhanced with any of the great salsas or dips in this book.

Tips

Broiler Method: After removing chicken from marinade, place in a lightly greased 9-inch (23 cm) square baking pan and pour in marinade. Broil, turning once, for 5 to 6 minutes per side or until chicken is no longer pink inside and has reached an internal temperature of 170°F (77°C).

Extra cooked chicken is always useful to add a quick protein boost to salads, stir-fries and soups.

2 tbsp	freshly squeezed lemon juice	30 mL
2 tsp	minced garlic	10 mL
2 tsp	minced gingerroot	10 mL
2 tsp	olive oil	10 mL
1 tsp	ground cumin	5 mL
4	boneless skinless chicken breasts (1 lb/500 g total)	4
	Freshly ground black pepper	

1. In a shallow dish, whisk together lemon juice, garlic, ginger, olive oil and cumin. Add chicken and turn to coat. Let stand at room temperature for 10 minutes, or cover and refrigerate for up to 4 hours. Preheat barbecue to medium.

2. Remove chicken from marinade and discard marinade. Place chicken on barbecue and cook, turning once, for 3 to 5 minutes per side or until chicken is no longer pink inside and has reached an internal temperature of 170°F (77°C). Season to taste with pepper.

This recipe courtesy of dietitian Judy Jenkins.

Nutrients per serving	
Calories	145
Fat	3 g
Carbohydrate	1 g
Protein	26 g

Broiled Rosemary Thighs

Makes 4 servings

This very simple recipe creates wonderfully moist and delicious chicken.

Tip

Lemon has low histamine levels. Occasional or small amounts are unlikely to trigger headaches.

- Preheat broiler
- Foil-lined broiling pan

8	chicken thighs	8
1/2 tsp	grated lemon zest	2 mL
3 tbsp	fresh lemon juice	45 mL
3 tbsp	olive oil	45 mL
1 tbsp	chopped fresh rosemary (or 1 tsp/5 mL dried rosemary, crumbled)	15 mL
	Salt and freshly ground black pepper	

1. Place chicken thighs in a glass dish just big enough to hold them in a single layer. In a bowl, whisk together the lemon zest, lemon juice, olive oil and rosemary. Pour over chicken and turn to coat well. Cover and let stand at room temperature for 30 minutes.

2. Reserving the marinade, arrange chicken thighs skin-side down on prepared pan; sprinkle with salt and pepper. Broil 4 inches (10 cm) from heat for 7 minutes, basting occasionally.

3. Turn, baste and broil 5 to 8 minutes longer, or until chicken is no longer pink inside.

Nutrients per serving	
Calories	498
Fat	10 g
Carbohydrate	1 g
Protein	29 g

Grilled Chicken Kabobs

Makes 4 servings

Put the chicken in the fridge to marinate first thing in the morning. Then, at suppertime, all you have to do is thread the chicken onto skewers and grill the kabobs. Serve with tzatziki on the side.

Tip

To bake these kabobs instead of grilling them, place them on a rimmed baking sheet lined with parchment paper and bake in a 350°F (180°C) oven, turning once, for 20 minutes or until chicken is no longer pink inside.

- Four 8- or 9-inch (20 or 23 cm) metal or wooden skewers

2 to 3	cloves garlic, minced	2 to 3
1 1/2 tbsp	olive oil	22 mL
1 tsp	dried parsley	5 mL
1/2 tsp	dried oregano	2 mL
1 lb	boneless skinless chicken breasts, cut into 1 1/2-inch (4 cm) cubes	500 g
	Salt and freshly ground black pepper	

1. In a large sealable plastic bag, combine garlic to taste, oil, parsley and oregano. Add chicken, seal and toss to coat. Refrigerate for at least 6 hours or overnight.

2. Preheat barbecue grill to medium. If using wooden skewers, soak them in water for 10 minutes.

3. Remove chicken from marinade, discarding marinade. Thread chicken onto skewers, leaving space between pieces. Grill chicken, turning often, for 7 to 10 minutes per side or until chicken is no longer pink inside. Season to taste with salt and pepper.

Nutrients per serving	
Calories	180
Fat	7 g
Carbohydrate	1 g
Protein	26 g

Chicken and Vegetable Stew

Makes 4 servings

Even if you don't have a lot of time to spend in the kitchen, you can rustle up a great-tasting stew using boneless chicken thighs and convenient frozen vegetables. This satisfying dish does away with browning the chicken. You'll save time but not lose any flavor. Serve over noodles.

Tip

Use 5 cups (1.25 L) fresh vegetables instead of frozen, if you wish. Cut them into bite-size pieces. For slower-cooking vegetables, such as carrots and celery, add them along with the chicken. For faster-cooking ones, such as broccoli and zucchini, add in the last 10 minutes of cooking.

1 tbsp	butter	15 mL
1	large onion, chopped	1
2	cloves garlic, finely chopped	2
1 tsp	dried Italian herbs or fines herbes	5 mL
1 lb	boneless skinless chicken thighs (about 8), cut into 1-inch (2.5 cm) cubes	500 g
3 tbsp	all-purpose flour	45 mL
2 cups	ready-to-use chicken broth	500 mL
1	package (1 lb/500 g) frozen mixed vegetables	1
	Salt and freshly ground black pepper	

1. In a Dutch oven or large saucepan, melt butter over medium heat. Add onion, garlic and Italian herbs; cook, stirring, for 4 minutes or until lightly colored.

2. In a bowl, toss chicken with flour until well coated. Add to pan along with any remaining flour; stir in broth. Bring to a boil and cook, stirring, until sauce thickens. Reduce heat, cover and simmer, stirring occasionally, for 20 minutes.

3. Add frozen vegetables; return to a boil. Season with salt and pepper to taste. Reduce heat, cover and simmer for 10 minutes or until chicken and vegetables are tender.

Reduce the Histamine

Replace the dried Italian herbs with 1 tbsp (15 mL) chopped fresh herbs, such as marjoram, thyme, rosemary, sage, oregano and/or basil. Add the fresh herbs at the end of step 3.

If serving over noodles, choose gluten-free noodles.

Replace the all-purpose flour with all-purpose gluten-free flour mix.

Nutrients per serving	
Calories	326
Fat	10 g
Carbohydrate	26 g
Protein	33 g

Oven-Baked Beef Stew

This stew is full of flavor, including the woodsy taste of thyme. Serve it up with mashed potatoes or over cooked rice, GF pasta or quinoa.

Tip

Onion has low levels of histamine. Eating it occasionally is unlikely to trigger headaches. You could replace it with an equal amount of chopped shallots, if desired.

- Preheat oven to 350°F (180°C)
- 8-inch (20 cm) glass baking dish

1 tbsp	grapeseed oil	15 mL
1 lb	lean stewing beef, cut into bite-size pieces	500 g
3	cloves garlic, minced	3
½ cup	chopped onion	125 mL
2 tsp	dried parsley	10 mL
1 tsp	dried thyme	5 mL
1 tbsp	white rice flour	15 mL
1¼ cups	ready-to-use reduced-sodium vegetable broth	300 mL
2 tsp	butter	10 mL
	Salt and freshly ground black pepper	

1. In a large skillet, heat oil over medium-high heat. Cook beef for 5 minutes or until browned on all sides. Using a slotted spoon, transfer to baking dish.

2. Reduce heat to medium. Add garlic, onion, parsley and thyme to skillet; sauté for 3 to 4 minutes or until onion is softened. Sprinkle with flour and cook, stirring, for 1 minute. Gradually stir in broth and bring to a boil, scraping up any brown bits from pan. Stir in butter until melted. Pour over beef.

3. Cover and bake in preheated oven for 1 hour or until meat is fork-tender. Season to taste with salt and pepper.

Nutrients per serving	
Calories	230
Fat	11 g
Carbohydrate	6 g
Protein	26 g

Bistecca alla Florentine

Simplicity itself — since its only partners are salt, pepper and very good olive oil — the T-bone must be of the absolute best quality, preferably prime, and as thick as 3 inches (7.5 cm). Traditionally, this steak is served rare.

● **Preheat barbecue grill to high**

1	T-bone steak (3 to 3½ lbs/1.5 to 1.75 kg)	1
	Salt and freshly ground black pepper	
	Extra virgin olive oil	

1. Sprinkle steak with salt and pepper. Place on preheated grill. Cook undisturbed for about 5 minutes on first side.

2. Using tongs, flip steak; cook undisturbed for another 5 minutes, then continue to cook, turning every 5 minutes, for 10 to 12 minutes or according to taste.

3. Remove steak to a cutting board. Let rest for 5 minutes before carving. Arrange on serving platter; drizzle with olive oil. Serve immediately.

Nutrients per 1 of 6 servings	
Calories	282
Fat	14 g
Carbohydrate	0 g
Protein	36 g

Veal Braised with Onions

Richly flavored braised meats like veal are always a welcome choice for a family meal. Make them in advance, as their flavor improves when refrigerated and reheated the next day. Serve this simple dish with noodles or creamy mashed potatoes.

Tip

To brown meat without having to add a lot of oil, pat meat dry with paper towels before cooking. Add a bit of the oil to the pan and heat until hot but not smoking. Add a small amount of the meat at a time until nicely colored; remove. Add a bit more oil to pan if necessary and reheat before adding next batch of meat.

2 lbs	lean stewing veal, cut into ¾-inch (2 cm) cubes	1 kg
2 tbsp	olive oil (approx.), divided	30 mL
2	large onions, chopped	2
2	cloves garlic, finely chopped	2
2 tbsp	all-purpose flour	30 mL
1½ cups	ready-to-use chicken broth	375 mL
½ cup	dry white wine or additional broth	125 mL
2 tbsp	tomato paste	30 mL
1 tsp	salt	5 mL
½ tsp	freshly ground black pepper	2 mL
¼ cup	chopped fresh parsley	60 mL
1 tsp	grated lemon zest	5 mL

1. Pat veal dry with paper towels. In a Dutch oven or large saucepan, heat 1 tbsp (15 mL) oil over high heat. Brown veal, in batches, adding more oil as needed. Transfer to a plate as meat browns.

2. Reduce heat to medium; add remaining oil. Cook onions and garlic, stirring, for 5 minutes or until lightly colored. Blend in flour; stir in broth, wine and tomato paste. Add veal along with accumulated juices; season with salt and pepper. Bring to a boil.

3. Reduce heat, cover and simmer, stirring occasionally, for 50 minutes. Stir in parsley and lemon zest; cook, covered, for 10 minutes or until veal is tender.

Reduce the Histamine

Use additional broth instead of white wine.

Omit the tomato paste or, to replace some or all of it, try roasting red bell peppers, peeling off the charred skin and puréeing the peppers in a blender.

If serving with noodles, choose gluten-free noodles.

Nutrients per serving	
Calories	171
Fat	7 g
Carbohydrate	10 g
Protein	17 g

Veal Meatloaf

Ground meats are one of the best supermarket buys for budget-trimming meals. Serve this family favorite accompanied with fluffy mashed potatoes and glazed carrots for a delicious, economical supper.

Variations

Mini Veal Meatloaves: Divide into 12 balls; lightly press into muffin cups. Bake at 400°F (200°C) for 20 minutes or until no longer pink in center. Drain off juice.

Ground chicken can be substituted for the ground veal.

Reduce the Histamine

Have your butcher grind the veal for you so it's as fresh as possible. Cook it as soon as you can.

Use gluten-free bread crumbs.

- Preheat oven to 350°F (180°C)
- 9- by 5-inch (23 by 12.5 cm) loaf pan, greased

1 tbsp	olive oil	15 mL
1	onion, finely chopped	1
1	large clove garlic, finely chopped	1
½ tsp	dried thyme or marjoram	2 mL
¾ tsp	salt	3 mL
¼ tsp	freshly ground black pepper	1 mL
1	large egg	1
¼ cup	ready-to-use chicken broth	60 mL
1 tsp	grated lemon zest	5 mL
½ cup	dry seasoned bread crumbs	125 mL
2 tbsp	finely chopped fresh parsley	30 mL
1½ lbs	lean ground veal	750 g

1. In a large nonstick skillet, heat oil over medium heat; cook onion, garlic, thyme, salt and pepper, stirring often, for 3 minutes or until softened. Let cool slightly.

2. In a bowl, beat together egg, broth and lemon zest. Stir in onion mixture, bread crumbs, parsley and veal. Using a wooden spoon, gently mix until evenly combined.

3. Press mixture lightly into prepared loaf pan. Bake in preheated oven for 1 hour or until meat thermometer registers 170°F (77°C). Let stand for 5 minutes. Drain pan juices; turn out onto a plate and cut into thick slices.

Nutrients per serving	
Calories	201
Fat	9 g
Carbohydrate	9 g
Protein	21 g

Side Dishes

Braised Baby Bok Choy

You're sure to enjoy this delicious, slightly sweet side dish.

Reduce the Histamine

If you have a histamine response to hot pepper flakes, omit them from the recipe. Place hot pepper sauce or hot pepper flakes on the table so diners can add heat to taste.

2	cloves garlic, minced	2
$\frac{1}{8}$ tsp	hot pepper flakes	0.5 mL
$1\frac{1}{2}$ cups	ready-to-use reduced-sodium vegetable or chicken broth	375 mL
$1\frac{1}{2}$ lbs	baby bok choy, trimmed	750 g
$\frac{1}{4}$ tsp	freshly ground black pepper	1 mL
1 tsp	toasted sesame oil	5 mL

1. In a large skillet, combine garlic, hot pepper flakes and broth. Bring to a simmer over medium-high heat. Arrange bok choy evenly in skillet. Reduce heat to medium-low, cover and simmer for about 5 minutes or until tender. Using tongs, transfer bok choy to a serving dish, cover and keep warm.

2. Increase heat to medium-high and boil broth mixture until reduced to about $\frac{1}{4}$ cup (60 mL), then stir in black pepper and sesame oil. Pour over bok choy.

Nutrients per serving	
Calories	40
Fat	2 g
Carbohydrate	5 g
Protein	3 g

Lemon-Glazed Baby Carrots

This is a good choice to accompany a holiday roast or turkey. Packages of ready-to-cook, peeled whole baby carrots are widely available in supermarkets. They certainly make a cook's life easier — especially when you're preparing a mammoth family dinner and plan to serve several dishes.

Tips

If doubling the recipe, glaze vegetables in a large nonstick skillet to evaporate the broth quickly.

Try this tasty treatment with a combination of blanched carrots, rutabaga and parsnip strips too.

Lemon has low histamine levels. Occasional or small amounts are unlikely to trigger headaches.

1 lb	peeled baby carrots	500 g
¼ cup	ready-to-use reduced-sodium chicken or vegetable broth	60 mL
2 tsp	butter	10 mL
1 tbsp	packed brown sugar	15 mL
½ tsp	grated lemon zest	2 mL
1 tbsp	freshly squeezed lemon juice	15 mL
¼ tsp	salt	1 mL
	Freshly ground black pepper	
1 tbsp	finely chopped fresh parsley or chives	15 mL

1. In a medium saucepan, cook carrots in boiling salted water for 5 to 7 minutes (start timing when water returns to a boil) or until just tender-crisp; drain and return to saucepan.

2. Add broth, butter, brown sugar, lemon zest and juice, salt and pepper to taste. Cook, stirring often, for 3 to 5 minutes or until liquid has evaporated and carrots are nicely glazed.

3. Sprinkle with parsley or chives and serve.

Nutrients per serving	
Calories	102
Fat	6 g
Carbohydrate	11 g
Protein	1 g

Ginger Carrots

Makes 4 to 6 servings

Mmmmmmm good — a delicious way to enjoy carrots. Kids love them.

Tip

Use the side of a spoon to scrape the skin off gingerroot before chopping or grating. Gingerroot keeps well in the freezer for up to 3 months and can be grated from frozen.

4 cups	chopped carrots	1 L
½ cup	ready-to-use vegetable or chicken broth	125 mL
2 tsp	minced gingerroot	10 mL
1 tsp	minced garlic	5 mL
1 tsp	packed brown sugar	5 mL
¼ tsp	freshly squeezed lemon juice	1 mL

1. In a large saucepan, combine carrots, broth, ginger, garlic, brown sugar and lemon juice. Bring to a boil, then reduce heat, cover and simmer for about 20 minutes or until carrots are tender-crisp and liquid is absorbed.

This recipe courtesy of dietitian Roberta Lowcay.

Nutrients per 1 of 6 servings	
Calories	34
Fat	0 g
Carbohydrate	8 g
Protein	1 g

Garlicky Cauliflower Purée

Makes 6 servings

This side dish makes a great match for steak or chicken.

- Steamer basket
- Food processor

4	cloves garlic	4
1	head cauliflower (2 to 2½ lbs/ 1 to 1.25 kg), broken into florets	1
¼ tsp	fine sea salt	1 mL
⅛ tsp	freshly ground black pepper	0.5 mL
¾ cup	ready-to-use reduced-sodium vegetable or chicken broth	175 mL
1 tbsp	extra virgin olive oil	15 mL

1. Place garlic and cauliflower in a steamer basket set over a large pot of boiling water. Cover and steam for 7 to 9 minutes or until cauliflower is tender. Reserve steaming water.

2. In food processor, combine half the cauliflower mixture, salt, pepper, broth and oil; purée until smooth. Add the remaining cauliflower mixture and purée until smooth, adding a bit of the steaming water as needed to moisten.

Nutrients per serving	
Calories	44
Fat	3 g
Carbohydrate	5 g
Protein	2 g

Fennel Gratin

Makes 4 servings

Fennel adds versatility to any recipe and goes particularly well with fish.

Tips

The stalks and bulbs of fennel should be firm.

If fennel is unavailable, replace with 1 large sliced zucchini or half a small sliced eggplant.

Make Ahead

Prepare and refrigerate early in day. Bake just before eating. This tastes great reheated.

Reduce the Histamine

To replace all or some of the tomato sauce, try roasting red bell peppers, peeling off the charred skin and puréeing the peppers in a blender.

- Preheat oven to 350°F (180°C)
- 8-inch (20 cm) square baking dish

1	fennel bulb, trimmed and thinly sliced	1
1½ tsp	vegetable oil	7 mL
2 tsp	crushed garlic	10 mL
½ cup	chopped onion	125 mL
2 cups	tomato sauce	500 mL
2 tbsp	chopped fresh dill (or 1 tsp/5 mL dried dillweed)	30 mL
½ cup	shredded mozzarella cheese	125 mL

1. In saucepan of boiling water, cook fennel just until tender, 5 to 8 minutes. Drain and set aside.

2. In nonstick skillet, heat oil; sauté garlic and onion until softened. Add tomato sauce and dill.

3. Add half of the tomato sauce mixture to baking dish. Add fennel; pour remaining sauce over top. Top with cheese.

4. Bake in preheated oven for 20 minutes or until hot and cheese melts.

Nutrients per serving	
Calories	122
Fat	4 g
Carbohydrate	16 g
Protein	7 g

Braised Green Beans and Fennel

This recipe works beautifully as a warm-up starter salad, or as a side vegetable to grilled meat or fish. Green beans provide the bulk, but it is the fresh fennel that gives it character.

Tip

The fennel bulb always comes attached to woody branches and thin leaves that look like dill. You'll need the leaves for the final garnish, so cut them off and set them aside. Cut off and discard the woody branches. Quarter the bulb vertically, then cut out and discard the hard triangular sections of core. What remains is the usable part of the fennel.

Reduce the Histamine

Replace the balsamic vinegar with cider vinegar.

1/4 cup	olive oil	60 mL
1/2 tsp	salt	2 mL
1/4 tsp	freshly ground black pepper	1 mL
1 tsp	whole fennel seeds	5 mL
12 oz	green beans, trimmed	375 g
1	large or 2 small fennel bulbs, trimmed, cored and cut into 1/2-inch (1 cm) slices (see tip, at left)	1
1	small carrot, peeled and sliced into 1/4-inch (0.5 cm) rounds	1
6	cloves garlic, thinly sliced	6
1 cup	water	250 mL
1 tbsp	balsamic vinegar	15 mL
	Few sprigs fennel greens, chopped	

1. In a large, deep frying pan, heat olive oil, salt and pepper over high heat for 1 minute. Add fennel seeds; stir-fry 1 minute or until just browning. Add green beans, fennel and carrots; stir-fry 3 minutes or until all the vegetables are shiny and beginning to sizzle. Add garlic; stir-fry for 1 more minute.

2. Immediately add water and vinegar; cook for 2 minutes or until bubbling. Reduce heat to medium-low, cover pan tightly and cook for 20 minutes.

3. Place a strainer over a bowl and strain contents of the pan. Transfer the strained vegetables onto a platter and keep warm. Transfer the liquid that has collected in the bowl back into the pan; bring to a boil and cook for 6 to 7 minutes or until thick and syrupy.

4. Spoon the reduced sauce over the vegetables, garnish with the chopped fennel greens and serve immediately.

Nutrients per serving	
Calories	144
Fat	11 g
Carbohydrate	11 g
Protein	2 g

Quick Sautéed Kale

Serve this nutrient-charged side dish alongside your favorite meals.

- Steamer basket

1 lb	kale, tough stems and ribs removed, leaves cut into ¼-inch (0.5 cm) wide strips (about 8 cups/2 L)	500 g
1 tbsp	extra virgin olive oil	15 mL
1 cup	thinly sliced red onion	250 mL
2	cloves garlic, minced	2
Pinch	hot pepper flakes	Pinch
¼ tsp	fine sea salt	1 mL
1 tbsp	red wine vinegar	15 mL

1. Place kale in a steamer basket set over a large pot of boiling water. Cover and steam for 8 to 10 minutes or until tender.

2. In a large skillet, heat oil over medium-high heat. Add red onion and cook, stirring, for 6 to 8 minutes or until golden. Add garlic and hot pepper flakes; cook, stirring, for 1 minute. Add kale, reduce heat to medium and cook, stirring occasionally, for 1 to 2 minutes or until heated through. Remove from heat and stir in salt and vinegar.

Nutrients per serving	
Calories	86
Fat	3 g
Carbohydrate	14 g
Protein	4 g

Sautéed Swiss Chard

Earthy, grassy Swiss chard makes a gorgeous, incredibly tasty side dish. It needs little adornment beyond a bit of olive oil and garlic.

Tip

Onion has low levels of histamine. Eating it occasionally is unlikely to trigger headaches. You could replace it with an equal amount of chopped shallots, if desired.

3 lbs	Swiss chard (about 2 large bunches)	1.5 kg
1 tbsp	extra virgin olive oil	15 mL
2	onions, halved, then thinly sliced	2
3	cloves garlic, minced	3
1/4 tsp	fine sea salt	1 mL
1/4 tsp	freshly ground black pepper	1 mL

1. Trim stems and center ribs from Swiss chard, then cut stems and ribs crosswise into 1-inch (2.5 cm) pieces. Stack chard leaves, roll them up crosswise into a tight cylinder and cut the cylinder crosswise into 1-inch (2.5 cm) thick slices.

2. In a large, heavy pot, heat oil over medium heat. Add onions and cook, stirring, for 8 to 9 minutes or until golden. Stir in chard stems and ribs, garlic, salt and pepper. Cover and cook, stirring occasionally, for 8 to 10 minutes or until stems are tender.

3. Add half the chard leaves and cook, stirring, for 1 minute or until slightly wilted. Add the remaining leaves, cover and cook, stirring occasionally, for 4 to 6 minutes or until leaves are tender. Using a slotted spoon, transfer Swiss chard mixture to plates or a serving bowl.

Nutrients per serving	
Calories	52
Fat	1 g
Carbohydrate	10 g
Protein	4 g

Herbed Parsnips

Once you try these appetizing parsnips, you are sure to make them often.

Tips

Chop parsnips into 1-inch (2.5 cm) pieces.

To make a simple parsnip soup, transfer the cooked parsnips to a blender and add 1 cup (250 mL) Vegetable Stock (page 218) or ready-to-use reduced-sodium vegetable broth; purée until smooth. Transfer to a saucepan and simmer over low heat until warmed through.

Variation

Substitute carrots for the parsnips.

- Preheat oven to 425°F (220°C)
- 4-cup (1 L) baking dish, lightly sprayed with light nonstick cooking spray

8 oz	parsnips, chopped (about 1⅓ cups/325 mL)	250 g
1	clove garlic, minced	1
½ tsp	dried thyme	2 mL
½ tsp	canola oil	2 mL
	Salt and freshly ground black pepper (optional)	
1 tsp	no-sugar-added maple-flavored syrup	5 mL

1. In prepared baking dish, combine parsnips, garlic, thyme and oil, tossing to coat. If desired, season to taste with salt and pepper.

2. Cover and bake in preheated oven for 30 minutes or until parsnips are almost tender. Carefully turn parsnips and stir in syrup. Bake, uncovered, for 10 minutes or until golden brown and tender.

Nutrients per serving	
Calories	56
Fat	1 g
Carbohydrate	13 g
Protein	1 g

Summer Zucchini

This side dish is a terrific use for zucchini at its peak of freshness.

Tips

Lemon has low histamine levels. Occasional or small amounts are unlikely to trigger headaches.

Adding leafy herbs to recipes reduces histamine levels.

4	young zucchini, preferably 2 each of green and yellow, less than 6 inches (15 cm) in length	4
3 tbsp	olive oil	45 mL
$\frac{1}{4}$ tsp	salt	1 mL
$\frac{1}{4}$ tsp	freshly ground black pepper	1 mL
1	red bell pepper, cut into thick strips	1
3	green onions, chopped	3
1 tbsp	freshly squeezed lemon juice	15 mL
	Few sprigs fresh basil and/or parsley, chopped	

1. Trim ends of zucchini and cut into $\frac{3}{4}$-inch (2 cm) chunks. Set aside.

2. In a large frying pan, heat olive oil over high heat for 30 seconds. Add salt and pepper and stir. Add zucchini chunks and red pepper strips. Stir-fry for 4 to 6 minutes until the zucchini chunks have browned on both sides and the red pepper has softened. Add green onions and stir-fry for 30 seconds. Transfer to a serving dish and drizzle evenly with lemon juice. Garnish with basil and/ or parsley and serve immediately.

Nutrients per serving	
Calories	121
Fat	10 g
Carbohydrate	7 g
Protein	2 g

Company Vegetables with Toasted Almonds

Makes 6 to 8 servings

Put your microwave oven to good use when preparing vegetables to serve a crowd. Arrange vegetables in dish, ready to pop in the microwave shortly before serving.

Tips

Test first to see if the dish called for fits comfortably in your microwave oven. If not, divide vegetable mixture among two 9-inch (23 cm) microwave-safe pie plates. Cover with inverted plate or plastic wrap with one corner turned back to vent. Microwave each plate on High for 4 to 6 minutes.

Serve almond butter with other steamed vegetables, such as Brussels sprouts.

- 10-cup (2.5 L) shallow baking dish or large (12-inch/30 cm) microwave-safe platter (see tip, at left)

4 cups	cauliflower florets (1/2 head)	1 L
4 cups	broccoli florets	1 L
1	red bell pepper, cut into squares	1
1	yellow or orange bell pepper, cut into squares	1

Topping

3 tbsp	butter, divided	45 mL
1/3 cup	sliced almonds	75 mL
1	clove garlic, minced	1
1 tbsp	freshly squeezed lemon juice	15 mL
2 tbsp	chopped fresh parsley	30 mL
	Salt and freshly ground black pepper	

1. In baking dish or platter, alternately arrange cauliflower and broccoli, with broccoli stalks toward the outside, around outer edge of dish. Mound pepper cubes in center. Add 1/3 cup (75 mL) water. Cover with lid or plastic wrap and turn back one corner to vent. Microwave on High for 6 to 9 minutes or until vegetables are tender-crisp. Let stand, covered, while preparing topping.

2. *Topping:* In a small microwave-safe glass bowl, combine 2 tbsp (30 mL) of the butter and almonds. Microwave, uncovered, on High for 1 1/2 to 3 minutes or until almonds are lightly toasted, stirring twice. (Can be done up to 4 hours ahead, if desired.)

3. Just before serving, add remaining butter and garlic to toasted almonds. Microwave, uncovered, on High for 45 to 60 seconds or until fragrant. Stir in lemon juice. Carefully drain water from vegetables (a plate set on top will hold vegetables in place).

4. Pour almond butter over top. Sprinkle with parsley. Season with salt and pepper to taste. Serve immediately.

Nutrients per 1 of 8 servings	
Calories	112
Fat	8 g
Carbohydrate	10 g
Protein	4 g

Butternut Squash with Snow Peas and Red Pepper

If the soft texture of a squash purée doesn't appeal to you, try this easy stir-fry instead.

Tips

To prepare squash, peel using a vegetable peeler or paring knife. Cut into lengthwise quarters and seed. Cut into ¼-inch (0.5 cm) wide by 1½-inch (4 cm) long pieces.

Warning: Snow peas may be a trigger for migraines for some people.

1 tbsp	vegetable oil	15 mL
5 cups	prepared butternut squash (see tip, at left)	1.25 L
4 oz	snow peas, ends trimmed	125 g
1	red bell pepper, cut into thin strips	1
1 tbsp	packed brown sugar	15 mL
1½ tsp	grated gingerroot	7 mL
	Freshly ground black pepper	

1. In a large nonstick skillet, heat oil over medium-high heat. Cook squash, stirring, for 3 to 4 minutes or until almost tender.

2. Add snow peas, red pepper, brown sugar and ginger. Cook, stirring often, for 2 minutes or until vegetables are tender-crisp. Season with pepper to taste.

Nutrients per serving	
Calories	47
Fat	3 g
Carbohydrate	3 g
Protein	2 g

Mashed Sweet Potatoes with Rosemary

Here's a healthy twist on traditional mashed potatoes.

	Nutrients per serving	
Calories		102
Fat		2 g
Carbohydrate		25 g
Protein		2 g

2 lbs	sweet potatoes, peeled and diced	1 kg
2½ tsp	minced fresh rosemary	12 mL
¼ tsp	fine sea salt	1 mL
¼ tsp	freshly ground black pepper	1 mL
2 tsp	extra virgin olive oil	10 mL

1. Place sweet potatoes in a medium saucepan and cover with water. Bring to a boil over high heat. Boil for 8 minutes or until tender. Drain, reserving ⅓ cup (75 mL) of the cooking water.

2. In a large bowl, using an electric mixer on medium speed, beat sweet potatoes and reserved cooking liquid until smooth. Beat in rosemary, salt and pepper. Spoon into a bowl and drizzle with oil.

Sweet Potato Fries

Sweet potatoes become incredibly tasty when roasted at a high temperature.

	Nutrients per serving	
Calories		86
Fat		3 g
Carbohydrate		14 g
Protein		1 g

- Preheat oven to 450°F (230°C)
- Large rimmed baking sheet, lined with foil and sprayed with nonstick cooking spray

4	sweet potatoes (each about 8 oz/250 g), peeled and cut into 3-inch (7.5 cm) long by ¼-inch (0.5 cm) thick sticks	4
½ tsp	fine sea salt	2 mL
¼ tsp	freshly ground black pepper	1 mL
4 tsp	vegetable oil	20 mL

1. In a large bowl, combine sweet potatoes, salt, pepper and oil, tossing to coat. Spread in a single layer on prepared baking sheet.

2. Bake in preheated oven for 20 minutes. Gently turn sweet potatoes over and bake for 12 to 17 minutes or until crisp. Serve immediately.

Baked Parsnip Fries

Makes 4 servings

When you're tired of the same old flavors, try introducing your family to this new twist on home fries.

Nutrients per serving	
Calories	95
Fat	3 g
Carbohydrate	20 g
Protein	1 g

- Preheat oven to 400°F (200°C)
- Large rimmed baking sheet, lined with foil and sprayed with nonstick cooking spray

1 lb	parsnips, cut into 3-inch (7.5 cm) long by 1/4-inch (0.5 cm) thick sticks	500 g
1/4 tsp	fine sea salt	1 mL
1/8 tsp	freshly ground black pepper	0.5 mL
1 tbsp	extra virgin olive oil	15 mL
1 tbsp	chopped fresh flat-leaf (Italian) parsley	15 mL

1. In a large bowl, combine parsnips, salt, pepper and oil, tossing to coat. Spread in a single layer on prepared baking sheet.

2. Bake in preheated oven for 15 minutes. Gently turn parsnips over and bake for 12 to 17 minutes or until crisp. Serve immediately, sprinkled with parsley.

Rutabaga Fries

Makes 8 servings

Crispy with a bite, these fries will quickly become your favorite side dish.

Variation
Use any herb or spice of your choice, such as dried oregano, ground turmeric, paprika, dried herbes de Provence or Chinese five-spice powder, in place of the garlic powder.

Nutrients per serving	
Calories	26
Fat	1 g
Carbohydrate	5 g
Protein	1 g

- Preheat oven to 400°F (200°C)
- Steamer basket
- Large rimmed baking sheet, lightly sprayed with light nonstick cooking spray

1 lb	rutabaga, peeled and cut into 1/2-inch (1 cm) thick spears	500 g
1/8 tsp	garlic powder	0.5 mL
1 tsp	olive oil	5 mL
1/8 tsp	coarse sea salt (or to taste)	0.5 mL

1. In a pot, bring 1 inch (2.5 cm) of water to a boil over high heat. Place rutabaga in steamer basket and set over boiling water. Cover and steam for 10 minutes or until starting to soften.

2. Transfer to a large bowl and, using a paper towel, pat rutabaga dry. Add garlic powder and oil; toss to coat. Spread out in a single layer on prepared baking sheet.

3. Bake in preheated oven for 30 minutes, turning halfway through, until golden brown and tender. Season with up to 1/8 tsp (0.5 mL) salt.

Basic Polenta and Grits

Polenta, the Italian version of cornmeal mush, is a magnificent way to add whole grains to your diet. When properly cooked, it is a soothing comfort food that functions like a bowl of steaming mashed potatoes, the yummy basis upon which more elaborate dishes can strut their stuff.

Tips

If you prefer, substitute ready-to-use vegetable or chicken broth for the water.

Grits, which are more coarsely ground than cornmeal, are even more delicious if you can find artisanal versions being produced in the southern U.S. They are prepared just like stone-ground cornmeal, but take longer to cook.

Grits are very sticky. Greasing the saucepan or using one with a nonstick finish helps with cleanup.

4½ cups	water (see tip, at left)	1.125 L
¼ tsp	salt	1 mL
1 cup	coarse stone-ground cornmeal or coarse stone-ground grits	250 mL

1. In a saucepan over medium heat, bring water and salt to a boil. Gradually stir in cornmeal in a steady stream. Cook, stirring constantly, until smooth and blended and mixture bubbles like lava, about 5 minutes.

2. Reduce heat to low (placing a heat diffuser under the pot if your stove doesn't have a true simmer). Continue cooking, stirring frequently, while the mixture bubbles and thickens, until the grains are tender and creamy, about 30 minutes for polenta; about 1 hour for grits. Serve immediately.

Variations

Creamy Polenta: Substitute 2½ cups (625 mL) milk or cream and 2 cups (500 mL) water or broth for the liquid. If you like, stir in 2 tbsp (30 mL) freshly grated Parmesan cheese after the cornmeal has been added to the liquid.

Polenta Squares: Transfer the hot cooked polenta into a greased baking pan or dish (depending upon the thickness you want), using the back of a spoon to even the top. Set aside to cool (it will solidify during the process) and cut into squares.

Cheesy Baked Grits: Complete step 1. Remove from heat and stir in 2 cups (500 mL) shredded Cheddar or Jack cheese and 2 beaten eggs. You can also add a finely chopped roasted red bell pepper or half of a chipotle pepper in adobo sauce, if you prefer. Stir well and transfer to a greased 6-cup (1.5 L) baking dish. Bake at 350°F (180°C) until grits are tender and pudding is set, about 1 hour.

Nutrients per serving	
Calories	73
Fat	1 g
Carbohydrate	16 g
Protein	1 g

Basic Brown Rice Pilaf

Even whole-grain skeptics will love this simple yet flavorful brown rice dish.

Tip

Onion has low levels of histamine. Eating it occasionally is unlikely to trigger headaches. You could replace it with an equal amount of chopped shallots, if desired.

2 tsp	extra virgin olive oil	10 mL
1 cup	finely chopped celery	250 mL
½ cup	finely chopped onion	125 mL
1 cup	long-grain brown rice	250 mL
⅛ tsp	freshly ground black pepper	0.5 mL
2 cups	ready-to-use reduced-sodium chicken or vegetable broth	500 mL

1. In a large saucepan, heat oil over medium-high heat. Add celery and onion; cook, stirring, for 3 minutes. Add rice and cook, stirring, for 2 minutes.

2. Stir in pepper and broth. Bring to a boil. Reduce heat to low, cover and simmer for 40 to 45 minutes or until broth is absorbed. Let stand, covered, for 5 minutes, then fluff with a fork.

Nutrients per serving	
Calories	140
Fat	3 g
Carbohydrate	27 g
Protein	3 g

Bulgur Pilaf

Bulgur makes a particularly nice pilaf. It has a pleasantly mild flavor that complements just about anything.

Tips

When making this pilaf, use water or a broth that complements the main dish it will accompany.

Onion has low levels of histamine. Eating it occasionally is unlikely to trigger headaches. You could replace it with an equal amount of chopped shallots, if desired.

Reduce the Histamine

Omit the tomato paste or, to replace some or all of it, try roasting red bell peppers, peeling off the charred skin and puréeing the peppers in a blender.

1 tbsp	olive oil	15 mL
1	onion, finely chopped	1
2	cloves garlic, minced	2
	Salt and freshly ground black pepper	
1 cup	coarse bulgur	250 mL
1 tbsp	tomato paste (optional)	15 mL
1½ cups	water or ready-to-use reduced-sodium vegetable, chicken or beef broth (see tip, at left)	375 mL

1. In a saucepan with a tight-fitting lid, heat oil over medium heat for 30 seconds. Add onion and cook, stirring, until softened, about 3 minutes. Add garlic and salt and pepper to taste and cook, stirring, for 1 minute.

2. Add bulgur, tomato paste (if using) and water. Stir well and bring to a boil. Reduce heat to low. Cover and simmer for 10 minutes. Remove from heat. Stir well, cover and let stand until all the liquid is absorbed, about 10 minutes.

Variations

Bulgur Chickpea Pilaf: Stir in 1 cup (250 mL) drained, rinsed cooked or canned chickpeas along with the bulgur.

Beef and Bulgur Pilaf: This can be a light main course. Cook 8 oz (250 g) extra-lean ground beef along with onions, until meat is no longer pink, about 5 minutes. Use beef broth for the liquid in step 2.

Cabbage and Bulgur Pilaf: This is a great way to use up extra cabbage. Add 1 tsp (5 mL) sweet paprika and 2 cups (500 mL) finely shredded cabbage along with garlic. Cook, stirring, for 1 minute. Then add 1 can (14 oz/398 mL) diced tomatoes with juice. Bring to a boil. Cover and cook for 5 minutes. Continue with step 2, omitting tomato paste and using only 1 cup (250 mL) of liquid.

Nutrients per serving	
Calories	109
Fat	3 g
Carbohydrate	20 g
Protein	3 g

Desserts

Quinoa Flake Pie or Tart Crust

Makes one 9-inch (23 cm) pie or tart crust

This fantastic pie crust gives graham cracker crusts a run for their money. Light and crispy, it works especially well with sweet custard- or fruit-filled pies.

- Preheat oven to 350°F (180°C)
- 9-inch (23 cm) pie plate or fluted tart pan with removable bottom

1½ cups	quinoa flakes or quick-cooking rolled oats (certified GF, if needed)	375 mL
¾ cup	quinoa flour	175 mL
⅓ cup	natural cane sugar or packed light brown sugar	75 mL
¼ tsp	fine sea salt	1 mL
6 tbsp	unsalted butter, melted and cooled slightly	90 mL
6 tbsp	milk or plain non-dairy milk (such as soy, almond, rice or hemp)	90 mL

1. In a large bowl, combine quinoa flakes, quinoa flour, sugar and salt. Stir in butter and milk until blended.

2. Transfer quinoa mixture to pie plate. Using moist fingers, press mixture over bottom and up sides of plate. Place pie plate on a large baking sheet.

To Parbake

3. Bake in preheated oven for 12 to 15 minutes or until golden. Let cool slightly on a wire rack, then fill and bake as directed in the recipe.

To Bake Completely

3. Bake in preheated oven for 23 to 27 minutes or until golden brown and set at the edges. Let cool completely on a wire rack. Fill as desired.

Nutrients per ⅙th pie crust	
Calories	139
Fat	3 g
Carbohydrate	25 g
Protein	3 g

Fresh Fruit Tart

This simple yet elegant dessert will delight both family and company.

Reduce the Histamine
Use a gluten-free pastry shell.

Nutrients per serving	
Calories	220
Fat	4 g
Carbohydrate	44 g
Protein	1 g

1 cup	skim milk	250 mL
2 tbsp	granulated sugar	30 mL
1 tsp	grated lemon zest	5 mL
1 tsp	grated orange zest	5 mL
1/2 tsp	vanilla extract	2 mL
1	large egg, beaten	1
1 tbsp	cornstarch	15 mL
1	8-inch (20 cm) pastry shell, baked	1
	Fresh berries and/or sliced fruit	
2 tbsp	red currant jelly	30 mL

1. In a saucepan, heat milk over medium heat until hot. Stir in sugar, lemon zest, orange zest and vanilla. In a bowl, beat egg with cornstarch until blended. Whisk a little of the hot milk into egg mixture, then pour back into remaining milk. Whisk constantly until mixture is thick enough to coat a spoon; do not boil. Chill.

2. Spread filling over baked shell. Decorate with fruit and berries. In a saucepan, melt jelly. Brush over fruit.

Ricotta Cheese with Pear

Makes 2 servings

Sweet pear and rich ricotta cheese combine to create a mouth-watering dessert or snack.

Variation
Use grated apple instead of pear and sprinkle the mixture with some ground cinnamon and/or nutmeg.

Nutrients per serving	
Calories	92
Fat	3 g
Carbohydrate	11 g
Protein	7 g

1/2	pear, grated	1/2
1/2 cup	low-fat ricotta cheese	125 mL
2 tbsp	granulated sucralose artificial sweetener, such as Splenda	30 mL

1. In a bowl, combine pear, ricotta and sweetener. Serve immediately.

Reduce the Histamine
Replace the artificial sweetener with sugar.

Be aware that adding cinnamon and/or nutmeg, as suggested in the variation, may increase histamine levels.

Blueberry Honey Cake

Makes 6 to 8 servings

This tantalizingly moist cake is so delicious, no one will care that it's also a healthy choice!

- Preheat oven to 350°F (180°C)
- 9-inch (23 cm) round cake pan sprayed with baking spray

1 cup	fresh or frozen blueberries	250 mL
⅔ cup	liquid honey, divided	150 mL
⅓ cup	water	75 mL
1 tbsp	cornstarch or arrowroot	15 mL
1 tbsp	water	15 mL
1½ cups	whole wheat flour	375 mL
1 tsp	baking powder	5 mL
1 cup	2% milk	250 mL
1 tbsp	vegetable oil	15 mL

1. In a saucepan, combine blueberries, half the honey and ⅓ cup (75 mL) water; bring to a boil over medium heat. Stir together cornstarch and 1 tbsp (15 mL) water; add to simmering blueberry mixture. Cook, stirring constantly, until thickened. Remove from heat; set aside.

2. In a large bowl, stir together flour and baking powder. In another bowl, whisk together milk, the remaining honey and oil until smooth; add to flour mixture, stirring to combine. Pour into prepared pan. Pour blueberry mixture on top of batter.

3. Bake in preheated oven for 25 to 35 minutes or until tester inserted in center comes out clean.

Nutrients per 1 of 8 servings	
Calories	176
Fat	3 g
Carbohydrate	36 g
Protein	5 g

Date Cake with Coconut Topping

This date cake has a moist, buttery flavor and is a good source of iron.

Tips

To chop dates easily, use kitchen shears. Whole pitted dates can be used, but then use a food processor to finely chop dates after they are cooked.

Chopped pitted prunes can replace dates.

Make Ahead

Prepare up to 2 days ahead, or freeze for up to 6 weeks. The dates keep this cake moist.

- Preheat oven to 350°F (180°C)
- 9-inch (23 cm) square cake pan, sprayed with vegetable spray

Cake

12 oz	chopped, pitted dried dates	375 g
1¾ cups	water	425 mL
¼ cup	margarine or butter	60 mL
1 cup	granulated sugar	250 mL
2	large eggs	2
1½ cups	all-purpose flour	375 mL
1½ tsp	baking powder	7 mL
1 tsp	baking soda	5 mL

Topping

⅓ cup	unsweetened coconut	75 mL
¼ cup	brown sugar	60 mL
3 tbsp	2% milk	45 mL
2 tbsp	margarine or butter	30 mL

1. *Cake:* Put dates and water in saucepan; bring to a boil, cover and reduce heat to low. Cook for 10 minutes, stirring often, or until dates are soft and most of the liquid has been absorbed. Set aside to cool for 10 minutes.

2. In a large bowl or food processor, beat together margarine and sugar. Add eggs and mix well. Add cooled date mixture and mix well.

3. In a small bowl, combine flour, baking powder and baking soda. Stir into date mixture just until blended. Pour into prepared cake pan.

4. Bake in preheated oven for 35 to 40 minutes or until cake tester inserted in center comes out dry.

5. *Topping:* In a small saucepan, combine coconut, brown sugar, milk and margarine; cook over medium heat, stirring, for 2 minutes, or until sugar dissolves. Pour over cake.

Nutrients per serving	
Calories	217
Fat	5 g
Carbohydrate	41 g
Protein	3 g

Berry Cheesecake Bars

These bars offer the decadent taste of cheesecake without all the calories. Enjoy after dinner or with afternoon tea.

Tips

When lining the baking pan, make sure the foil extends 1 inch (2.5 cm) beyond the edge for easy removal.

Try these bars with raspberries, blueberries or mixed berries. All versions taste great.

Reduce the Histamine

Use an all-purpose gluten-free flour mix in the crumb mixture.

Replace the orange zest with lemon zest.

- Preheat oven to 350°F (180°C)
- 13- by 9-inch (33 by 23 cm) baking pan, lined with greased foil

Crumb Mixture

1 cup	all-purpose flour	250 mL
1 cup	packed brown sugar	250 mL
½ cup	ground almonds	125 mL
¼ cup	melted butter	60 mL
2 tbsp	cold water	30 mL

Filling

2	large eggs	2
1	large egg white	1
1	package (8 oz/250 g) light cream cheese, softened	1
¾ cup	granulated sugar	175 mL
½ cup	low-fat plain yogurt	125 mL
1½ tsp	almond extract	7 mL
1 tsp	grated orange zest	5 mL
1½ cups	fresh or frozen berries (see tip, at left)	375 mL

1. *Crumb Mixture:* In a medium bowl, combine flour, brown sugar, almonds, butter and water.

2. *Filling:* In a large bowl, using an electric mixer on high speed, beat eggs, egg white, cream cheese, sugar, yogurt, almond extract and orange zest until fluffy.

3. Press half of the crumb mixture into prepared pan. Pour in filling and spread evenly. Sprinkle with berries. Drop remaining crumb mixture by tablespoonfuls (15 mL) over berries. Using a knife, swirl filling, berries and crumb mixture.

4. Bake in preheated oven for 35 minutes or until a tester inserted in the center comes out clean. Let cool completely in pan on a wire rack. Remove from pan by lifting foil and transfer to a cutting board. Remove foil and cut into bars.

This recipe courtesy of Eileen Campbell.

Nutrients per bar	
Calories	163
Fat	4 g
Carbohydrate	28 g
Protein	4 g

Crispy Brown Rice Treats

It's always a good idea to have a few no-nonsense recipes in your repertoire. Crispy rice treats are just that, and with some simple ingredient swaps and additions, this variation on the classic offers good health and great taste in equal measure.

Tip

For the dried fruit, try raisins, cranberries, cherries or chopped apricots. For the nut or seed butter, try almond butter, peanut butter or sunflower butter.

Make Ahead

Store the rice treats in an airtight container at room temperature for up to 3 days.

Reduce the Histamine

Replace the vanilla with almond extract.

- 9-inch (23 cm) square metal baking pan, sprayed with nonstick cooking spray

4 cups	crisp brown rice cereal	1 L
½ cup	finely chopped dried fruit	125 mL
½ cup	unsweetened natural nut or seed butter	125 mL
⅓ cup	brown rice syrup or liquid honey	75 mL
2 tsp	vanilla extract	10 mL

1. In a large bowl, combine rice cereal and dried fruit.

2. In a small saucepan, over medium-low heat, heat nut butter and brown rice syrup for 2 to 3 minutes or until warm and blended. Remove from heat and stir in vanilla.

3. Add the nut butter mixture to the cereal mixture, stirring until combined. Spread in prepared baking pan. Cover and refrigerate for 1 hour or until set. Cut into 16 bars.

Nutrients per bar	
Calories	92
Fat	4 g
Carbohydrate	14 g
Protein	2 g

Oatmeal Raisin Cookies

These old-fashioned,
healthy, chewy cookies are
sure to be a hit!

Reduce the Histamine

Replace the vanilla extract
with almond extract.

Replace the wheat germ
with ground buckwheat
groats.

- Preheat oven to 375°F (190°C)
- Baking sheet sprayed with baking spray

6 tbsp	packed brown sugar	90 mL
1/4 cup	butter, softened	60 mL
1	large egg	1
1 tsp	vanilla extract	5 mL
1/2 cup	rolled oats	125 mL
1/2 cup	raisins	125 mL
1/4 cup	whole wheat flour	60 mL
1/4 cup	wheat germ	60 mL
1/2 tsp	baking powder	2 mL

1. In a bowl, cream brown sugar with butter. Beat in egg and vanilla.

2. In another bowl, stir together oats, raisins, whole wheat flour, wheat germ and baking powder. Stir into creamed mixture just until blended.

3. Drop batter by teaspoonfuls (5 mL) onto prepared baking sheet, leaving 2 inches (5 cm) between cookies.

4. Bake in preheated oven for 10 to 12 minutes or until golden. Cool on wire racks.

Nutrients per cookie	
Calories	49
Fat	2 g
Carbohydrate	6 g
Protein	1 g

Lemon Almond Biscotti

Makes about 36 cookies	

These crunchy cookies have a lemony fragrance and are great with tea or coffee.

Reduce the Histamine
Replace the vanilla extract with almond extract.

- Preheat oven to 325°F (160°C)
- Greased baking sheet

1¾ cups	all-purpose flour	425 mL
¾ cup	granulated sugar	175 mL
1 tbsp	baking powder	15 mL
2 tbsp	finely grated lemon zest	30 mL
¾ cup	coarsely chopped almonds	175 mL
2	large eggs	2
⅓ cup	olive oil	75 mL
1 tsp	vanilla extract	5 mL
½ tsp	almond extract	2 mL

1. In a bowl, mix together flour, sugar, baking powder, lemon zest and almonds. Make a well in the center.

2. In another bowl, whisk eggs, oil, vanilla and almond extract. Pour into well and mix until a soft, sticky dough forms.

3. Divide dough in half. Shape into two rolls about 10 inches (25 cm) long. Place about 2 inches (5 cm) apart on prepared baking sheet.

4. Bake in preheated oven for 20 minutes. Cool on sheet for 5 minutes, then cut into ½-inch (1 cm) thick slices. Return to sheet and bake for 10 minutes. Turn slices over and bake for 10 minutes more. Immediately transfer to wire racks.

Nutrients per cookie	
Calories	78
Fat	4 g
Carbohydrate	10 g
Protein	2 g

Baked Granola Apples

This is a very speedy dessert that you can prepare and cook while making the rest of a meal.

Tips

The best apples for baking are Spartan, Empire, Golden Delicious and Cortland, as they will keep their shape while cooking.

When using margarine, choose a non-hydrogenated version to limit consumption of trans fats.

Make this dessert on a night when the oven is already on for another recipe.

Variations

These also bake quickly in the microwave. Place on a microwave-safe plate and cover with microwave-safe plastic wrap. Cook on High for 2 to 3 minutes or until apples are tender.

Pears can be prepared the same way.

- Preheat oven to 350°F (180°C)
- 9-inch (23 cm) glass pie plate, ungreased

4	apples	4
¾ cup	low-fat granola	175 mL
2 tsp	margarine	10 mL
½ cup	low-fat plain yogurt	125 mL
1 tbsp	pure maple syrup	15 mL

1. Core apples, creating a large hollow. Firmly pack with granola and dot with margarine. Place on pie plate.

2. Bake, uncovered, in preheated oven for 30 minutes or until apples are tender.

3. Meanwhile, in a small bowl, combine yogurt and maple syrup; set aside.

4. Place each apple in a dessert bowl and garnish with maple-flavored yogurt.

This recipe courtesy of Eileen Campbell.

Nutrients per serving	
Calories	192
Fat	4 g
Carbohydrate	37 g
Protein	4 g

Pears in Tosca Sauce

You can't get simpler than this quick dessert made with canned pear halves. It tastes rich and decadent. Enjoy it on its own or with a scoop of fruit sorbet or frozen yogurt.

Tip

This is a pretty dessert to serve directly from the dish, so use a glass or ceramic baking dish rather than a metal pan.

Reduce the Histamine

Replace the vanilla extract with almond extract.

Replace the all-purpose flour with all-purpose gluten-free flour mix.

- Preheat oven to 350°F (180°C)
- 8-inch (20 cm) square glass baking dish

1/2 cup	sliced almonds	125 mL
1/3 cup	packed brown sugar	75 mL
1/3 cup	milk	75 mL
2 tbsp	unsalted butter	30 mL
1 tbsp	all-purpose flour	15 mL
1 tsp	vanilla extract	5 mL
1	can (28 oz/796 mL) pear halves, drained	1

1. In a small saucepan, over medium-high heat, combine almonds, brown sugar, milk, butter, flour and vanilla. Bring to a boil and cook until sauce thickens, about 5 minutes.

2. Place pears in baking dish and pour sauce over top.

3. Bake in preheated oven until browned on top, about 15 minutes.

This recipe courtesy of Eileen Campbell.

Nutrients per serving	
Calories	177
Fat	8 g
Carbohydrate	25 g
Protein	3 g

Lemon Blueberry Panna Cotta

This traditional Italian dessert means "cooked cream," and, indeed, the original is made with whipping cream. This version has the same silky texture but is a lighter end to a meal. It is a great make-ahead dessert, as it can be stored in the refrigerator for several days.

Reduce the Histamine

Replace the evaporated milk with an equal amount of half-and-half (10%) cream.

- Eight ¾-cup (175 mL) custard cups or ramekins, sprayed with vegetable cooking spray

1 cup	milk	250 mL
1½ tbsp	unflavored gelatin	22 mL
¾ cup	granulated sugar	175 mL
3 cups	evaporated milk	750 mL
1 tsp	grated lemon zest	5 mL
2 cups	fresh blueberries, divided	500 mL

1. Pour milk into a small saucepan and sprinkle with gelatin; let stand for 10 minutes. Cook over medium-low heat, stirring constantly with a whisk, until gelatin dissolves, about 2 minutes. Increase heat to medium and add sugar. Continue whisking until sugar dissolves, about 2 minutes. Remove from heat. Stir in evaporated milk and lemon zest, stirring well to combine.

2. Divide mixture evenly among prepared custard cups and add 2 tbsp (30 mL) blueberries to each cup. Cover and refrigerate for at least 4 hours or overnight.

3. To serve, slide a knife around the edge of each cup to loosen the panna cotta. Invert onto a dessert plate and spoon 2 tbsp (30 mL) blueberries onto the side of each plate.

This recipe courtesy of Eileen Campbell.

Nutrients per serving	
Calories	219
Fat	5 g
Carbohydrate	36 g
Protein	9 g

Cold Maple Mousse

This tasty dessert is particularly good served with fresh fruit.

Tip

To toast almonds: In a nonstick skillet over medium heat, toast almonds, stirring constantly, for 3 to 4 minutes or until golden brown. Alternatively, microwave on High for 3 to 5 minutes, stirring at 1-minute intervals.

- Double boiler
- 6-cup (1.5 L) soufflé dish

1 tbsp	unflavored gelatin (1 package)	15 mL
2 tbsp	cold water	30 mL
1 cup	pure maple syrup	250 mL
1	large egg, beaten	1
1/8 tsp	salt	0.5 mL
2 cups	heavy or whipping (35%) cream	500 mL
1/2 cup	toasted slivered almonds (optional)	125 mL

1. In a small bowl, soak gelatin in cold water.

2. Meanwhile, in a double boiler over medium-low heat, whisk together maple syrup, egg and salt; cook, stirring constantly, for 5 to 8 minutes or until slightly thickened. Remove from heat and whisk in gelatin mixture. Refrigerate mixture until cool.

3. In a bowl and using electric mixer, whip cream until stiff. Add one-third of the cream to maple mixture; beat until well blended. (This gives the mousse a bit more volume.) Gently fold in the remaining cream. Pour into soufflé dish. Chill until set. Garnish with almonds, if desired.

This recipe courtesy of Ingrid Ermanovics.

Nutrients per serving	
Calories	244
Fat	17 g
Carbohydrate	21 g
Protein	2 g

Lemon Pudding

This is a less sweet version of an old-fashioned family favorite. What's old is new again! Consider this recipe for days when your headache triggers are low.

Tips

Placing puddings in a water bath to bake helps them to stay moist and cook evenly.

Serve with fresh berries to add vitamins and antioxidants.

Lemon has low histamine levels. Occasional or small amounts are unlikely to trigger headaches.

Reduce the Histamine

Replace the all-purpose flour with all-purpose gluten-free flour mix.

- Preheat oven to 350°F (180°C)
- 4-cup (1 L) baking dish, lightly greased

1	medium lemon	1
1/3 cup	granulated sugar	75 mL
2 tbsp	all-purpose flour	30 mL
Pinch	salt	Pinch
2	large eggs, separated	2
1 cup	2% milk	250 mL

1. With a lemon zester or grater, remove zest from lemon. Squeeze juice; set juice and zest aside.

2. In a mixing bowl, combine sugar, flour and salt. Stir in lemon juice, zest, beaten egg yolks and milk. Beat egg whites until stiff but not dry; fold into lemon mixture.

3. Pour into lightly greased 4-cup (1 L) baking dish. Place in larger pan; pour in hot water to about 1-inch (2.5 cm) depth. Bake in preheated oven for about 30 minutes or until topping is set and golden brown. Serve warm.

This recipe courtesy of Valerie Caldicott.

Nutrients per serving	
Calories	150
Fat	4 g
Carbohydrate	24 g
Protein	5 g

Black Sticky Rice Pudding

This delightful concoction is so good you don't even need the fruit. Although it's high in saturated fat, it comes from the coconut milk, which may have healthful benefits.

Tips

Thai black sticky rice is available in Asian markets.

Try using piloncillo, unrefined Mexican sugar, which is sold in cones in Latin markets. Use a 4-oz (125 g) cone in this recipe.

Reduce the Histamine

Use chopped mango or pear in place of strawberries, kiwis or peaches.

1	can (14 oz/400 mL) coconut milk	1
½ cup	packed Demerara or other raw cane sugar	125 mL
½ tsp	salt	2 mL
2 cups	cooked Thai black sticky rice	500 mL
1 cup	sliced strawberries or kiwifruit or chopped peaches or mango	250 mL
¼ cup	toasted shredded sweetened coconut	60 mL
	Finely chopped mint (optional)	

1. In a saucepan, combine coconut milk, brown sugar and salt. Bring to a boil over medium heat and cook, stirring, until sugar dissolves. Stir in rice and cook, stirring, until thickened, about 10 minutes. Transfer to a serving bowl and chill, if desired.

2. When you're ready to serve, top with fruit and garnish with coconut and mint, if desired.

Nutrients per serving	
Calories	305
Fat	15 g
Carbohydrate	41 g
Protein	3 g

Rhubarb Bread Pudding

An interesting twist to an old favorite. Cold leftovers are good too!

Tip

Leftovers can be stored in an airtight container in the fridge for up to 3 days or in the freezer for up to 3 months.

Variation

Try making this pudding with another fruit, such as frozen berries or peaches.

Reduce the Histamine

Replace the white and whole wheat bread with gluten-free bread.

Use lemon zest in place of orange zest.

Replace the vanilla extract with almond extract.

Omit the cinnamon.

- Preheat oven to 350°F (180°C)
- 8-inch (20 cm) square baking dish

2 cups	chopped fresh or frozen rhubarb, thawed	500 mL
3 cups	torn stale white and whole wheat bread	750 mL
1	can (14 oz/385 mL) evaporated milk	1
2	large eggs	2
¼ cup	granulated sugar	60 mL
1 tsp	vanilla extract	5 mL
1 tsp	ground cinnamon	5 mL
	Grated zest of 1 orange	

1. Place rhubarb in prepared baking dish and cover with bread pieces.

2. In a medium bowl, beat evaporated milk, eggs, sugar, vanilla, cinnamon and orange zest. Pour over bread. Let stand for 10 minutes.

3. Bake in preheated oven for 40 to 45 minutes or until a tester inserted in the center comes out clean. Serve warm.

This recipe courtesy of dietitian Helen Haresign.

Nutrients per serving	
Calories	175
Fat	4 g
Carbohydrate	27 g
Protein	9 g

Date Paste

This versatile recipe is a rich whole-food sweetener that makes a perfect alternative to refined sugar. It can be used as a replacement for agave nectar in many recipes and is a great finish for many desserts.

Tip

If you are sensitive to sulfites, make sure the dates are free of added sulfites.

Variation

For a sweeter paste, substitute the water with freshly squeezed orange juice, or use half of each.

- Food processor

10	chopped pitted dates	10
2 cups	water	500 mL
1 cup	filtered water	250 mL

1. Place dates in a bowl and add 2 cups (500 mL) water. Cover and set aside for 20 minutes. Drain, discarding soaking water.

2. In food processor, process soaked dates and filtered water until smooth. Use immediately or transfer to an airtight container and refrigerate for up to 1 week.

Nutrients per 2 tbsp (30 mL)	
Calories	25
Fat	0 g
Carbohydrate	7 g
Protein	0 g

Lemon Sherbet

Make this light, lower-calorie, low-fat dessert a staple in your recipe repertoire. Not only does it complement any meal, it is rich in vitamins C and A as well as in calcium from the skim-milk powder.

Tips

This recipe contains raw eggs. If you are concerned about the food safety of raw eggs, substitute pasteurized eggs in the shell or ½ cup (125 mL) pasteurized liquid whole eggs.

Consider this recipe for days when your headache triggers are low, since egg whites and lemon juice may increase histamine levels.

Reduce the Histamine

Use ⅔ cup (150 mL) skim milk to replace the skim milk powder and cold water.

- **8 small custard cups**

½ cup	granulated sugar	125 mL
2 tsp	grated lemon zest	10 mL
⅓ cup	lemon juice	75 mL
2	large eggs, separated	2
⅔ cup	skim milk powder	150 mL
⅔ cup	cold water	150 mL

1. Whisk together sugar, lemon zest, lemon juice and egg yolks; set aside.

2. Using an electric mixer on high speed, beat egg whites, skim milk powder and water for 3 to 5 minutes or until stiff peaks form. Fold in lemon mixture.

3. Pour into custard cups, cover and freeze for about 3 hours or until firm. Transfer from freezer to refrigerator about 15 minutes before serving.

This recipe courtesy of dietitian Joan Gallant.

Nutrients per serving	
Calories	90
Fat	1 g
Carbohydrate	17 g
Protein	4 g

Blueberry Yogurt Pops

Blue heaven. Why restrict delectable blueberries to muffins and pies? Here, they shine in cool, creamy ice pops guaranteed to thrill.

Tip

You can use 4-oz (125 mL) paper cups as ice-pop molds. Place them on a baking sheet, then fill until almost full. Cover with foil, then make a small slit to insert ice-pop sticks or small bamboo skewers and freeze as directed.

Variation

Peaches and Cream Pops: Substitute chopped peeled peaches for the blueberries, and freshly squeezed orange juice for the apple juice.

Reduce the Histamine

Replace the vanilla extract with almond extract.

- Blender
- 8-serving ice-pop mold

1 cup	fresh or thawed frozen blueberries	250 mL
2/3 cup	unsweetened apple juice	150 mL
2/3 cup	nonfat plain yogurt	150 mL
1/2 tsp	vanilla extract	2 mL

1. In blender, combine blueberries, apple juice, yogurt and vanilla; purée until smooth.

2. Pour blueberry mixture into ice-pop molds, insert sticks and freeze for 4 to 6 hours, until solid, or for up to 3 days. If necessary, briefly dip bases of mold in hot water to loosen and unmold.

Nutrients per pop	
Calories	28
Fat	0 g
Carbohydrate	6 g
Protein	1 g

Contributing Authors

**Alexandra Anca with
  Theresa Santandrea-Cull**
Complete Gluten-Free Diet & Nutrition Guide
Recipes from this book are found on pages 184,
  190, 197, 202, 233, 247, 260, 279 and 281.

**Byron Ayanoglu with contributions from
  Algis Kemezys**
125 Best Vegetarian Recipes
Recipes from this book are found on pages 248,
  291 and 295.

Esther Brody
The 250 Best Cookie Recipes
A recipe from this book is found on page 311.

Esther Brody
Another 250 Best Muffin Recipes
A recipe from this book is found on page 201.

Johanna Burkhard
125 Best Microwave Oven Recipes
A recipe from this book is found on page 296.

Johanna Burkhard
500 Best Comfort Food Recipes
A recipe from this book is found on page 230.

Johanna Burkhard
Diabetes Comfort Food
Recipes from this book are found on pages 264,
  273, 274, 287 and 297.

Dietitians of Canada
Cook Great Food
Recipes from this book are found on pages 177,
  187, 206, 219, 240, 241, 257, 258, 262, 267,
  270, 275, 315, 316 and 320.

Dietitians of Canada
Simply Great Food
Recipes from this book are found on pages 174,
  181, 182, 186, 188, 204, 207 (both), 214
  (bottom), 215, 226, 236, 252, 259, 266, 272,
  277, 308, 312, 313, 314 and 318.

Sue Ekserci with Dr. Laz Klein
*The Complete Weight-Loss Surgery Guide &
  Diet Program*
Recipes from this book are found on pages 178
  (bottom), 294, 299 (bottom) and 305 (bottom).

Judith Finlayson
The Complete Whole Grains Cookbook
Recipes from this book are found on pages 194,
  196, 234, 300, 302 and 317.

Judith Finlayson
The Convenience Cook
A recipe from this book is found on page 179.

Margaret Howard
The 250 Best 4-Ingredient Recipes
Recipes from this book are found on pages 180,
  238 (top), 249 (top), 254 and 256.

Douglas McNish
Eat Raw, Eat Well
Recipes from this book are found on pages 214
  (top), 216 (both) and 319.

Rose Murray
125 Best Chicken Recipes
A recipe from this book is found on page 278.

from Robert Rose Inc.
The Best Low-Carb Cookbook
A recipe from this book is found on page 310.

Lynn Roblin, Nutrition Editor
500 Best Healthy Recipes
Recipes from this book are found on pages
  203, 220–22, 224, 225, 227, 231, 242, 245,
  263, 276, 280, 283, 284, 290, 305 (top), 306
  and 307.

Camilla V. Saulsbury
5 Easy Steps to Healthy Cooking
Recipes from this book are found on pages
  200, 211 (top), 223, 238 (bottom), 243, 244,
  246, 255, 261, 265, 268, 269, 286, 289,
  292, 293, 298 (both), 299 (top), 301, 309
  and 321.

Camilla V. Saulsbury
500 Best Quinoa Recipes
Recipes from this book are found on pages 175,
  176, 178 (top), 183, 185, 191–93, 195, 198,
  199, 209, 210, 228, 239 and 304.

Kathleen Sloan-McIntosh
100 Best Grilling Recipes
A recipe from this book is found on page 282.

Kathleen Sloan-McIntosh
125 Best Italian Recipes
A recipe from this book is found on page 208.

Carla Snyder & Meredith Deeds
300 Sensational Soups
Recipes from this book are found on pages
211 (bottom), 212 (both), 232, 249 (bottom)
and 250.

Dr. Jillian Stansbury with Dr. Sheila Mitchell
The PCOS Health & Nutrition Guide
A recipe from this book is found on page 213.

Katherine E. Younker, Editor
America's Complete Diabetes Cookbook
Recipes from this book are found on pages 218,
229 and 253.

Acknowledgments

The authors would like to express their appreciation of the dedication, skill and patience of each of the members of the Robert Rose team. Special thanks to Sue Sumeraj for everything she does.

Recommended Resources

Here is a sampling of some reliable headache and health sites on the Internet.

Headache

The American Headache Society:
http://www.achenet.org/
Headache Group, UCL Institute of Neurology:
www.ucl.ac.uk/ion/departments/repair/
themes/headache
International Headache Society:
http://www.ihs-headache.org
The Migraine Trust: www.migrainetrust.org

General Health

Mayo Clinic: www.mayoclinic.com
World Health Organization: www.who.int

Diet

Centers for Disease Control and Prevention,
Nutrition for Everyone: www.cdc.gov/
nutrition/everyone/basics/index.html
Centers for Disease Control and Prevention,
Improving Your Eating Habits: www.cdc.gov/
healthyweight/losing_weight/eating_habits.
html
Health Canada, Canada's Food Guide:
http://hc-sc.gc.ca/fn-an/food-guide-aliment/
index-eng.php
Office of Dietary Supplements/National
Institutes of Health/Dietary Supplement fact
sheet: Magnesium, http://ods.od.nih.gov/
factsheets/Magnesium-HealthProfessional/
United States Department of Agriculture (USDA)
ChooseMyPlate: www.choosemyplate.gov

References

Articles

Adams J, Barbery G, Lui CW. Complementary and alternative medicine use for headache and migraine: A critical review of the literature. *Headache: J Head Face Pain*, 2013 Mar;53(3):459–73.

Aguggia M, Cavallini M, Divito N, et al. Sleep and primary headaches. *Neurol Sci*, 2011 May;32 Suppl 1:S51–54.

Alehan F, Ozçay F, Erol I, et al. Increased risk for coeliac disease in paediatric patients with migraine. *Cephalalgia*, 2008 Sep;28(9): 945–49.

Armstrong LE, Ganio MS, Casa DJ, et al. Mild dehydration affects mood in healthy young women. *J Nutr*, 2012 Feb;142(2):382–88.

Arroyave Hernández CM, Echavarría Pinto M, Hernández Montiel HL. Food allergy mediated by IgG antibodies associated with migraine in adults. *Rev Alerg Mex*, 2007 Sep–Oct;54(5):162–68.

Ashina S, Bendtsen L, Ashina M. Pathophysiology of tension-type headache. *Curr Pain Headache Rep*, 2005 Dec;9(6):415–22.

Bezov D, Ashina S, Jensen R, Bendtsen L. Pain perception studies in tension-type headache. *Headache: J Head Face Pain*, 2011 Feb;51(2):262–71.

Bigal ME, Kurth T, Santanello N, et al. Migraine and cardiovascular disease: A population-based study. *Neurology*, 2010 Feb 23;74(8):628–35.

Bigal ME, Liberman JN, Lipton RB. Obesity and migraine: A population study. *Neurology*, 2006 Feb 28;66(4):545–50.

Bonakdar R, Jackson C. *Integrative Approaches to Headache Management*. A publication based on a plenary presentation from the 20th Annual Clinical Meeting of Scripps Center for Integrative Medicine, October 2009. Available at: www.scripps.org/assets/documents/robert_bonakdar_md_10-13-10_handout.pdf. Accessed January 20, 2013.

Bonavita V, De Simone R. Towards a definition of comorbidity in the light of clinical complexity. *Neurol Sci*, 2008 May;29 Suppl 1:S99–102.

Brennan KC, Charles A. Sleep and headache. *Semin Neurol*, 2009 Sep;29(4):406–18.

Bromberg J, Wood ME, Black RA, et al. A randomized trial of a web-based intervention to improve migraine self-management and coping. *Headache: J Head Face Pain*, 2012 Feb;52(2):244–61.

Cady RK, Farmer K, Dexter JK, Hall J. The bowel and migraine: Update on celiac disease and irritable bowel syndrome. *Curr Pain Headache Rep*, 2012 Jun;16(3):278–86.

Carville S, Padhi S, Reason T, Underwood M. Guideline Development Group. Diagnosis and management of headaches in young people and adults: Summary of NICE guidance. *BMJ*, 2012 Sep 19;345:e5765.

Chaibi A, Tuchin PJ, Russell MB. Manual therapies for migraine: A systematic review. *J Headache Pain*, 2011 Apr;12(2):127–33.

Chen PK, Fuh JL, Chen SP, Wang SJ. Association between restless legs syndrome and migraine. *J Neurol Neurosurg Psychiatry*, 2010 May; 81(5):524–28.

Chen YC, Tang CH, Ng K, Wang SJ. Comorbidity profiles of chronic migraine sufferers in a national database in Taiwan. *J Headache Pain*, 2012 Jun;13(4):311–19.

Chung BY, Cho SI, Ahn IS, et al. Treatment of atopic dermatitis with a low-histamine diet. *Ann Dermatol*, 2011 Sep;23 Suppl 1:S91–95.

Clarke T, Baskurt Z, Strug LJ, Pal DK. Evidence of shared genetic risk factors for migraine and rolandic epilepsy. *Epilepsia*, 2009 Nov; 50(11):2428–33.

DaSilva AF, Goadsby PJ, Borsook D. The Headache Group, UCL Institute of Neurology. Cluster headache: A review of neuroimaging findings. *Curr Pain Headache Rep*, 2007 Apr;11(2):131–36. Available at: www.ucl.ac.uk/ion/departments/repair/themes/headache. Accessed January 4, 2013.

de Tommaso M, Sardaro M, Serpino C, et al. Fibromyalgia comorbidity in primary headaches. *Cephalalgia*, 2009 Apr;29(4):453–64.

Deprez L, Peeters K, Van Paesschen W, et al. Familial occipitotemporal lobe epilepsy and migraine with visual aura: Linkage to chromosome 9q. *Neurology*, 2007 Jun 5;68(23):1995–2002.

d'Onofrio F, Bussone G, Cologno D, et al. Restless legs syndrome and primary headaches: A clinical study. *Neurol Sci*, 2008 May;29(Suppl 1):S169–72.

EFSA Panel on Biological Hazards (BIOHAZ). Scientific Opinion on risk based control of biogenic amine formation in fermented foods. Technical University of Denmark, National Food Institute, Division of Microbiology and Risk Assessment. *The EFSA Journal*, 2011;9(11):2393.

Elkind MS. Endothelial repair capacity and migraine: The fix is in. *Neurology*, 2008 Apr 22;70(17):1506–7.

Evers S. Headache and sleep: The missing links. *Cephalalgia*, 2011 Apr;31(6):643–44.

Fernández-de-las-Peñas C, Hernández-Barrera V, Carrasco-Garrido P, et al. Population-based study of migraine in Spanish adults: Relation to socio-demographic factors, lifestyle and co-morbidity with other conditions. *Headache: J Head Face Pain*, 2010 Apr;11(2):97–104.

Fischera M, Marziniak M, Gralow I, Evers S. The incidence and prevalence of cluster headache: A meta-analysis of population-based studies. *Cephalalgia*, 2008 Jun;28(6):614–18.

Fogel WA, Lewinski A, Jochem J. Histamine in food: Is there anything to worry about? *Biochem Soc Trans*, 2007 Apr;35(Pt 2): 349–52.

Ford ES, Li C, Pearson WS, et al. Body mass index and headaches: Findings from a national sample of US adults. *Cephalalgia*, 2008 Dec;28(12):1270–76.

Francis GJ, Becker WJ, Pringsheim TM. Acute and preventive pharmacologic treatment of cluster headache. *Neurology*, 2010 Aug 3;75(5):463–73.

Freitag FG. The cycle of migraine: Patients' quality of life during and between migraine attacks. *Clin Ther*, 2007 May;29(5):939–49.

Friedman DI, De ver Dye T. Migraine and the environment. *Headache*, Jun 2009;49(6): 941–52.

Gaul C, Visscher CM, Bhola R, et al. Team players against headache: Multidisciplinary treatment of primary headaches and medication overuse headache. *J Headache Pain*, 2011 Oct;12(5):511–19.

Gee ME, Bienek A, Campbell NR, et al. Prevalence of, and barriers to, preventive lifestyle behaviors in hypertension (from a national survey of Canadians with hypertension). *Am J Cardiol*, 2012 Feb;109(4):570–75.

Gupta S, Mehrotra S, Villalón CM, et al. Potential role of female sex hormones in the pathophysiology of migraine. *Pharmacol Ther*, 2007 Feb;113(2):321–40.

Hauge AW, Kirchmann M, Olesen J. Trigger factors in migraine with aura. *Cephalalgia*, 2010 Mar;30(3):346–53.

Hedborg K, Anderberg UM, Muhr C. Stress in migraine: Personality-dependent vulnerability, life events, and gender are of significance. *Ups J Med Sci*, 2011 Aug;116(3):187–99.

Houle TT, Butschek RA, Turner DP, et al. Stress and sleep duration predict headache severity in chronic headache sufferers. *Pain*, 2012 Dec;153(12):2432–40.

Ifergane G, Buskila D, Simiseshvely N, et al. Prevalence of fibromyalgia syndrome in migraine patients. *Cephalalgia*, 2006 Apr;26(4):451–56.

Janis JE, Dhanik A, Howard JH. Validation of the peripheral trigger point theory of migraine headaches: Single-surgeon experience using botulinum toxin and surgical decompression. *Plast Reconstr Surg*, 2011 Jul:128(1):123–31.

Jones BL, Kearns GL. Histamine: New thoughts about a familiar mediator. *Clin Pharmacol Ther*, 2011 Feb;89(2):189–97.

Kano H, Kondziolka D, Mathieu D, et al. Stereotactic radiosurgery for intractable cluster headache: An initial report from the North American Gamma Knife Consortium. *J Neurosurg*, 2011 Jun;114(6):1736–43.

Kapur K, Kapur A, Ramachandran S, et al. Barriers to changing dietary behavior. *J Assoc Physicians India*, 2008 Jan;56:29–32.

Kofler H, Aberer W, Deibi M, et al. Diamine oxidase (DAO) serum activity: Not a useful marker for diagnosis of histamine intolerance. *Allergologie*, 2009 Jan;32(3),105–9.

Kofler L, Ulmer H, Kofler H. Histamine 50-skin-prick test: A tool to diagnose histamine intolerance. *ISRN Allergy*, 2011 Feb 22; 2011:353045.

Kung TA, Pannucci CJ, Chamberlain JL, Cederna PS. Migraine surgery practice patterns and attitudes. *Plast Reconstr Surg*, 2012 Mar;129(3):623–28.

Kurth T, Schürks M, Logroscino G, et al. Migraine, vascular risk, and cardiovascular events in women: Prospective cohort study. *BMJ*, 2008 Aug 7;337:a636.

Kurth T, Slomke MA, Kase CS, et al. Migraine, headache, and the risk of stroke in women: A prospective study. *Neurology*, 2005 Mar 22;64:1020–26.

Ladero V, Calles-Enriquez M, Fernández M, Alvarez MA. Toxicological effects of dietary biogenic amines. *Curr Nutr Food Sci*, 2010 May;6(2):145–56.

Lafrenière RG, Cader ZM, Poulin JF, et al. A dominant-negative mutation in the TRESK potassium channel is linked to familial migraine with aura. *Nat Med*, 2010 Oct;16(10):1157–60.

Lagiou P, Sandin S, Lof M, et al. Low carbohydrate-high protein diet and incidence of cardiovascular diseases in Swedish women: Prospective cohort study. *BMJ*, 2012 Jun;344:e4026.

Lee ST, Chu K, Jung KH, et al. Decreased number and function of endothelial progenitor cells in patients with migraine. *Neurology*, 2008 Apr;70(17):1510–17.

Liang JF, Chen YT, Fuh JL, et al. Cluster headache is associated with an increased risk of depression: A nationwide population-based cohort study. *Cephalalgia*, 2013 Feb;33(3):182–89.

Liebman TN, Crystal SC. What is the evidence that riboflavin can be used for medical prophylaxis? *Einstein J Biol Med*, 2011;27(1):7–9.

Lovati C, D'Amico D, Raimondi E, et al. Sleep and headache: A bidirectional relationship. *Expert Rev Neurother*, 2010 Jan;10(1):105–17.

Maintz L, Benfadal S, Allam JP, et al. Evidence for a reduced histamine degradation capacity in a subgroup of patients with atopic eczema. *J Allergy Clin Immunol*, 2006 May;117(5):1106–12.

Maintz L, Novak N. Histamine and histamine intolerance. *Am J Clin Nutr*, 2007 May;85(5):1185–96.

Maintz L, Yu CF, Rodriguez E, et al. Association of single nucleotide polymorphisms in the diamine oxidase gene with diamine oxidase serum activities. *Allergy*, 2011 Jul;66(7):893–902.

Maizels M, Aurora S, Heinricher M. Beyond neurovascular: Migraine as a dysfunctional neurolimbic pain network. *Headache*, 2012 Jul;52(10):1553–65.

Martin PR. Behavioral management of migraine headache triggers: Learning to cope with triggers. *Curr Pain Headache Rep*, 2010 Jun;14(3):221–27.

Martin VT, Behbehani M. Ovarian hormones and migraine headache: Understanding mechanisms and pathogenesis — Part I. *Headache*, 2006 Jan;46(1):3–23.

Merikangas KR. Update on the genetics of migraine. *Headache: J Head Face Pain*, 2012 Mar;52(3):521–22.

Mollaoğlu M. Trigger factors in migraine patients. *J Health Psychol*, 2012 Oct 26. doi: 10.1177/1359105312446773.

Mušič E, Korošec P, Šilar M, et al. Serum diamine oxidase activity as a diagnostic test for histamine intolerance. *Wien Klin Wochenschr*, 2013 May;125(9–10):239–43.

Naila A, Flint S, Fletcher G, et al. Control of biogenic amines in food — Existing and emerging approaches. *J Food Sci*, 2010 Sep;75(7):R139–50.

Nash JM, Thebarge RW. Understanding psychological stress, its biological processes, and impact on primary headache. *Headache: J Head Face Pain*, 2006 Oct;46(9):1377–86.

Oh T. Riboflavin: An alternative approach to managing migraine attacks in the adult population. *Nutrition Bytes*, 2010;14(1), Article 2. Available at: http://escholarship.ucop.edu/uc/item/2rd9m4j0.

Ospina MB, Bond K, Karkhaneh M, et al. Meditation practices for health: State of the research. *Evid Rep Technol Assess*, 2007 Jun;155:1–263.

Ossipov MH, Dussor GO, Porreca F. Central modulation of pain. *J Clin Invest*, 2010 Nov;120(11):3779–87.

Ottman R, Lipton RB, Ettinger AB, et al. Comorbidities of epilepsy: Results from the Epilepsy Comorbidities and Health (EPIC) survey. *Epilepsia*, 2011 Feb;52(2):308–15.

Park KR, Kim SY, Park HS, Jung YS. Surgery-first approach on patients with temporomandibular joint disease by intraoral vertical ramus osteotomy. *Oral Surg Oral Med Oral Pathol Oral Radiol*, 2012 Jul 6. Available at: http://dx.doi.org/10.1016/j.oooo.2011.11.038.

Penzien DB, Rains JC, Lipchik GL, Creer TL. Behavioral interventions for tension-type headache: Overview of current therapies and recommendation for a self-management model for chronic headache. *Curr Pain Headache Rep*, 2004 Dec;8(6):489–99.

Peterlin BL, Rosso AL, Rapoport AM, Scher AI. Obesity and migraine: The effect of age, gender and adipose tissue distribution. *Headache*, 2010 Jan;50(1):52–62.

Plessas S, Bosnea L, Alexopoulos A, Bezirtzoglou E. Potential effects of probiotics in cheese and yogurt production: A review. *Eng Life Sci*, 2012 Aug;12(4):433–40.

Prakash VB, Chandurkar N, Sanghavi T. Case studies on prophylactic Ayurvedic therapy in migraine patients. *TANG In J Genuine Trad Med*, 2012;2(2):e17.

Prester L. Biogenic amines in fish, fish products and shellfish: A review. *Food Addit Contam Part A Chem Anal Control Expo Risk Assess*, 2011 Nov;28(11):1547–60.

Rainero I, Rubino E, Gallone S, et al. Cluster headache is associated with the alcohol dehydrogenase 4 (ADH4) gene. *Headache: J Head Face Pain*, 2010 Jan;50(1):92–98.

Ringeisen AL, Harrison AR, Lee MS. Ocular and orbital pain for the headache specialist. *Curr Neurol Neurosci Rep*, 2011 Apr;11(2):156–63.

Robin O, Chiomento A. Prevalence of risk factors for temporomandibular disorders: A retrospective survey from 300 consecutive patients seeking care for TMD in a French dental school. *Int J Stomatol Occlusion Med*, 2010 Dec;3(4):179–86.

Rosser BA, Eccleston C. Smartphone applications for pain management. *J Telemed Telecare*, 2011;17(6):308–12.

Rozen TD, Fishman RS. Cluster headache in the United States of America: Demographics, clinical characteristics, triggers, suicidality, and personal burden. *Headache: J Head Face Pain*, 2012 Jan;52(1):99–113.

Russell MB. Genetics of tension-type headache. *J Headache Pain*, 2007 Apr;8(2):71–76.

Sances G, Catarci T. Management of headache patients (flow chart of the management of headache patient, amended from Chapter 9). *Handb Clin Neurol*, 2010;97:127–35.

Sarchielli P, Granella F, Prudenzano MP, et al. Italian guidelines for primary headaches: 2012 revised version. *Headache: J Head Face Pain*, 2012 May;13 Suppl 2:S31–70.

Schafer AM, Rains JC, Penzien DB, et al. Direct costs of preventive headache treatments: Comparison of behavioral and pharmacologic approaches. *Headache: J Head Face Pain*, 2011 Jun;51(6):985–91.

Scher AI, Gudmundsson LS, Sigurdsson S, et al. Migraine headache in middle age and late-life brain infarcts. *JAMA*, 2009 Jun;301(24):2563–70.

Scher AI, Stewart WF, Lipton RB. The comorbidity of headache with other pain syndromes. *Headache: J Head Face Pain*, 2006 Oct;46(9):1416–23.

Schürks M, Kurth T, Buring JE, Zee RY. A candidate gene association study of 77 polymorphisms in migraine. *J Pain*, 2009 Jul;10(7):759–66.

Schwedt TJ, Demaerschalk BM, Dodick DW. Patent foramen ovale and migraine: A quantitative systematic review. *Cephalalgia*, 2008 May;28(5):531–40.

Schwelberger HG. Histamine intolerance: A metabolic disease? *Inflamm Res*, 2010 Mar; 59 Suppl 2:S219–21.

Sekhar MS, Sasidharan S, Joseph S, Kumar A. Migraine management: How do the adult and paediatric migraines differ? *Saudi Pharm J*, 2012 Jan;20(1):1–7.

Shahid M, Tripathi T, Khardori N, Khan RA. An overview of histamine synthesis, regulation and metabolism, and its clinical aspects in biological system. *Biom Aspects Histamine*, published by Springer Netherlands, 2011:3–13.

Silberstein SD, Dodick DW, Saper J, et al. Safety and efficacy of peripheral nerve stimulation of the occipital nerves for the management of chronic migraine: Results from a randomized, multicenter, double-blinded, controlled study. *Cephalalgia*, 2012 Dec;32(16):1165–79.

Sun-Edelstein C, Mauskop A. Alternative headache treatments: Nutraceuticals, behavioral and physical treatments. *Headache: J Head Face Pain*, 2011 Mar;51(3):469–83.

Tikka-Kleemola P, Artto V, Vepsäläinen S, et al. A visual migraine aura locus maps to 9q21-q22. *Neurology*, 2010 Apr 13;74(15):1171–77.

Tiwari G, Tiwari R, Pandey S, Pandey P. Promising future of probiotics for human health: Current scenario. *Chron Young Sci*, 2012 Jan;3(1):17–28.

Tonini MC, Giordano L, Atzeni L, et al. Primary headache and epilepsy: A multicenter cross-sectional study. *Epilepsy Behav*, 2012 Mar;23(3):342–47.

Ungari C, Quarato D, Gennaro P, et al. A retrospective analysis of the headache associated with temporomandibular joint disorder. *Eur Rev Med Pharmacol Sci*, 2012 Nov;16(13):1878–81.

Vaidya PB, Vaidya BS, Vaidya SK. Response to Ayurvedic therapy in the treatment of migraine without aura. *Int J Ayurveda Res*, 2010 Jan;1(1):30–36.

Valent P, Akin C, Arock M, et al. Definitions, criteria and global classification of mast cell disorders with special reference to mast cell activation syndromes: A consensus proposal. *Int Arch Allergy Immunol*, 2012;157(3):215–25.

Varkey E, Linde M, Henoch I. "It's a balance between letting it influence life completely and not letting it influence life at all" — A qualitative study of migraine prevention from patients' perspective. *Disabil Rehabil*, 2013 May;35(10):835–44.

Wang SJ, Chen PK, Fuh JL. Comorbidities of migraine. *Front Neurol*, 2010 Aug 23;1:16.

Wang SJ, Fuh JL, Juang KD, Lu SR. Migraine
and suicidal ideation in adolescents aged
13 to 15 years old. *Neurology*, 2009 May
31;72(13):1146–52.

Wantke F, Götz M, Jarisch R. Histamine-free diet:
Treatment of choice for histamine-induced
food intolerance and supporting treatment for
chronic headaches. *Clin Exp Allergy*, 1993
Dec;23(12):982–85.

Winter AC, Berger K, Buring JE, Kurth T. Body
mass index, migraine, migraine frequency
and migraine features in women. *Cephalalgia*,
2009 Feb;29(2):269–78.

Zidverc-Trajkovic JJ, Pekmezovic TD, Sundic
AL, et al. Comorbidities in cluster headache
and migraine. *Acta Neurol Belg*, 2011
Mar;111(1):50–55.

Books

Ansari M, Rafiee K, Emamgholipour S, Fallah
MS. Migraine: Molecular basis and herbal
medicine. In Chen KS, ed. *Advanced Topics
in Neurological Disorders*. New York: InTech,
2012: 187–214.

DeLaune V. *Trigger Point Therapy for Headaches
& Migraines: Your Self-Treatment Workbook
for Pain Relief*. Oakland, CA: New Harbinger
Publications, 2008.

Longo D, Fauci A, Kasper D, et al, eds. *Harrison's
Principles of Internal Medicine*, 18th ed. New
York: McGraw Hill Professional, 2011.

Prousky J. *Principles & Practices of Naturopathic
Clinical Nutrition*. Toronto: CCNM Press,
2008.

Rogawski MA. Migraine and epilepsy — Shared
mechanisms within the family of episodic
disorders. In Noebels JL, Avoli M, Rogawski
MA, Olsen RW, Delgado-Escueta AV, eds.
Jasper's Basic Mechanisms of the Epilepsies, 4th
ed. New York: Oxford University Press, 2012:
928–42.

Ropper AH, Samuels MA. Headache and other
craniofacial pains. In *Adams and Victor's
Principles of Neurology*, 9th ed. New York:
McGraw-Hill, 2009:174–76.

Smith F. *An Introduction to Principles & Practices
of Naturopathic Medicine*. Toronto: CCNM
Press, 2008.

Vickerstaff J. *Dietary Management of Food Allergies
& Intolerances: A Comprehensive Guide*.
Vancouver: J.A. Hall Publications, 1998.

Websites

Centers for Disease Control and Prevention,
Division of Nutrition, Physical Activity, and
Obesity: www.cdc.gov/healthyweight/losing_
weight/eating_habits.html

Headache Group, UCL Institute of Neurology:
www.ucl.ac.uk/ion/departments/repair/
themes/headache

International Chronic Urticaria Society:
http://chronichives.com

International Headache Society: www.ihs-
headache.org

John Hopkins Medicine, Health Library,
Headache: www.hopkinsmedicine.org/
healthlibrary/conditions/adult/nervous_
system_disorders/headache_85,P00784

Mount Sinai Hospital: www.mountsinai.org/
patient-care/health-library/diseases-and-
conditions/tension-headache

National Center for Complementary and
Alternative Medicine (NCCAM), Headaches
and Complementary Health Approaches:
http://nccam.nih.gov/health/pain/
headachefacts.htm

Nutrition for Everyone, by Centers for Disease
Control and Prevention: www.cdc.gov/
nutrition/everyone/basics/index.html

The Migraine Trust: www.migrainetrust.org

USDA National Nutrient Database for Standard
Reference, National Agriculture Library:
http://ndb.nal.usda.gov

World Health Organization, Atlas of Headache
Disorders and Resources in the World 2011:
www.who.int/mental_health/management/
atlas_headache_disorders/en

Index

329

T

Tabbouleh, 248
tai chi, 110
T cells, 30
Tea Biscuits, Traditional, 197
teeth, 98–99
temporomandibular joint (TMJ), 98–99
tension-type headaches (TTHs), 15, 17, 19, 21
  diagnostic criteria, 47
  emergency care, 93
  inflammation and, 37
  lifestyle remedies, 65
  manual therapies, 96–97
  medications for, 81
  triggers, 28, 38
TENS (transcutaneous electrical nerve stimulation), 99
Thai-Style Squash Soup, 226
therapeutic touch, 109–10
tomatoes and tomato sauces
  Bulgur Pilaf (variation), 302
  Fennel Gratin, 290
  Quinoa and Black Bean Salad, 246
  Red Pepper and Goat Cheese Pizza, 270
  Tabbouleh, 248
  Zucchini Stuffed with Rice and Mushrooms, 263
topiramate, 82
Toradol (ketorolac), 90
traditional Chinese medicine (TCM), 105–6
Traditional Tea Biscuits, 197
trans fats, 127
Treximet, 88
trigeminal nerve surgery, 102, 103
trigger point injection (TPI), 98
triggers
  avoiding, 63–64, 67
  common, 26–28

  exercise as, 75
  foods as, 42, 116–17
  hormones as, 36, 38, 43
  stress as, 38–39
  of tension headaches, 28, 38
triptans, 84, 88, 90
  cautions for, 94
Tylenol (acetaminophen), 86
tyramine, 139

U

unsaturated fats, 127

V

vasodilation, 31
Veal Braised with Onions, 283
Veal Meatloaf, 284
vegetables, 123, 134. See also greens; specific vegetables
  Chicken and Vegetable Stew, 280
  Grilled Vegetable Salad, 242
  Kasha with Summer Vegetables, 265
  Lemon-Thyme Roast Chicken (variation), 272
  Pasta with Roasted Vegetables and Goat Cheese, 267
  Salmon with Roasted Vegetables, 257
  Spanish Vegetable Paella, 264
  Vegetable Stock, 218
  Veggie Sandwich, 207
verapamil (Verelan), 84, 86
vitamin B3 (niacin), 114
vitamin B2 (riboflavin), 84, 113
vitamin B12, 113
vitamin therapy, 84
Voltaren (diclofenac sodium), 90

W

Watercress, Carrots and Almonds, Capellini with, 268
white blood cells, 30
wild rice. See rice

willow, 115
Winter Squash Quinoa Bisque, 228
wisdom teeth, 99

X

Xylocaine (lidocaine), 93

Y

yoga, 110
yogurt
  Apple Berry Muesli, 174
  Baked Granola Apples, 312
  Berry Cheesecake Bars, 308
  Blueberry Lemon Cornmeal Muffins, 203
  Blueberry Yogurt Pops, 321
  Cool Cucumber Salad, 240
  Mango Lassi, 215
  Mint Yogurt Dip, 207
yo-yo dieting, 62

Z

zolmitriptan (Zomig), 84, 90, 93
zucchini
  Crustless Zucchini Quiche, 182
  Fennel Gratin (tip), 290
  Grilled Vegetable Salad, 242
  Harvest Vegetable Barley Soup, 230
  Kasha with Summer Vegetables, 265
  Pasta with Roasted Vegetables and Goat Cheese, 267
  Red Pepper and Goat Cheese Pizza (substitute), 270
  Salmon with Roasted Vegetables, 257
  Summer Zucchini, 295
  Zucchini and Chickpea Salad, 244
  Zucchini Frittata, 262
  Zucchini Stuffed with Rice and Mushrooms, 263

Library and Archives Canada Cataloguing in Publication

Hannah, Susan, 1956-, author
    The complete migraine health, diet guide & cookbook : practical solutions for managing migraine and headache pain + 150 recipes / Susan Hannah, BA, BScH, with Dr. Lawrence Leung, Medical Advisor, MBBChir, BChinMed, FRCGP, CCFP, and Elizabeth Dares-Dobbie, BSc, BEd, RD, MA.

Includes index.
ISBN 978-0-7788-0454-3 (pbk.)

    1. Migraine. 2. Migraine—Diet therapy—Recipes. I. Leung, Lawrence, 1965-, author II. Dares-Dobbie, Elizabeth, author III. Title.

RC392.H363 2013   641.5'631   C2013-903331-9